HEALTH CARE MANAGEMENT

Strategy, Structure & Process

Edited by

Montague Brown, MBA, DrPH, JD
Editor, *Health Care Management Review*
and
Chairman
Strategic Management Services, Inc.
Washington, D.C. and
Shawnee Mission, Kansas

HEALTH CARE MANAGEMENT REVIEW

AN ASPEN PUBLICATION®
Aspen Publishers, Inc.
Gaithersburg, Maryland
1992

Library of Congress Cataloging-in-Publication Data

Health care management : strategy, structure & process / edited by Montague Brown.

p. cm.
Collection of reprints of articles previously published in Health care management review.
Includes bibliographical references and index.
ISBN: 0-8342-0299-9

1. Hospitals—Administration. I. Brown, Montague. II. Health care management review.
[DNLM: 1. Health Services—organization & administration—collected works.
2. Hospital Administration—collected works.
WX 150 H4342]
RA971.H3855 1992
362.1'1'068—dc20
DNLM/DLC
for Library of Congress
92-7149
CIP

Aspen Publishers, Inc., grants permission for photocopying for limited personal or internal use. This consent does not extend to other kinds of copying, such as copying for general distribution, for advertising or promotional purposes, for creating new collective works, or for resale. For information, address Aspen Publishers, Inc., Permissions Department, 200 Orchard Ridge Drive, Suite 200, Gaithersburg, Maryland 20878.

Editorial Services: Ruth Bloom

Library of Congress Catalog Card Number: 92-7149
ISBN: 0-8342-0299-9

Printed in the United States of America

1 2 3 4 5

Contents

III   Process

Preface

OVERVIEW

Health Care Management Review's principal thrust continues to bring the best of management thinking to our readers. The articles in this volume focus on enduring themes central to the role of chief executive officers, their management teams and policy makers who seek to understand and influence the overall direction of the industry.

CEOs need a core strategy; they must elaborate a structure that supports that strategy and evolve a process by which the organization sets its patterns in motion, keeps them going and determines the necessary course corrections that keep them on track. Files offers a definition and elaboration which captures the core of concern in the development of strategic policy formulation. "... strategy formulation is the process of determining an activity map or pattern that guides an organization's deliberate moves from here to there."

The articles in this volume deal with many aspects of issues inherent in strategy formulation, its impact on organization, and the methods by which managers harness the necessary human energy to make it work better and better. Some articles deal principally with the concept of strategy while others feature issues related to the structuring of organizational systems to achieve desired goals. A smaller set of articles deals with the emerging issues of how total quality management fits into the organizational life of health care organizations. Fewer articles have emerged on quality process, not because of its potential importance, but because we are only now seeing widespread attempts to try this approach to health care management. Whether quality process becomes routine or proves to be but another fad remains to be seen.

STRATEGY

Files ("Strategy Formulation in Hospitals") sets the stage for this section with a thorough review which aids executives in harnessing the tools of strategy for use in the field of health care. Pointer ("Offering-Level Strategy Formulation in Health Service Organizations") brings the marketing concepts of segmentation to bear on outlining a number of factors that lead to a topology of six principal strategic alternatives for the strategist. Rhyne and Jupp ("Health Care Requirements Planning: A Conceptual Framework") offers a method that moves planning from the strategic level to materials management planning requirements. Unlike Files and Pointer who focus on major theoretical elements of planning,

Rhyne and Jupp offer the reader a method for mastering the immense detail and analysis that inevitably follow from even the more modest schemes of the strategy level of planning.

Still another approach to strategy and planning is outlined by Harrell and Fors in "Planning Evolution in Hospital Management." Here the authors range over an evolutionary process that distinguishes financial planning and control systems, environment-based planning, project market planning, strategic business unit portfolio development and strategic portfolio applications. Of the many ways to conceptually consider strategic policy, each is sufficient for some purposes.

Strategic policy formulation ultimately stems from, leads to, or otherwise is related to the mission for which it seeks to maximize opportunities—a fact that makes "An Empirical Investigation of the Nature of Hospital Mission Statements" (Kendrick Gibson, Newton, and Cochran) a must read. Ultimately, the strategist needs to anchor strategies to a particular point of view. Consultants, researchers and executive practitioners recognize the area of mission statements as fertile ground for aiding organizations to achieve that which they purport to accomplish. Questioning and probing a mission statement adds great value to any strategic policy development. Such statements can produce great insight into the motives and sustaining values of an organization, or lack thereof. Burns and Mauet ("Patrolling the Turbulent Borderland: Managerial Strategies for a Changing Health Care Environment") discuss a number of problems organizations face (resource dependency) and strategies (internal needs assessment, etc.) which they can employ to deal with the issues.

STRUCTURE

The structure articles deal extensively with vertical integration, diversification, interorganizational linkages, partnership versus competition, acquisition and other means for or against greater integration of the industry. "Vertical Integration: Exploration of a Popular Strategic Concept" (Brown and McCool) lays out much of the historical antecedents of the concept as applied to health care, recent trends and the likely evolution of the concept. In "Vertical Integration in Health Services: Theory and Managerial Implications," Conrad and Dowling zero in on the underlying theory, management implications and offer suggestions on how to analyze, decide about and bring controls to bear on making the concept

of vertical integration work. Longest ("Inter-Organizational Linkages in the Health Sector") focuses on the generic problem of organizational linkages and the mechanism through which such mechanisms are managed.

Fox ("Vertical Integration Strategies: More Promising Than Diversification"), and Clement ("Corporate Diversification: Expectations and Outcomes") deal with one or more aspects of diversification and vertical integration. Clement focuses on financial success and Fox outlines approaches used in other industries to choose between diversification and vertical integration. In "The Case for Hospital Diversification into Long-Term Care," Giardina, Fottler, Shewchuk, and Hill make the case for diversification into long-term care. Schwartz and Stone ("Strategic Acquisitions by Academic Medical Centers: The Jefferson Experience As Operational Paradigm") outline the experience of a hospital acquisition by Thomas Jefferson University as a diversification strategy. Anyone interested in the cultural issues inherent in pulling organizations together, especially where academic medical centers are involved, will enjoy this article.

Morrisey and Alexander ("Hospital Acquisition or Management Contract: A Theory of Strategic Choice") illustrate a strategic alternative to blending cultures through acquisition—namely contract management. With the many mergers, acquisitions and extensive use of contract management as a way to transport management to needy organizations, this article offers insights into a broader range of choice than might have seemed possible or desirable in the mid-1970s when both trends rapidly gained momentum.

Zuckerman and D'Aunno ("Hospital Alliances: Cooperative Strategy in a Competitive Environment") lay out the major rationale for hospital alliances and their growth and ways in which one might analyze such alliances. Given the changes in such alliances and their changing prospects as regional system building takes on greater meaning than what might be gained from national efforts, one can appreciate the humor and deep insights offered by Kinzer in "Twelve Laws of Hospital Interaction." Kinzer passed away in 1990 leaving this as one of his last insightful critiques on our profession and the industry. A complementary piece to Kinzer's contribution is MacStravic's "Warfare or Partnership: Which Way for Health Care?" which presents a case for seeking partnerships instead of building more competitive warfare between organizations.

PROCESS

The articles here delve into a relatively new subject for health care journals: total quality management. It took *Health Care Management Review* nearly three years to find its first such article. We searched for possibilities, we sought out possible authors and we turned away many before selecting the path breaking piece entitled "Total Quality Management in Health: Making It Work" by McLaughlin and Kaluzny. They clearly recognize TQM as path breaking. They perform the difficult task of trying to determine just how this new cultural paradigm fits into the culture, norm and behavior of people in the health care industry before trying to see if and how TQM might fit. Nelson and Goldstein ("Health Care Quality: The New Marketing Challenge") make the case to consider TQM as a way to relate to buyers and others in the market who are looking for TQM as a way to get better value—at lower cost, we suspect. Milakovich ("Creating a Total Quality Health Care Environment") examines many of the details and methods for building a TQM program.

Other articles on process and the managing side of the business are covered in greater depth in other books in this series. The TQM papers were selected here due, in large part, to the fact that many see TQM as a paradigm and major strategic change in providing health care in the country.

CONCLUSION

The decade of the 1980s generated much debate over the strategic directions of vertical integration and diversification. Both strategies can count failures, both successes. Which to use and when will need to be grounded in a solid understanding of the environment, the particular organization, and the person power and capital resources available to carry out the work. Few observers, especially those whose profession is strategic thinking, can quibble with the idea that under some circumstances either or neither strategy will work. On the other hand, anyone seriously studying this collection of articles will have a much greater probability of choosing the right strategy for any particular situation.

—Montague Brown

Acknowledgments

Editors of volumes such as this get principal billing on the cover although as the readers quickly discover, the real feast is in the articles themselves. The real authors are those whose names appear on each article.

But it takes many people to make such articles possible. Before submission, authors typically have many others read and comment on their writings. When it arrives on the editor's desk, two or more outside reviewers are assigned to read and critique the article using criteria established by *Health Care Management Review*. These anonymous readers spend countless hours to provide insights and suggestions that often greatly strengthen the authors' initial efforts. Frequently, authors revise their articles. Once accepted at this level, Aspen editors copyedit the article to fit *HCMR* style requirements.

Thus, each article here represents the work of the named authors and the work of countless others who make substantial contributions to the final product.

This book is dedicated to the unpaid editorial board members and other reviewers who served *HCMR* during the period when these papers were originally published.

Dedicated to

Associate Editors

Barbara P. McCool, Ph.D.
President
Strategic Management Services, Inc.

B. Jon Jaeger, Ph.D.
Professor
Duke University Medical Center

HCMR Past and Present Board Members

F.K. Ackerman, Jr.	R. Mark Herring
Gary D. Aden	Sagar C. Jain
Paul Anderson	Donald E.L. Johnson
Don L. Arnwine	Everett A. Johnson
Alexander Balc, Jr.	John C. Johnson
H. David Banta	Arnold D. Kaluzny
Thomas W. Bice	Frank Karel
Jan E. Blanpain	Karl S. Klicka
Phillip Caper	Richard M. Knapp
Raymond G. Davis	Anthony R. Kovner
Carole E. Esley	John Kralewski
A.A. Gavazzi	Lowell C. Kruse
John R. Griffith	John J. Laverty
William Hejna	Samuel Levey

Stephen H. Lipson   Robert A. Milch   David Pitts   C. Thomas Smith
Wallace Lonergan   William F. Moreland   Dennis D. Pointer   David B. Starkweather
James E. Ludlam   Anthony T. Mott   Lawrence D. Prybil   Donald C. Wegmiller
Robert O. Lunn   Duncan Neuhauser   John H. Renner   M. Keith Weikel
J. Joel May   Harry A. Nurkin   Carolyn C. Roberts   Thomas P. Weil
Carol M. McCarthy   Robert J. O'Brien   Gerald Rosenthal   John H. Westerman
John P. McDaniels   Nora O'Malley   Lou Rossiter   Richard D. Wittrup
Curtis P. McLaughlin   Barry A. Passett   William R. Roy   G. Rodney Wolford
Matthew F. McNulty, Jr.   David A. Pearson   Stephen M. Shortell   Janice B. Wyatt

In addition, *HCMR* wishes to thank the many ad hoc reviewers for their exemplary service in bringing out the best in the articles presented here.

Part I

STRATEGY

Strategy formulation in hospitals

Laurel A. Files

By acknowledging the inherent antagonism between strategic planning and the structure and function of hospitals, and explicitly integrating and adapting existing models, hospital administrators can develop a strategy formulation process into an operational tool.

Simply put, strategy formulation is the process of determining an activity map or pattern that guides an organization's deliberate moves from here to there. The growing recognition of the importance of strategy formulation to hospitals' survival is reflected in the current proliferation of conferences and workshops offered by professional associations and independent consultants to those in hospital administration. The focus on this topic in print media is another barometer of this interest, with entire journals or issues of journals devoted to strategic planning (e.g., *Health Care Strategic Management* and *Strategic Management Journal; Hospitals*, vol. 56, no. 12, 1982; and *Hospital & Health Services Administration*, vol. 29, no. 4, 1984).

There should be no question that the hospital's determination of an appropriate map to guide its activities in getting from here to there is important.[1] As the total number of its component parts, stakeholders and constituencies, environments, and actors increases, the hospital's mission, goals, and objectives become increasingly complex and filled with contradictions. In fact, primary actors may not agree about where here and there are located. Therefore, an explicit, structured, and institutionalized process of strategic decision making, programmed for contingencies, is needed to provide a buffer for the organization between its predominantly routine, slowly changing, maintenance-level, internal decision-making processes and the demands made by conflicting internal dynamics, as well as the turbulent external environment.

This article reviews the art and practice of strategy formulation in hospitals today, as revealed in the recent journal literature, in order to identify some of the significant management and research issues currently facing the hospital industry in its quest for strategic sophistication.

Laurel A. Files, *Ph.D., is Associate Professor, Acting Chairman, and Director of the Master's Program, Department of Health Policy and Administration, School of Public Health, University of North Carolina at Chapel Hill.*

This article was adapted with permission from Files, L.A. "Strategy Formulation in Hospitals: Where Are We? What Next?" In *Strategic Management in the Health Care Sector: Towards the Year 2000* , edited by F. Simyar and J. Lloyd-Jones, Englewood Cliffs, N.J.: Prentice-Hall, 1988.

DEFINING STRATEGY FORMULATION

The concept of strategy has been described as elusive, both in terms of its definition and its operationalization for purposes of more systematic study.[2] Strategies may be intended or unintended and realized or unrealized,[3] while approaches to studying strategy may be normative or descriptive, analytical or hypothesis testing, or problem solving.

Determining *whether* an organization has a strategy is difficult, in part because managers and researchers conceptualize strategy from different perspectives. Researchers tend to narrow the definition of strategy to render it measurable. Managers, as a protective tactic, often will not explicitly articulate their strategy even if one does exist.[4]

Following the advice of Mintzberg[5] and Miles and Snow,[6] the departure point here will be to define strategy as a *"pattern* in the organization's important decisions and actions,"[7] the process that guides the organization's deliberate moves from here to there.

Focusing on process, and on its concrete and discrete components, enables attention to be directed to those aspects of the organization that are more easily observable to an outsider. The limitation of this definition is that while it distinguishes strategy formulation from a random and irregularly patterned decision-making process, it reveals nothing of the quality of the decision pattern, that is, whether the strategy is better, or more effective, than an aggregation of impulsive decisions. Nevertheless, it provides a framework for an initial examination of strategy.

Snow and Hambrick report a general consensus among researchers on the distinction between strategy formulation (the cognitive aspects of strategy) and strategy implementation (the action components). They further observe that this distinction is built on the assumption that strategy development is conscious and purposeful, an assumption with which they feel some would argue.[8] Since the definition adopted for this article assumes rational decision-making behavior, the dichotomy is appropriate and should be inferred throughout the discussion.

The distinction should be qualified, nonetheless, in that it is an artifact of the level of the organization from which the activity is addressed. Determining mode of competition and management strategies for functional and operating areas, for instance, moves the process from corporate-level strategy formulation to "map making" at a smaller unit of analysis. Such lower-level decision making would be considered to be an implementation activity from the perspective of the corporate decision maker, but might be considered to be strategy formulation by the smaller unit, particularly if a corporate-level strategic planning process was not in place.

With this distinction in mind, it is possible to examine the process of strategy formulation. An individual-level example of strategy formulation is the way in which most people select the means and route taken to work in the morning, the process of choice among transportation and travel options. That process includes *identification of issues* (e.g., cost, availability, and accessibility of different forms of transportation; weather; possible speed and available time); *generation of alternatives* (e.g., bus, car, train; crosstown, uptown route); *evaluation of alternatives* (e.g., cost–time analysis); and *choice among alternatives.*[9]

In hospitals, most decisions are the result of at least implicit strategy formulation. For example, a decision to expand emergency services will probably include (1) consideration of cost, community need, availability of personnel, space requirements, competition, and market potential (identification of issues); (2) consideration of using contract physicians versus hiring new full-time staff versus reassigning existing staff, increasing emergency nursing staff versus hiring physician's assistants, and building new emergency facilities or reallocating old space (generation of alternatives); (3) comparing cost and effectiveness of contract physicians versus new hires, and capital expansion versus space reassignment (evaluation of alternatives); and (4) choice among alternatives.

In hospitals, most decisions are the result of at least implicit strategy formulation.

Even when the decision maker proceeds on instinct, that instinct is usually rooted in a prior consideration of issues and alternatives that determines later choices. Similarly, a logical thought process will often yield a strategic path, even if it was not the conscious intention of the decision maker to define such a path. The distinction between implicit and explicit strategy formulation is that between taking the four steps above intuitively at the time a decision must be made (implicit strategy formulation), and intentionally making an observable effort to work systematically through this integrated series of decisions (explicit strategy formulation).

If the decision process is explicit, structured, and institutionalized (i.e., key decision makers in the organization follow an established, known, and observable procedure for identifying issues, generating and evaluating alternatives, and making a choice), the process is usually referred to as strategic planning.[10,11]

DETERMINING STRATEGY

Andrews identifies four components that influence the determination of a strategy: market opportunity, corporate competence and resources, personal values and aspirations, and acknowledged obligations to society.[12] Andrews's conceptualization is relevant for generating appropriate questions during a hospital's strategy formulation process, such as the following:

1. *Marketing opportunity:* Is the target population changing? For example, is there an increasing number of elderly, industrial workers, and infants and children in the population served? Have other providers departed from, or arrived on, the scene? Has the introduction of new technology enabled the hospital to offer current services at new sites or new services at the same site?
2. *Corporate competence and resources:* What are the size and specialties of the hospital's administrative and medical staff? What are the size, location, and condition of the physical plant? What are the current sources of funding and likely opportunities for new revenue generation?
3. *Personal values and aspirations:* Does the hospital want to provide all aspects of health care to all consumers? Is preventive care as important as curative care? Is provision of care for children a higher priority than attention to the elderly? Is ability to pay a significant criterion for receiving care? Do personal or institutional values (e.g., in church-run hospitals) prevent the hospital from providing abortion services? How are handicapped infants to be treated?[13]
4. *Societal obligations:* Is health care a right or a privilege? Does the hospital have a historical obligation to the city or county, for example, is charity care provided for indigent residents while indigent nonresidents are referred elsewhere?

General Electric has described strategy as "a statement of how what resources are going to be used to take advantage of which opportunities to minimize which threats to produce a desired result,"[14] and has crystallized four managerial issues involved in developing this statement: how to respond to changing conditions, how to allocate resources, how to compete, and how to manage the major functional areas and operating departments. These issues are relevant to the hospital's decision-making process. Examples of important questions related to each issue include the following:

1. *How to respond to changing conditions:* How does the hospital plan to care for the medically indigent if Medicaid and Medicare subsidies are cut back?
2. *How to allocate resources:* How does the hospital decide whether to provide revenue-generating services versus critically needed services? To provide increased outpatient care versus increased inpatient care?
3. *How to compete:* How does the hospital decide whether to increase or cut back services and hours, whether to buy equipment independently or share with other providers, and whether to provide new services by reassigning existing personnel or by hiring people?
4. *How to manage the major functional areas and operating departments:* How does the hospital manage planning, finance, dietary, and maintenance functions? How does the hospital manage the emergency department, the outpatient clinic, the medical-surgical department, and the obstetrics and gynecology departments?

The components identified by Andrews and the issues identified by General Electric can be used as normative guides to the strategy formulation process for practitioners, as well as suggesting benchmarks, or variables, for operationalizing studies of the process for researchers.

Thompson and Strickland further elaborate strategy formulation as "inherently situational and evolutionary," involving "goodness of fit" between the chosen strategy and the internal and external situations, and "incremental adjustments to unfolding events."[15] In other words, in developing and adopting a strategy formulation process, the organization engages in a process of activity selection that will discriminate between, and respond accordingly to, restrictive and unconstrained external environments, adversarial and supportive stakeholder situations, and times of strong and weak leadership, for instance. The process is programmed to reformulate when regulations change, stakeholders multiply, and leaders are replaced. It is an iterative and self-correcting process, which involves a continuing reidentification of issues and the generation and assessment of new sets of alternatives.

An additional critical task to be addressed by organizations and managers in this regard is to integrate the analytical aspects of the strategy formulation process (gathering intelligence, maintaining organizational balance between centralization and decentralization, and carrying out systematic quantitative and qualitative analysis) with the intuitive aspects (innovation, proactivity, and risk taking);

> [T]he three analytical issues impose structure (or understanding) on the unstructured, ill-defined, internal and external environments and identify arrays of alternatives for the firm to consider . . . the intuitive issues allow the firm to exploit the insights developed by the analytical issues, and thus create opportunities and develop appropriate strategies that will enable the firm to exploit the results of its analytical capabilities.[16]

Such integration is difficult to operationalize. McGinnis suggests organizational mechanisms that rely on the awareness and proactive capabilities of individual managers: Strategic planning must be conducted as an ongoing process. There needs to be a free flow of information, vertically and horizontally. Managers must be sensitive to identifying and rejecting unimaginative strategies. Underlying assumptions must be questioned. McGinnis sees these tasks as the responsibility of both managers and the educators who train these managers. Clearly this integration requires not just the implementation of appropriate management tools and organization structures[17] but also the adjustment of managerial mindsets—a much more time-consuming process.

STRATEGIC PLANNING IN HOSPITALS: STATE OF THE ART

The current external environment is such that hospitals cannot afford to parallel each other's trials and errors in strategy formulation. Ideally, they need to learn from, and build on, each other's experiences. Consequently, the professional publications should provide information on the key elements of strategy formulation as practiced in the health care industry, relative to

- the process of strategy formulation;
- the elements that influence strategy formulation; and
- the issues that are critical to the decision-making process.

Literature review

A review of the dozens of journal articles addressing the issue of strategic planning in hospitals over the past five years reveals that the literature is primarily descriptive or prescriptive, and is based at best on only limited systematically gathered empirical data.[18-27] One subset of these recent articles equates strategic planning with marketing and focuses predominantly on marketing and marketing techniques.[28-32]

Another significant subset addresses the application of the strategy formulation process to circumscribed functional or program areas. This includes, for example, application of strategy formulation to human resources planning and the interrelations of overall strategy formulation with this process,[33,34] information planning and operations research,[35-37] purchasing,[38] financial planning and management,[39-41] and multihospital systems planning.[42]

There is also in this literature a strategic planning consciousness-raising effort for a wide array of specialists active in hospitals, such as osteopaths,[43] medical technologists,[44] nurses,[45] pharmacists,[46] respiratory therapists,[47] pathologists,[48,49] and radiologists,[50] as well as applications to geriatrics,[51] burn care,[52] psychiatry,[53] and surgery.[54]

Relevant studies

At least five major studies are exceptional in that they provide more insight into strategic planning in hospitals, either by an intensive analysis of multiple cases or by an examination of a respectably sized sample of hospitals. Bander's study reported that 80 percent of the institutions examined focused their planning efforts on the short term (one to three years), and only one hospital was modeled at all according to the available literature. Her study was limited, however, to a review of the planning approach of ten urban, voluntary, nonprofit teaching hospitals with 450 or more beds. She herself concluded that her findings were influenced by the nature of teaching hospitals and were not necessarily generalizable beyond that population.[55]

Bander's hospitals might be expected to be more progressive, in some ways, than the typical community hospital, so it might be assumed that even less strategic planning is occurring in the latter. On the other hand, proprietary hospitals and members of multihospital systems may be closer in structure and functioning to typical businesses, so it might be assumed that these hospitals would be more likely to adopt strategic planning. It will take hypothesis-testing empirical research to begin to suggest better answers to these questions.

Kropf and Goldsmith worked with a larger and somewhat more representative sample than did Bander (32 hospitals), although it was a sample limited to those with whom there had been significant previous contact on the part of the researchers—none were investor owned, and only one was located in the Southwest. The authors analyzed actual plans provided by the hospitals, only three of which they defined as strategic plans and nine of which were long-range plans. Fifteen of the institutions had a plan in progress, but only two of these hospitals were working against a deadline to finalize the plans.

Kropf and Goldsmith's analysis of the three plans they classified as strategic revealed that there was an embracing of marketing concepts and techniques, incorporation of quantitative utilization trend analysis, and a tendency to apply the term "strategic" to what would probably more accurately be described as facility plans. Reviewing all the plans, they found that several important dimensions of the strategic or long-range planning process were often not included and there was "minimal use of sophisticated analytical techniques" in terms of market analysis, quantitative trend analysis, and forecasting.[56]

Proprietary hospitals and members of multi-hospital systems may be closer in structure and functioning to typical businesses, so it might be assumed that these hospitals would be more likely to adopt strategic planning.

The Peters and Tseng study was limited to ten hospitals undergoing or having recently completed important strategic change; these hospitals were carefully selected for the study based on their success in meeting the challenges of their environment. Theirs is an in-depth piece of research, important for its focus on strategy implementation, however, rather than on strategy formulation.[57]

Zallocco, Joseph, and Furey reported on a national survey of 209 hospitals (with a 45 percent usable response rate) that they described as representative, al-

though there was a disproportionate number of large hospitals and several of the findings were correlated with size. The authors projected that approximately one-half of all hospitals have formalized strategic planning, although "strategic planning practices are still in an embryonic or immature stage of development."[58]

Scotti conducted survey research of 101 smaller (100-299 beds) not-for-profit community hospitals in Pennsylvania (usable response rate of 60 percent). Based on his scheme for classifying the hospitals according to the process of strategic planning, 20 hospitals were "progressive strategic planners," meeting all the criteria typically considered to comprise the strategic planning process. Another 24 hospitals had long-range plans and had formulated strategies, although the latter were not necessarily in writing.

Scotti's conclusions, based on the characteristics of the hospitals studied but generally consistent with the recommendations of hospitals' planning authorities were that a supportive organizational framework includes board-level strategic planning committees, with technical responsibilities vested in the hands of top management rather than lower-level administrative personnel or outside consultants.[59]

Models of strategy

Chaffee describes three models of strategy, based on a synthesis of the general management literature: linear, adaptive, and interpretive. She distinguishes them as follows:

In linear strategy, leaders of the organization plan how they will deal with competitors to achieve their organization's goals. In adaptive strategy, the organization and its parts change, proactively or reactively, in order to be aligned with consumer preferences. In interpretive strategy, organizational representatives convey meanings that are intended to motivate stakeholders in ways that favor the organization.[60]

This article has addressed strategy formulation only in the sense of the first two models, linear ("the methodical, directed, sequential action involved in planning") and adaptive (an assessment of internal and external conditions, leading to "adjustments in the organization or in its relevant environment" that would lead to an alignment of environmental opportunities and threats with organizational capabilities and resources).[61] This delimitation is a consequence of the relative ease of determining the existence and extent of linear and adaptive strategies, as compared to interpretive strategy, which still has unclear parameters and which demands that the organization "deal with the environment through symbolic actions and communication."[62]

Given that Chaffee's literature search was rather broad based and was not limited to hospitals or health care, it would be unrealistic to expect her framework to provide much insight for specifically assessing the performance of hospitals, because the application of strategic planning is a relatively recent focus for hospitals. The hierarchical nature of Chaffee's conceptualization, however, does imply that, compared to other organizations, hospitals are in the very early stages of effective strategy formulation and even that involvement is limited.

Furthermore, the literature review presented here reveals that even at the linear and adaptive levels, few hospitals incorporate strategic planning as an integral part of the day-to-day executive management process. What does appear to prevail is a disjointed strategic planning process, with strategy formulation and implementation taking place in some functional or operational pockets of the hospital, but not necessarily as part of an integrated, pervasive, institutionwide process.

Hofer and Schendel have described a four-tiered planning process, with different questions to be addressed at each level: *corporate* (what business are we in?), *strategic business unit* (how should we compete in that business?), *functional area* (how do we maximize resource productivity?), and *operational* (how do we implement the strategy efficiently?)[63] The usefulness of this conceptualization is that it emphasizes the multilevel and hierarchical nature of strategy formulation and the necessary interconnectedness of these decision-making levels. There is little evidence that this kind of strategy formulation is taking place or even evolving, to any significant extent, in hospitals.

Research and management issues

Shortell, Morrison, and Robbins, in their extensive review of strategy formulation, content, and implementation, identify four areas of research on strategy formulation that they feel are both important and interesting: initiating the process; defining goals; achieving analytical comprehensiveness; and achieving integrative comprehensiveness. They suggest several sample hypotheses to be tested in each area. They further suggest that because of the immaturity of the field, as well as the

nature of the questions, the research design of choice for studying strategy formulation is "well-done qualitative case studies."[64] On the basis of the review here, the case study methodology appears to be the only viable way to examine strategy formulation in hospitals because currently there is insufficient activity to warrant broader statistical studies.

The primary research issues at this time, however, might more appropriately be directed toward determining why so little significant strategy development is actually taking place in hospitals.

- Why is the strategic planning process in hospitals more lip service than strategic activity?
- Does the pluralism of decision-making power in hospitals among trustees, administrators, and physicians mitigate against the centralized control needed to initiate an effective strategic planning process?
- Is the rational basis of the strategy formulation process inconsistent with the demands of the hospital's typically value-laden mission?
- Are the hospital's products too intangible to be effectively manipulated through strategic planning?

In summary, both practitioners and researchers must pay more attention to the nature of the antagonism between strategic planning and the structure and functioning of hospitals before real progress can be expected in the adaptation of the strategy formulation process to the hospital setting.

REFERENCES

1. Files, L.A. "Strategy Formulation and Strategic Planning in Hospitals." *Hospital & Health Services Administration* 28, no. 6 (1983): 9-20.
2. Hambrick, D.C. "Operationalizing the Concept of Business-level Strategy in Research." *Academy of Management Review* 5 (1980): 567-75.
3. Mintzberg, H. "Patterns in Strategy Formulation." *Management Science* 24 (1978): 934-48.
4. Snow, C.C., and Hambrick, D.C. "Measuring Organizational Strategies: Some Theoretical and Methodological Problems." *Academy of Management Review* 5 (1980): 527-38.
5. Mintzberg, "Patterns in Strategy Formulation."
6. Miles, R.E., and Snow, C.C. *Organizational Strategy, Structure, and Process.* New York: McGraw-Hill, 1978.

7. Snow and Hambrick, "Measuring Organizational Strategies," 528.
8. Ibid.
9. Hofer, C.W., and Schendel, D. *Strategy Formulation: Analytical Concepts*. St. Paul, Minn.: West, 1978.
10. Ibid.
11. Lorange, P., and Vancil, R.F. "How to Design a Strategic Planning System." *Harvard Business Review* 54, no. 5 (1976): 75-81.
12. Andrews, K.R. *The Concept of Corporate Strategy*. Homewood, Ill.: Richard D. Irwin, 1980.
13. Peters, J.P., and Wacker, R.C. "Hospital Strategic Planning Must Be Rooted in Values and Ethics." *Hospitals* 56, no. 12 (1982): 90-92, 95, 97-98.
14. Thompson, A.A., Jr., and Strickland, A.J. III. *Strategy Formulation and Implementation: Tasks of the General Manager*. Plano , Tex.: Business Publications, 1983, p. 31.
15. Ibid., 35.
16. McGinnis, M.A. "The Key to Strategic Planning: Integrating Analysis and Intuition." *Sloan Management Review* 26, no. 1 (1984): 49.
17. Karger, D.W., and Vora, J.A. "Integrated Planning for Health Care Organizations, Especially Hospitals." *Long Range Planning* 12, no. 2 (1979): 91-96.
18. Talle, M.A. "Strategic Planning." *Issues in Health Care* 4, no. 1 (1983): 39-41.
19. Eresian, J.G. "Skills Trustees and CEOs Will Need to Go to Bat for the Hospital." *Trustee* 36, no. 4 (1983): 18, 20-22.
20. Sinioris, M.E., and Butler, P.W. "Basic Business Strategy." *Hospitals* 57, no. 11 (1983): 68-73.
21. Berger, S. "Strategic Planning Plots a Steady Business Approach to Restructuring." *Modern Healthcare* 13, no. 7 (1983): 196-98.
22. Nauert, R.C. "Jumping the Hurdles to Strategic Planning." *Healthcare Financial Management* 37, no. 8 (1983): 26-30.
23. Katz, G., Zavodnick, L., and Markezin, E. "Strategic Planning in a Restrictive and Competitive Environment." *Health Care Management Review* 8, no. 4 (1983): 7-12.
24. Rontal, R.A. "External Environmental Analysis: Theory and Practice." *Health Care Strategic Management* 1, no. 2 (1983): 16-20.
25. Scammon, D., and Kennard, L. "Incorrect Perception of Public Opinion May Skew Strategic Planning." *Hospital Management Quarterly* (Spring 1984): 14-15.
26. Coddington, D.C., Palmquist, L.E., and Trollinger, W.V. "Strategies for Survival in the Hospital Industry." *Harvard Business Review* 63, no. 3 (1985): 129-38.
27. Buller, P., and Timpson, L. "The Strategic Management of Hospitals: Toward an Integrative Approach." *Health Care Management Review* 11, no. 2 (1986): 7-13.
28. Craig, T.T. "Integrating Institutional Long Range Strategic Planning." *Hospital & Health Services Administration* 28, no. 3 (1983): 16-26.
29. Gregory, D., and Klegon, D. "The Value of Strategic Marketing to the Hospital." *Healthcare Financial Management* 37, no. 12 (1983): 16-22.
30. Oliphant, C.A. "Strengthening the Marketing Program through Strategic Planning." *Health Marketing* 2, no. 2 (1983): 2-4.
31. Fontana, J.P. "Hospital Marketing is Here to Stay." *Hospital Topics* 62, no. 3 (1984): 12-13.
32. Muller, A. "Consumer Research and Strategic Planning for Hospitals: A Second Opinion." *Hospital & Health Services Administration* 29, no. 4 (1984): 21-29.
33. Baird, J., Meshonlam, I., and Degive, G. "Meshing Human Resources Planning with Strategic Business Planning: A Model Approach." *Personnel* 60, no. 5 (1983): 14-25.
34. Ulrich, D., Geller, A., and DeSouza, G. "A Strategy, Structure, and Human Resource Database: OASIS." *Human Resource Management* 23, no. 1 (1984): 77-90.
35. Tomlinson, R., and Dyson, R. "Some Systems Aspects of Strategic Planning." *Journal of the Operational Research Society* 34 (1983): 765-78.
36. Collier, D.J. "Using MIS Data for Strategic Planning." *Health Care Strategic Management* 2, no. 7 (1984): 8-11.
37. Macies, J.S. "Strategic Information Planning for the 1990s." *Health Care* 26, no. 1 (1984): 22-23.
38. Krumenacker, J., and Gray, S.P. "Strategic Planning: Key to Survival for Purchasing Groups." *Hospital Purchasing Management* 7, no. 10 (1982): 3-5.
39. Cleverley, W.O. "Using FAS in Strategic Planning." *Healthcare Financial Management* 38, no. 6 (1984): 72-73.
40. Costello, W.A. "Establishing a Framework for Strategic Planning Under DRGs." *Issues in Health Care* 5, no. 1 (1984): 21-22.
41. Zuckerman, A.M. "The Impact of DRG Reimbursement on Strategic Planning." *Hospital & Health Services Administration* 29, no. 4 (1984): 40-49.
42. Longo, D.R. "Strategic Planning: Is a Multihospital System the Answer?" *Urban Health* 12, no. 9 (1983): 20-21.
43. Abel, J.L. "A Primer on Strategic Planning." *Osteopathic Hospitals* 26, no. 2 (1982): 15-18.
44. Albers, J., and Vice, J.L. "Strategic Planning." *American Journal of Medical Technology* 49 (1983): 411-414.
45. Lukacs, J.L. "Strategic Planning in Hospitals. Applications for Nurse Executives." *Journal of Nursing Administration* 14, no. 9 (1984): 11-17.
46. Jones, R.H. "PERT/CPM Network Analysis: A Management Tool for Hospital Pharmacists Involved in Strategic Planning." *Hospital Pharmacy* 19, no. 2 (1984): 89-90, 94-97.
47. Nicol, J., et al. "Strategies for Developing a Cost Effective Pulmonary Rehabilitation Program." *Respiratory Care* 28 (1983): 1451-65.
48. Palmquist, L.E. "Strategic Planning—Issues for Hospitals in the 1980s." *Pathologist* 37 (1983): 474-76.
49. Portugal, B. "Strategic Planning for Outreach Laboratory Services." *Pathologist* 37 (1983): 537-40.

50. "Strategic Planning." *Radiology Management* 5, no. 2 (1983): 15-19.

51. Cahn, B.W., and Rapoport, M.I. "A Strategic Planning Model for a Geriatric Initiative in a School of Medicine." *Health Care Management Review* 7, no. 1 (1982): 75-80.

52. Caro, D.H. "Strategic Planning of Burn Care Services and the Role of Information Systems." *Burns* 8, no. 4 (1982): 227-30.

53. DeVore, R.W. "Strategic Management: Key to the Implementation of Strategic Planning." *Psychiatric Hospital* 14, no. 4 (1983): 219-24.

54. Jitsukawa, S. "Trend Analysis of Surgery Revenues at Osaka University Hospital." *Medical Instrumentation* 18, no. 1 (1984): 84-85.

55. Bander, K.W. "Strategic Planning: Reality Versus Literature." *Hospital & Health Services Administration* 25, special issue no. 1 (1980): 7-22.

56. Kropf, R., and Goldsmith, S.B. "Innovation in Hospital Plans." *Health Care Management Review* 8, no. 2 (1983): 7-16.

57. Peters, J.P., and Tseng, S. *Managing Strategic Change in Hospitals: Ten Success Stories.* Chicago: American Hospital Publishing, 1983.

58. Zallocco, R., Joseph, B., and Furey, N. "Do Hospitals Practice Strategic Planning? An Empirical Study." *Health Care Strategic Management* 2, no. 2 (1984): 19.

59. Scotti, D.J. "Organizing for Strategic Planning in Smaller Not-For-Profit Community Hospitals." *Hospital & Health Services Administration* 29, no. 4 (1984): 50-63.

60. Chaffee, E.E. "Three Models of Strategy." *Academy of Management Review* 10, no. 1 (1985): 89-98.

61. Ibid., 90-91.

62. Ibid., 93-94.

63. Hofer and Schendel, *Strategy Formulation.*

64. Shortell, S.M., Morrison, E.M., and Robbins, S. "Strategy-making in Health Care Organizations: A Framework and Agenda for Research." *Medical Care Review* 42 (1985): 219-66.

Offering-level strategy formulation in health service organizations

Dennis D. Pointer

One of six different strategies must be selected for a health service offering to provide consumers with distinctive value and achieve sustainable competitive advantage in a market or market segment. Decisions must be made regarding objectives sought, market segmentation, market scope, and the customer-value proposition that will be pursued.

Competition in the health care industry occurs at two levels: among organizations and among individual offerings. Health service organizations compete for prestige, vertical and horizontal linkages, capital, franchises, and factor inputs, to cite only several examples. Health care organizations with comparable offerings compete with one another for customers in specific markets. Two hospitals may be offering-level competitors in one market (e.g., general medical-surgical inpatient care), avoid each other in another market (e.g., open heart surgery), and collaborate in a third (e.g., mobile diagnostic imaging). Both organizational and offering-level competition necessitate the formulation of strategy to gain and sustain advantage. Although considerable attention has been accorded to organization-level strategy,[1-7] relatively little has been paid to the formulation of strategy for individual offerings. (Among several exceptions to this generalization is an article by J.X. Reynolds.[8])

This article identifies and discusses alternative offering-level strategies that can be employed to gain competitive advantage in markets and market segments. The sections that follow provide a brief description of the distinctive attributes of health service offerings; a model of the offering-level strategic alternatives; and a discussion of the decisions regarding objectives, segmentation, scope, and value proposition that must be made to formulate strategy for a health service offering. These topics lie midway between business strategy and marketing; concepts from both disciplines are utilized.

The offering-level strategic model presented here extends the work of MacStravic who, in a recent article, suggests that health care organizations must move from a functional and product orientation to a market orientation.[9] This model can assist an organization engaging in market administration (MA).

MA (and segment administration) focuses on the groups whose behavior determines the organization's success.... For its target markets and segments, it sets objectives and develops strategies aimed at achieving or maintaining a pattern of behavior that protects or enhances the organization's mission or survival, by making that behavior competitively attractive and worth repeating....[9(p.42)]

Health Care Manage Rev, 1990, 15(3), 15-23
© 1990 Aspen Publishers, Inc.

Dennis D. Pointer, *Ph.D., is the Arthur Graham Glasgow Professor, Department of Health Administration, Medical College of Virginia/Virginia Commonwealth University in Richmond, Virginia.*

HEALTH SERVICE OFFERINGS: DISTINCTIVE ATTRIBUTES

Strategy formulation for health service offerings is shaped by their attributes. The distinctive, although not totally unique, aspects of health care services flow from both the service and the health natures of the offering, which are summarized in Table 1.

Service attributes

First, health care is a service rather than a product.[10] Service offerings are intangible experiences, not tangible goods that can be possessed. They are performed, not produced. Service organizations face the challenge of designing and managing performance systems in which customers are intimately involved in the process, rather than production systems, which produce physical objects that are later consumed or used by the customer. Whereas the purchasers of products are separated from the production system, service customers are an integral part of it. Second, service offerings are purchased, then consumed and performed simultaneously. Products are produced, purchased, and then used. Accordingly, services cannot be inventoried; they are perfectly perishable. Performance capacity not used at a specific moment is lost forever. Third, in purchasing a service, it is the customer, not the offering, who moves through the distribution channel. Because customers must come to the organization, the markets for most services are geographically constrained and local in nature.

Health attributes

First, health care services focus on the person, not the person's possessions. Health care services are critical to one's existence and well-being. As a consequence, basic access takes on the status of a right. Second, health service use often accompanies life's most important marker events of birth, sickness, and death. Accordingly, they are imbued with great emotional and spiritual significance.

Not all health service offerings share these attributes to the same degree, and many others could be noted. However, the critical point is that services are different from products, and health care services are different from other service offerings.

OFFERING-LEVEL STRATEGY: MODEL AND ALTERNATIVES

Formulating a strategy for a health service offering entails making four decisions. These decisions, their interrelationships, and the resulting strategic alternatives are shown in Figure 1.

First, a decision must be made regarding objectives: What function will the offering maximize? A health care offering might seek to maximize service volume, revenue, profit or social benefit, to mention several examples. Offering-level objectives must be formulated in a way that furthers organizational goals.

Second, a decision must be made regarding segmentation: Is the market for the offering segmented? If the

TABLE 1

DISTINCTIVE ATTRIBUTES OF HEALTH SERVICE OFFERINGS

Offering	Attributes	Implications
Service	The offering is an intangible that is experienced, not possessed.	The offering is performed, not produced.
	The offering is purchased, then performed and consumed simultaneously.	The offering cannot be inventoried.
	The consumer, not the offering, moves through the distribution channel.	The market for the offering is spatially or geographically constrained (local in nature).
Health	The offering deals with the self, not the artifacts that surround the self.	The offering is critical to well-being and existence.
	The offering is consumed during life's marker events.	The consumption of the offering is emotionally and spiritually charged.

FIGURE 1

OFFERING-LEVEL STRATEGY: A DECISION MODEL

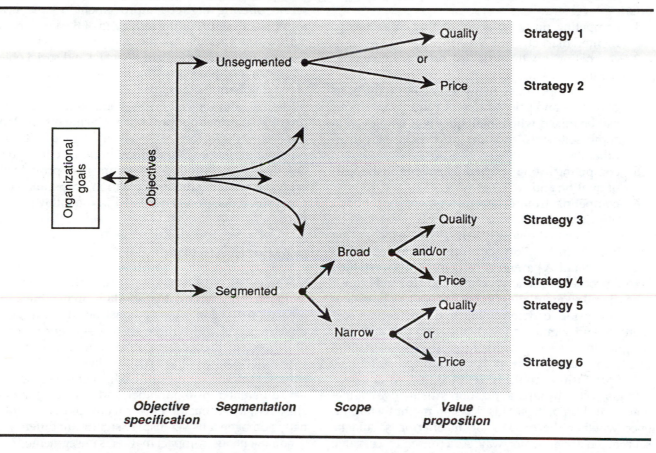

Objective specification	*Segmentation*	*Scope*	*Value proposition*

---

needs, wants, and characteristics of customers are similar, one offering can satisfy all; however, if they are dissimilar, then an array of offerings must be developed. For example, until the mid-1970s, the market for obstetrical service was relatively homogeneous. An offering composed of a physician-assisted birth under an anesthetic and a four-day hospital stay fulfilled the needs of most customers. This market is now segmented along several dimensions: preferences of the mother regarding whether anesthetic should be used and, if so, what type; the type of birth setting; the extent of the father's participation in the event; and the condition of the mother and child. The dimensions and their possible combinations are numerous.

Third, a decision must be made regarding scope: If the market is segmented, should the service be offered in a few or many of these segments? Which segments should be entered? For example, a hospital must decide whether it will develop offerings for all, or only some,

of these obstetrical segments. Possible offerings include neonatal intensive care units, birthing centers, short-stay delivery packages, and home birthing.

Fourth, a decision must be made regarding value proposition: On what basis should the offering compete with other offerings in the same market or market segment? Competitive advantage can be achieved in two different ways: low price or high quality. For example, a birthing center employing a high-quality value proposition could provide distinctive value to the customer by offering hotel-like suites, gourmet evening meals for the mother and father, and limousine trans-

---

In most instances, high quality and low price cannot be achieved simultaneously.

---

portation home at the end of the stay. In most instances, high quality and low price cannot be achieved simultaneously.

These four decisions interact to form the following six offering-level strategies:

1. competing on the basis of quality in an unsegmented market;
2. competing on the basis of price in an unsegmented market;
3 and 4.   competing in many segments on the basis of quality and price (different value propositions can be mixed where high quality is employed in some segments and low price is employed in others);
5. competing in one or several segments on the basis of quality; and
6. competing in one or several segments on the basis of price.

The sections that follow discuss decisions regarding objectives, segmentation, scope, and value proposition in greater detail. A parenthetical comment is warranted before proceeding. The decisions depicted in Figure 1 are ordered sequentially. Decisions about scope cannot be made prior to determining if the market is segmented, and segmentation depends on the objectives sought. However, in practice the process is iterative and less linear than portrayed. For example, an offering's value proposition could be selected first, as this decision is affected by an organization's distinctive competencies and capacities. This decision might then influence whether the market for an offering should be segmented and in which way. As a consequence, value proposition and segmentation decisions would actually precede rather than flow out of the formulation of objectives for the offering.

DECISIONS REGARDING OBJECTIVES

Objectives are statements about desired future states. Influenced by the preferences of both internal and external constituencies such as managers, physicians, staff, and the public, they are idiosyncratic. However, the offering-level objectives pursued by health service organizations can be conceptualized as growth, financial, and social.

Growth objectives seek to increase, or occasionally decrease, organizational mass. They generally focus on changes in offering sales volume, market share, or both. *Financial* objectives seek to maximize energy, dollars being the most fluid form. They could focus on revenue, profit, return, or some combination of the three. *Social*

objectives seek to maximize the public benefits that flow from consumption of the offering to society as a whole, the community, or specific populations. For example, social benefit objectives for a particular health service offering might be improvement in some measure of health status or the reduction of the incidence of a disease in a population served by the hospital.

At a minimum, growth of financial and social objectives for a health service offering must be quantifiable, specifying both the target and time frame for accomplishment, and logically consistent, so that achieving one objective does not prohibit achieving others. Most important, the objectives must be aligned with and promote the accomplishment of organizational goals. Offering-level objectives constrain and provide the context for making the segmentation, scope, and value proposition decisions addressed in the following sections.

SEGMENTATION DECISIONS

Segmentation decisions require a subtle combination of quantitative and qualitative skills. In making a segmentation decision, a map is constructed of a market's topography, of which there are three generic types (as illustrated in Figure 2): (1) homogeneous-compact, where all customers have roughly the same characteristics; (2) heterogeneous-diffused, where customers are very different from one another; and (3) heterogeneous-clustered, where customers form groups that are internally homogeneous yet display significant differences. A homogeneous-compact market is unsegmented, and a single offering can satisfy most customers. A heterogeneous-diffused market is also unsegmented, but a single offering can satisfy only a very small proportion of the total market. A heterogeneous-clustered market is segmented: Here offerings must have different features to meet the distinctive needs and wants of customers in each segment entered.

There are several quantitative approaches available for determining the topography of a market space and identifying the characteristics of specific segments.[11,12] The most frequently used techniques are perceptual mapping,[13] benefit segmentation,[14] and conjoint analysis.[15] Regardless of the technique employed, the process has two phases. First, information is collected regarding the extent to which customers prefer different offering attributes and the sociodemographic, psychographic, and purchase-behavior characteristics of the customers.[16] Second, these data are analyzed employing multivariate or factor analytic techniques. Which-

FIGURE 2

SEGMENTATION DECISIONS: ILLUSTRATIVE MARKET TOPOGRAPHICS

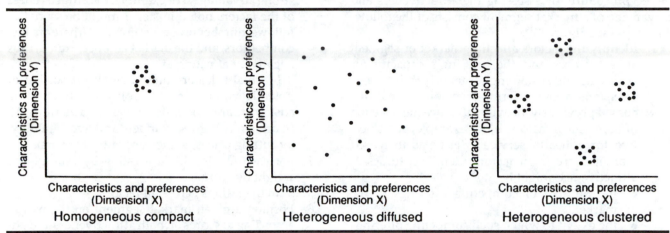

| Homogeneous compact | Heterogeneous diffused | Heterogeneous clustered |

ever technique is employed, the objective of the scope decision is to determine if a market is segmented, and, if so, the characteristics of each segment.

SCOPE DECISIONS

Scope decisions arise only if the market for an offering is segmented. The question addressed is, How many and which segments should be entered? Each segment entered necessitates the configuration of a different offering variation (or brand). Two factors affect such decisions: (1) *opportunity,* a function of the attractiveness of different market segments and the ability of the organization to achieve competitive advantage in them; and (2) *financial resources* available to the organization, recognizing that entering a segment requires an investment and entails opportunity costs.

The opportunity presented by different market segments can be assessed through portfolio analysis. Two such techniques, the Boston Consulting Group (BCG) growth/share matrix and the General Electric (GE) business screen, are among the most popular.[17,18] However, the BCG matrix uses only market growth rate to measure *attractiveness* and market share to measure competitive advantage. Because of the GE business screen's ability to incorporate a wider variety of factors, it will be employed as an example here.

Figure 3 portrays how a modified GE business screen can be adapted to make scope decisions. Each specific market segment, as identified in the segmentation decision, is assessed along two dimensions: (1) the intrinsic attractiveness of the segment, and (2) the

organization's capacity and competence to achieve and sustain competitive *advantage* in the segment. Both attractiveness and advantage are critical components of opportunity. A market segment may be extremely attractive, yet an organization's capacities and competencies might be such that the organization is unable to achieve or sustain competitive advantage in that seg-

FIGURE 3

SCOPE DECISIONS: SEGMENT ATTRACTIVENESS AND ADVANTAGE

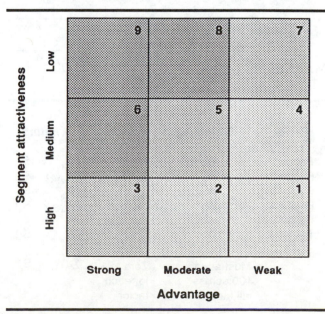

ment. On the other hand, an organization may be able to achieve advantage in a particular market segment, but the segment itself may be unattractive.

The procedure for assessing the attractiveness and advantage of a market segment consists of the following steps (see Figure 4)[19]:

1. Identify the factors affecting market or segment attractiveness and the offering's capacity for achieving and sustaining competitive advantage. Decisions about offering-level objectives, discussed previously, heavily influence the selection of both sets of factors. If, for example, one objective for a health service offering is increased market share, then factors identified to assess attractiveness might be
   - the number of competing offerings in the market,
   - the extent to which such competing offerings have penetrated the market (i.e., the ratio of actual sales to potential market volume),
   - consumer loyalty to competing offerings, and
   - the profit margins of competitors.
2. Weight the relative importance of each factor. One hundred points are distributed across the factors, with a larger number of points allocated to those deemed most important. The importance of the factors affecting market attractiveness identified above might be weighted as follows: number of competitors, 25; penetration, 40; customer loyalty, 20; and margins, 15.

3. Score each factor on a scale of 0 to 1.0: 0 for totally unattractive and 1.0 for extremely attractive, or 0 for weak advantage and 1.0 for an extremely strong advantage. For example, the attractiveness of the factors noted in step 1 might be scored as follows: number of competitors, 0.3 (there are few competitors, and the market is concentrated, thus negatively affecting attractiveness); penetration, 0.8 (actual sales are only a small proportion of potential volume); customer loyalty, 0.6 (existing customers are moderately loyal); and margins, 0.2 (margins are high, so competitors have the ability, by cutting prices, to increase entry barriers).
4. For each factor, obtain a rating by multiplying weight by score.
5. Sum the ratings across all factors.
6. Position a given market segment on the matrix according to scores on both attractiveness and advantage. For example, market segment A may have a summed attractiveness rating of 95 and a summed advantage rating of 90; it would occupy cell 9 of the matrix.

This process produces an opportunity map of all market segments. Everything else being equal, an organization would want to enter those market segments that are in cells 9, 8, and 6. Cells 7, 5, and 3 present only modest opportunities, and cells 4, 2, and 1 should usually be avoided.

The number of different segments that should be entered is a function not only of opportunity but also of
- the amount of resources available to an organization;
- the potential return on investment or some other measure of utility, depending on the objectives sought; and
- opportunity costs.

These considerations lie outside the scope of this article.

VALUE PROPOSITION DECISIONS

Decisions regarding value proposition must be made regardless of whether the market for the offering is segmented, and if segmented, regardless of the number of markets entered. Such decisions depend on the answers to two questions. First, from an organizational perspective, on what basis should the offering compete with other offerings in the market or segment, so it can achieve and sustain competitive advantage? Second, from a consumer-oriented perspective, how can the offering provide the customer with distinctive value? The answers to these questions are interrelated. Com-

FIGURE 4

MARKET SEGMENT ATTRACTIVENESS OR ADVANTAGE

Factor	Weighting	Score	Rating
Factor 1	W_1	S_1	$(W_1 \times S_1)$
Factor 2	W_2	S_2	$(W_2 \times S_2)$
Factor 3	W_3	S_3	$(W_3 \times S_3)$
Factor 4	W_4	S_4	$(W_4 \times S_4)$
Factor i	W_i	S_i	$(W_i \times S_i)$
Factor n	W_n	S_n	$(W_n \times S_n)$
	Must add to 100 across all factors	Zero to 1.0 for each factor	$\Sigma (W_i \times S_i)$

Value varies directly with the offering's quality and inversely with both price and other purchase expenses.

petitive advantage is attained by providing an offering that customers perceive to have greater value than competing offerings in the market or segment.

Value is a function of three factors: offering price, offering quality, and other expenses incurred by the customer in purchasing it. Value varies directly with the offering's quality and inversely with both price and other purchase expenses. An organization has most control over price and quality, because both are associated with costs. Figure 5 portrays these relationships.

Offering cost or price is depicted on the vertical axis; there is a theoretical maximum price beyond which customers will not pay for an offering regardless of its quality. Offering quality is depicted on the horizontal axis: There is a theoretical minimum quality below which customers will not purchase the offering regardless of its price. The quality and cost of an offering are directly related, although the relationship is curvilinear. Up to a point, quality-cost elasticity is less than 1; that is, a 1% increase in cost results in more than a 1% increase in quality. Beyond a point, increases in quality require more than proportional increases in costs.

An infinite number of value propositions (cost-price and quality combinations on curve OC) are possible. Porter has argued that two value propositions present the best opportunities for providing value to the customer and thus achieving competitive advantage for the offering.[5] These are represented by the points: C_1, P_1, a low–cost-price and low-quality value proposition, and C_2, P_2, a high-quality and high–cost-price value proposition. The relationships among cost, price, and quality make these value propositions mutually exclusive; in most instances, low cost-price and high quality cannot be achieved simultaneously.

Price

This value proposition assumes that some customers in an unsegmented market or those customers comprising one or more segments in a segmented market are willing to trade off high quality for a low price. The rationale underlying this value proposition is that the quality threshold below which customers are unwilling to purchase the offering can be determined, and cost-price can be reduced as service quality is held constant

above that threshold. This relationship is depicted below:

$$\frac{\text{Quality level (constraint)}}{\text{Cost-price} \downarrow} = \text{Value} \uparrow$$

Here, a level of quality is set above the minimum acceptable by customers and professionals performing the service. With this level of quality serving as a constant, costs are reduced, providing the opportunity to lower prices. Value is optimized by achieving a high quality–price ratio; that is, the numerator is held constant and the denominator is minimized.

Health care, like all service offerings, has two types of attributes: core and peripheral. Core attributes are those directly related to the performance of an effective outcome, such as cure or minimized dysfunction. Performance system features affecting these outcomes include professional skill level and the availability of necessary equipment and supplies. Peripherals are contextual features of the service offering; they are amenities that embellish the core but are not directly related to the accomplishment of effective outcomes. Examples are in-room video cassette recorders, better accommodations, gourmet meals, and a higher level of personal service. Eliminating peripherals reduces costs, and hence prices, without affecting outcomes. Other ways to pursue a low-price value proposition are reducing the costs of factor inputs, increasing productivity, and exploiting scale, learning, and experience effects.

Quality

This value proposition assumes that some customers in an unsegmented market, or the customers comprising one or more segments in a segmented market, prefer high quality to low price. The rationale underpinning this proposition is that the maximum price consumers are willing to pay can be determined, and price, at some point below the maximum, serves as a constraint as quality is increased. This relationship is noted below:

$$\frac{\text{Quality} \uparrow}{\text{Cost-price (constraint)}} = \text{Value} \uparrow$$

Here, an offering's price is set below the maximum acceptable to customers. With price serving as a con-

---

FIGURE 5

VALUE PROPOSITION DECISIONS: THE RELATIONSHIPS BETWEEN COST-PRICE AND QUALITY

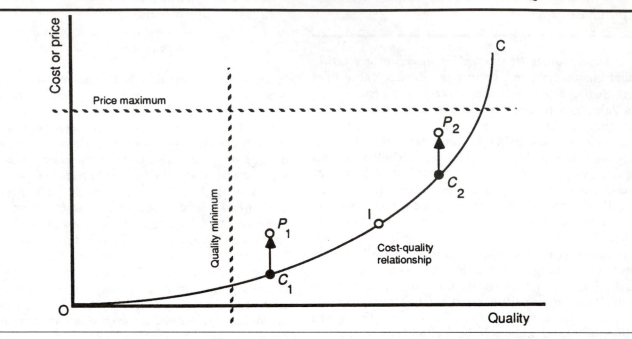

Based on concepts forwarded in Lele, M.M., and Sheth, J.N. *The Customer Is Key: Gaining an Unbeatable Advantage through Customer Satisfaction.* New York, N.Y.: Wiley, 1987.

---

straint, quality is maximized. Value is optimized through a high quality–price ratio; that is, the denominator is held constant and the numerator is maximized. The most straightforward tactic for pursuing this proposition is to increase the number and quality of amenities that embellish the core attributes of the health service offering.

Porter introduces a conceptual framework (the value chain) that can be employed to pursue either a low-price or high-quality value proposition. He notes that

Competitive advantage cannot be understood by looking at a firm as a whole. It stems from the many discrete activities a firm performs in designing, producing, marketing, delivering and supporting its product. Each of these activities can contribute to a firm's relative cost position [a low-price value proposition] and create a basis for differentiation [a high-quality value proposition].... The value chain disaggregates a firm into its strategically relevant activities in order to understand the behavior of cost [critical to executing a price value proposition] and the potential sources of differentiation [critical to executing a quality value proposition]. (Emphasis added.)[5(pp.33–34)]

He identifies two sets of value chain activities: primary and support. Primary activities include inbound logistics, operations, outbound logistics, marketing and sales, and service. Support activities include procurement, technology development, human resources management, and firm infrastructure. Porter presents a detailed discussion of how both primary and support activities of the value chain can be configured to implement either a low-price or a high-quality value proposition.[5]

Execution of a low-price or high-quality value proposition must be preceded by a decision regarding which proposition should be pursued in a specific market or segment. A complete discussion of contingency factors that influence this decision lies beyond the scope of this article. However, two sets of factors that must be considered (beyond those discussed previously, such as objectives and factors affecting scope) are customer price sensitivity and the value propositions of competing offerings in the market or segment.

•   •   •

Decisions regarding objectives, segmentation, scope, and value proposition link organizationwide strategies with the design and execution of an offering's tactical marketing mix (i.e., positioning, pricing, promotion, and distribution). As the health care industry has become far more competitive, both organizational strategy and marketing tactics have been elevated from obscurity to ritualistic preeminence. A hospital may have a beautifully crafted and adroitly executed organizationwide strategy and devote considerable energy and expense to developing marketing tactics for its array of offerings. However, if offering-level strategy is neglected or poorly formulated, organizational strategies cannot be translated into effective marketing tactics.

This article has presented a model of offering-level strategy that flows out of decisions that must be made regarding objectives, segmentation, scope, and value proposition. The interaction of such decisions produces a typology of six strategic alternatives. The model has immediate application for the health care strategist and marketer. It can be employed to rigorously specify, analyze, and evaluate the full range of offering-level strategic alternatives so that consumer value is maximized and competitive advantage is achieved and sustained. Both, accomplished simultaneously, equate with success in the marketplace.

REFERENCES

1. Hofer, C.W. "Toward a Contingency Theory of Business Strategy." *Academy of Management Journal* 18 (1975): 784–810.
2. Hofer, C.W., and Schendel, D. *Strategy Formulation: Analytical Concepts.* St. Paul, Minn.: West Publishing, 1978.
3. Miles, R.E., and Snow, C.C. *Organizational Strategy: Structure and Process.* New York, N.Y.: McGraw-Hill, 1978.
4. Porter, M.E. *Competitive Strategy: Techniques for Analyzing Industries and Competitors.* New York, N.Y.: Free Press, 1980.
5. Porter, M.E. *Competitive Advantage: Creating and Sustaining Superior Performance.* New York, N.Y.: Free Press, 1985.
6. Chrisman, J.J., Hofer, C.W., and Boulton, W.R. "Toward a System for Classifying Business Strategies." *Academy of Management Review* 13 (1988): 413–27.
7. Files, L.A. "Strategy Formulation in Hospitals." *Health Care Management Review* 13, no. 1 (1988): 9–15.
8. Reynolds, J.X. "Using DRGs for Competitive Positioning and Practical Business Planning." *Health Care Management Review* 11, no. 3 (1986): 37–55.
9. MacStravic, S. "Market Administration in Health Care Delivery." *Health Care Management Review* 14, no. 1 (1989): 41–48.
10. Mills, P., and Margulies, N. "Toward a Core Topology of Service Organizations." *Academy of Management Review* 5 (1980): 255–65.
11. Urban, G.L., and Hauser, J.R. *Designing and Marketing New Products.* Englewood Cliffs, N.J.: Prentice Hall, 1980.
12. Green, P.E., and Tull, D.S. *Research for Marketing Decisions.* 4th ed. Englewood Cliffs, N.J.: Prentice Hall, 1978.
13. Hauser, J.R., and Koppelman, F.S. "Alternative Perceptual Mapping Techniques: Relative Accuracy and Usefulness." *Journal of Marketing Research* 11 (1979): 495–506.
14. Haley, R.I. "Benefit Segmentation: A Decision Oriented Research Tool." *Journal of Marketing* 32 (1968): 30–35.
15. Green, P.E., and Srinivasan, V. "Conjoint Analysis in Consumer Research: Issues and Outlook." *Journal of Consumer Research* 5 (1978): 103–22.
16. Robertson, T.S., Zielinski, J., and Ward, S. *Consumer Behavior.* Glenview, Ill.: Scott, Foresman, 1984.
17. Abell, D.F., and Hammond, J.S. *Strategic Market Planning: Problems and Analytical Approaches.* Englewood Cliffs, N.J.: Prentice Hall, 1979.
18. Thomas, H., and Gardner, D. *Strategic Marketing and Management.* New York, N.Y.: Wiley, 1985.
19. Day, G.S. *Analysis for Strategic Marketing Decisions.* St. Paul, Minn.: West Publishing, 1986.

Health care requirements planning: A conceptual framework

David M. Rhyne
and
David Jupp

A clearly defined closed-loop operations management system comparable to the Manufacturing Resource Planning System (MRP-II) does not exist in the health care industry. Therefore, a study was conducted to evaluate the basic modules of MRP-II in terms of their applicability for developing a workable health care requirements planning system.

Health Care Manage Rev, 1988, 13(1), 17–27
© 1988 Aspen Publishers, Inc.

The health care industry is in the midst of significant changes. External forces such as government reimbursement programs and internal industry forces in the form of competition and changing market baskets have not had their final impact on the industry, but one thing is certain. The health care industry will never be the way it was before October 1, 1983, when fixed government reimbursement began. Today's environment calls for different organizational structures, different relationships between physicians and administrative personnel, and changes in the roles of the management team. The payoff for making these changes will include survival, profitability, increased control of operations, efficient delivery of services, and reductions in cost.

Many hospital boards of directors and administrative personnel are beginning to view their business in a different light. In an effort to gain more control of hospital operations and thereby control costs the following changes are occurring:

- development of physician-approved standard medical protocols for each diagnosis related group (DRG);
- tracking of staff physician compliance with DRG guidelines;
- product line management to determine which services offer the greatest financial potential;
- development of standard cost systems to determine allowed costs and to track actual costs of delivered services; and
- proliferation of productivity improvement systems that focus primarily on labor.

HOSPITALS IN A SYSTEMS PERSPECTIVE

Rather than isolating a specific component that is experiencing change, it is important to look at hospitals as a total health care system. The major system components and their interrelationships within the operational (hospital) setting as related to effective

David M. Rhyne, *Ph.D., PE, CPIM, is an Assistant Professor in the Department of Management, Auburn University, Auburn, Alabama. He has experience in manufacturing and services types of industries and has worked in the health care industry as a management engineer and consultant to hospitals.*

David Jupp, *B.Sc., is Vice-President of Marketing and Product Development for Accelerated Receivables Management, Chicago, Illinois, a health care services and consulting firm. He has had extensive experience in the health care and manufacturing sectors.*

resource planning and utilization must be identified. This total system analysis parallels the manufacturing resources planning system (MRP-II), which has been applied extensively in manufacturing systems. MRP-II, as employed in the manufacturing sector, is a closed-loop system, that is, a defined flow exists among system components. Furthermore, that flow is multilateral in providing information and receiving feedback. Ultimately each component is connected to some other component in a framework of a closed loop. The system described in this article is the health care requirements planning system (HCRPS), which will be discussed primarily as a hospital-type planning system. Its principal components include

- strategic planning;
- marketing planning;
- operations planning;
- master scheduling;
- capacity planning; and
- material requirements planning.

The need to handle these pieces of the health care business is due to both external and internal forces. In a recent speech before the Berks County of Pennsylvania Manufacturers Association, Mr. Donald Mazziotti, the executive director of the Business Council of Pennsylvania, stated that "the purchasers of health care buy wrong. Instead of purchasing from the lowest cost, highest quality sources, you buy from any and all providers and ignore their efficiency."[1] Industry, in general, has begun to emphasize the need to obtain the biggest purchase possible for the dollar in health care benefits programs. Mazziotti also stated that businesses in Pennsylvania could spend 20 to 30 percent less than they now spend on health care and maintain or improve quality and access to care for their employees. His assertion could be applied on a more national basis, and there is a tone of precision and credibility in what he says. Just as purchasing revolutions are occurring in industry with newly defined relationships between vendor and supplier for manufacturing materials, it seems certain that the same or similar changes are evolving or are destined to evolve regarding health care programs.

DISTINCTION AND APPLICABILITY

Before looking at manufacturing systems and hospital systems, it is important to understand the distinctions between them and the potential interchange of concepts and operational techniques between the two systems. The most obvious distinction is the nature of the two industries. Generally in a manufacturing environment, raw materials are purchased, component parts are produced or purchased, process operations are performed, and a product is produced. These manufactured products are inert (i.e., they are void of life). As such, product flow through a manufacturing cycle can be rigorously controlled without major consequences. The product flow may be increased, decreased, or even terminated. The product may be accepted, rejected, reworked, or scrapped.

Based on these characteristics of a manufacturing system, it is logical for someone in the health care field to develop an initial perception and position that there is no place for manufacturing operations management in health care or hospitals. This initial apprehension is understandable. After all, hospitals are in the people business and that is different from producing things. While this position makes sense, some aspects of the manufacturing planning system are transferable in modified form to hospital management and operations.

The applicability of the resource requirements planning concept to hospital operations may be seen by looking at some of the demand and process characteris-

TABLE 1

COMPARISON OF MANUFACTURING AND HOSPITAL OPERATIONS

Manufacturer	Hospital
Demand	
Production begins with receipt of a customer order.	Services are provided based on patient and mission.
Demand for finished goods is primarily independent.	Demand for services and materials is primarily independent.
Bill of materials is a minimum-level bill that does not emphasize assemblies or subassemblies and their relationships.	Bill of labor is a single-level listing of labor resources required.
Unexpected demands occur with a constantly changing product mix.	Emergency and urgent admissions occur with a fluctuating case mix.
Process	
Complex routings across different work centers may occur.	Services are provided by many ancillary departments.
Assembly operations for a particular product tend to flow in parallel and not sequentially.	The variety of services to be provided do not necessarily occur in a fixed sequence.

tics of a manufacturing company that is successfully using appropriate components of a manufacturing planning and control system. Table 1 shows a comparison of these characteristics to the operational features typically found in a hospital.

These comparisons could be extended, but with these some of the operational similarities can be detected even though the nature of the two businesses is significantly different.

MANUFACTURING RESOURCE PLANNING

During the late 1960s a tool for better management of inventories and scheduling systems was developed and referred to as material requirements planning (MRP). Those organizations strong enough to force MRP to work realized its intended purpose—reduced inventories and improved on-time customer delivery performance. The successor to the forward planning material requirements of MRP was MRP-II (See Figure 1). In this system the three principal components of manufacturing, marketing, and finance aggregate their resources to produce a manufacturing schedule designed to optimize the way in which the firm meets the demands placed on it. McSpadden cites the key functional areas of the total planning system entailed in MRP-II as

- business planning;
- production planning;
- master scheduling (demand management);
- material requirements planning; and
- capacity requirements planning.[2]

A portion of the specific activities that are required, achieved, and maintained in support of these key functional areas include the following:

1. establishing the financial objectives of the organization by top management;
2. identifying markets and products and forecasting demand;
3. determining and allocating resources to meet the forecasted demand;
4. developing time-phased schedules for building all products;
5. using bills of materials that define the structure of the product;
6. using routings that describe the sequence of the various operations involved in building the product;
7. maintaining accurate and timely status of all inventory items required to manufacture the product;

FIGURE 1

A CLOSED-LOOP MANUFACTURING RESOURCE PLANNING (MRP II) SYSTEM

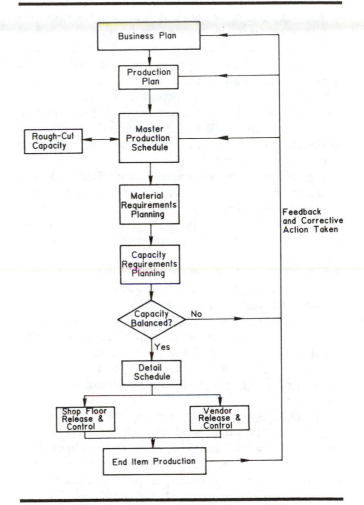

8. creating schedules for requirements of raw materials and component parts used to manufacture a product;
9. managing the capacity of each work center; and
10. using standard product costs to report operating results and measure performance according to plan at each step of the manufacturing process.

The bottom line effect of MRP-II, when all key functional areas and their applications are properly operating, is the ability to plan and control what, when, how much, and in which priority to manufacture. That is, what the business planning system planned to make will be made according to the assigned priority within the framework of available resources.

HEALTH CARE REQUIREMENTS PLANNING

Although it is heavily oriented toward the manufacturing of components and finished goods, the conceptual framework of MRP-II has significant applicability for health care delivery systems. Hospital operations is a specific application of the concepts of MRP-II. There is talk of MRP-III, which incorporates return on investments in the total business requirements planning system. This feature will be an additional incentive for hospitals to begin viewing their operations more from a total systems perspective.

The chief problem confronting hospitals today is how to achieve the most productive use of resources with the highest quality service in the shortest possible time at the lowest cost. Under the new prospective payment system (PPS) of DRG, the hospital will operate profitably if it can deliver the product (i.e., a healthy or recovering patient) at less cost than the government's DRG allowances. Length of patient stay and all the supporting activities (e.g., X-rays, laboratory tests, meals, pharmaceuticals) now have a different connotation. Rather than maximizing them for billing purposes, the hospital must minimize them. Time is of the essence, like a production order situation, in providing quicker or more timely deliveries, and thus maintaining a competitive edge.

The DRG is the primary driving mechanism of the HCRPS. It is the sun around which the planets revolve. In general, the DRG is analogous to the end item of the manufacturing company. In the manufacturing sector, each different product that a company manufactures is defined by a bill of materials (BOM). This BOM is a listing of each component (purchased or manufactured) that goes into the finished product.

So it is with DRGs. Each DRG can be defined in terms of the procedures, services, and materials that apply to it. This concept of DRGs implies that it is possible to develop a standard course of treatment for each DRG.

The diagnosis related group is the driving mechanism of the health care requirements planning system.

This does not imply that each patient must be treated exactly the same way, but it is essential to be able to forecast the resources required to fulfill the objective of efficient utilization of resources.

The framework of the HCRPS provides the principal pieces in a closed-loop fashion for streamlining hospital operations and improving their performance levels (see Figure 2). As with MRP-II these elements include:

1. strategic planning to review the mission of the hospital and to define the goals and objectives of the organization;
2. market research to identify the need for existing services, the development of new services, and the forecasting of customer demand for both;
3. operations planning to determine and allocate resources to meet anticipated demand over the life of the plan;
4. development of a short-term, time-phased plan for delivery of services and allocation of resources;
5. a database consisting of
   - bills of resources that define the services and procedures involved in the treatment of patients,
   - standard treatment profiles that describe the sequence of the various procedures and services involved in treating a patient with a specific diagnosis, and
   - a resources status file that maintains an accurate and timely status of all resource items required in the treatment of a patient;
6. schedules for required services and procedures involved in treating a patient;
7. management of capacity at each work or cost center; and
8. standard costs to report operating results and measure performance at each critical work center.

STRATEGIC PLANNING

In view of the hospital's mission the top administrators initiate the HCRPS process through strategic planning. As in manufacturing, the strategic plan covers a multi-year period; has specific, quantifiable, and measurable goals and objectives; and is usually expressed in financial terms. The need to thoroughly analyze the organizational mission is fundamental to all that follows in the plan's goals, objectives, strategy, and implementation. Peter Drucker's famous line, "What is the business of this business?"[3] cannot be minimized. Is the

FIGURE 2

THE HEALTH CARE REQUIREMENTS PLANNING SYSTEM

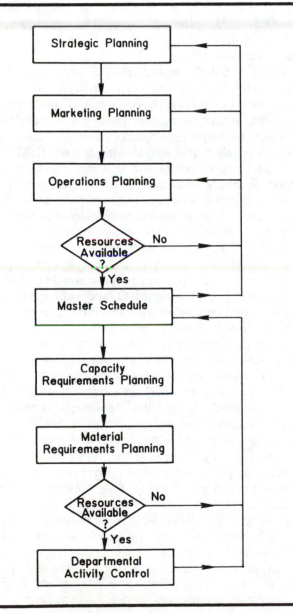

Rather, it considers the futurity of decisions that have to be made now to enable the hospital to be where it wants and needs to be operationally at specific points in the future.

MARKETING PLANNING

The hospital's marketing group will be responsible for transforming the goals and objectives of the strategic plan into a market basket assessment of what the hospital is producing and what the anticipated or forecasted demand is for the products or services. Demographic data analyses by an assortment of independent variables will be helpful. These include type of speciality and number of physicians, age of the local population, record of past treatment needs, and competition of other hospitals. Surveys of marketplace perception of needs and potential acceptance of new services will also be useful. New ventures are continuously being explored by aggressive hospitals as they attempt to expand their product line.

OPERATIONS PLANNING

The underlying principle on which the system is based is predictability. The more predictable a business's manufacturing operations, products, and sales, the more accurate is the forecasting. In this sense, the health care industry is not significantly different than many manufacturing companies. A hospital can readily identify its products, and it can do just as well as the manufacturing company in forecasting sales of these products. The hospital is much the same as the automobile manufacturer when it comes to forecasting demand. The automobile company does not attempt to forecast demand for all its products with a myriad of options; instead, it will forecast demand for the basic automobile, such as a two-door or four-door with a V-6 engine or a four-cylinder engine. Likewise, the hospital would not attempt a long-range forecast for all the various DRGs, but it could forecast demand by major diagnostic category.

Persons assigned to the key functional area of operations planning will then take the demand forecast and develop an operations plan. This plan is an itemization by major diagnostic category of what services (e.g., radiology procedures, laboratory tests, surgical procedures) the hospital should and will need to provide, and what quantities it will provide to meet the criteria of the strategic plan.

hospital to provide rehabilitation, prevention programs (emphasis on wellness), acute care, or some other type or level of service? Another aspect of Drucker's philosophy of strategic planning that is highly appropriate for hospitals today is that it is not performed in the future.[4]

At this point in the HCRPS the initial resource requirements analysis is performed to determine the effects of the anticipated demands on the hospital's resources—labor, capital, and facilities. It is essential to ascertain whether the objectives of the strategic plan are achievable, given the actual or anticipated resource levels of the hospital. Depending on the outcome of this resource analysis, the hospital may require no change, may have to redistribute resources, or may have to obtain additional resources.

The operations planning activity essentially completes the top management input to the system. As the balance of the framework loop provides feedback to the top management level, strategic planning and its ensuing activities are being continuously reviewed and modified. The remainder of the framework, including master scheduling of anticipated demand, detailed capacity planning, and material requirements planning, requires middle-level management participation. These activities comprise the day-to-day operations of a hospital.

ANTICIPATED DEMAND SCHEDULE

The anticipated demand schedule is a time-phased plan for the forthcoming delivery of services. In a manufacturing setting, it is typically a statement of production objectives for each end item or finished goods part number. In a hospital setting, it would be a statement of service objectives for each DRG category. In this sense it differs from the top management plan, which was described in terms of major diagnostic category.

Whereas the top management operations plan covered at least a one-year period, the anticipated demand schedule will typically cover a much shorter period of time. The length of the schedule, expressed in weeks or days, is at least as long as the longest lead time of a specific type of care being provided. In this context, lead time is the total time required to purchase materials and provide the necessary services to a patient in a specific DRG. By way of example, assume that a given hospital is a general acute care hospital and provides services ranging from normal labor and delivery to heart transplant, with heart transplant constituting an average length of stay of 30 days. The anticipated demand schedule for this hospital would cover a minimum of 30 days.

The anticipated demand schedule consists of DRGs of both scheduled and forecasted admissions. Scheduled admissions will constitute the majority of the near-term parts of the schedule, while forecasted admissions will dominate the far-term portion. The hospital's marketing department should provide the forecast of admissions to the scheduling department. The forecast would be based on a number of factors, including historical case mix data, statistical forecasting techniques, and estimates supplied by the medical staff of their anticipated admissions.

The anticipated demand schedule provides management with its first near-term preview of how the hospital's resources will be consumed. This weighing of available resources against projected demand is referred to as rough-cut capacity planning. Drawing on the bill of labor data file, looking at each DRG in the schedule, management can examine the number of standard hours of labor typically consumed by that DRG at each work center. The total projected demand hours are then matched against the demonstrated total capacity of the major work centers for each time period of the total time window covered by the schedule. There are two primary benefits to this rough-cut capacity analysis. First, periodic capacity overloads and underloads can be readily identified, and appropriate management actions relative to reallocation of resources can be developed. Second, where there are periods of underload, new elective admissions can be trial fitted to determine how the available capacity would be utilized. Thus, admission dates for purely elective procedures can be established so as not to overload the hospital's available capacity. Of course, this implies that a certain percentage of capacity must be held in reserve for non-scheduled admissions, and must not be committed without top management authorization.

Most hospitals have a few major work centers that supply the majority of the hospitals' resources. Usually these are nursing, laboratory, operating room, and radiology. If the workload in these major departments can be balanced so that total available capacity is neither overloaded or underloaded, the remaining less critical departments will tend to load accordingly and operate satisfactorily. At this point, a word of caution is in order. As Clark points out in his article on capacity management, there may be a tendency and a perceived need to try to develop a rough-cut capacity plan for all work centers.[5] However, at this level of planning, the effort would not be cost-effective or useful. Too much detail would be generated and the forest would be lost in the trees. Detailed capacity planning occurs later in the HCRPS.

A rough-cut capacity plan can be generated for the major departments by converting the master-scheduled DRG units into standard hours of work required in each major work center. This is a relatively simple procedure that uses a document of data called a bill of labor. An example is shown in Figure 3.

Next, the total hours of work required for all cases scheduled in a given period are compared to the total available capacity. This process assumes that all hours will be consumed in the period in which they are planned. This assumption may not be true; however, for planning purposes it can be assumed that freed capacity will equal committed capacity during any particular period. As an illustration, assume that a given hospital provides treatment only for cataracts. Furthermore, assume

- the anticipated demand schedule is for a 30-day period;
- the first week of the schedule is consumed by scheduled admissions;
- the balance of the schedule is loaded according to projections based on historical data and admissions forecasts from the medical staff; and
- only the nursing, surgery, and laboratory departments are considered critical work centers.

Table 2 shows a simplified anticipated demand schedule based on the previous assumptions. The next step in the rough-cut capacity planning process is to project the workload by period. This projection is shown in Table 3. Finally, the required department (work center) capacity in relationship to available capacity is shown in Table 4. Similar analyses will be

FIGURE 3

TYPICAL BILL OF LABOR

DRG XXX	
Work center	Total standard hours
010	15
020	2
030	3
040	8

TABLE 2

ANTICIPATED DEMAND SCHEDULE

DRG description	Cases per period				Critical work center load profile (standard hours/case)		
	1	2	3	4	Nursing	Surgery	Laboratory
Cataracts	100	70	90	120	8.7	2.0	1.0

performed for the other critical work centers over the projected time periods.

The results of these capacity comparisons to projected demand will be extremely valuable to hospital management in balancing departmental resource availability with projected demand. It should be noted too that the simple example presented addressed only the labor input requirement. Physical facilities such as patient rooms, surgery suites, and laboratory equipment could also be analyzed from the standpoint of resources available versus resources required.

The development of the anticipated demand schedule completes the planning phase of the HCRPS. The daily operations component of the system must be examined next.

CAPACITY PLANNING AND CONTROL

Capacity planning has been discussed in relation to the strategic plan and the anticipated demand schedule. The progression has moved from long-term capacity planning, which translates into resources that need to be acquired, to near-term rough-cut capacity planning, which focuses on the plan for consuming capacity re-

TABLE 3

PROJECTED LOAD BY PERIOD (STANDARD LABOR HOURS)

Department	Period			
	1	2	3	4
Nursing	870	609	783	996
Surgery	200	140	180	240
Laboratory	100	70	90	120

TABLE 4

COMPARISONS OF ANTICIPATED DEMAND
SCHEDULE TO CAPACITY RESOURCES

	Period			
	1	2	3	4
Cases scheduled, DRG-XXX-Cataracts	100	70	90	120
Departmental load profile				
Nursing				
Scheduled hours	1,000	1,000	1,000	1,000
Utilization	.85			
Efficiency	.95			
Net capacity	810			
Load (standard hours)	870			
Load percent	107			
Surgery				
Scheduled hours				
Utilization				
Efficiency				
Net capacity				
Load (standard hours)				
Load percent				
Laboratory				
Scheduled hours				
Utilization				
Efficiency				
Net capacity				
Load (standard hours)				
Load percent				

sources. Patients will not always enter facilities according to a forecast. In fact, hospitals are fortunate if their load has 50 percent elective admissions. Consequently, the daily consumption of resources is subject to a great deal of unknown demand. It is difficult to determine how to actually use the available resources, given the fact that a considerable portion of demand is unknown until patients are admitted to the hospital. The essence of this problem is how to accurately control priorities and capacities to use available resources efficiently. That is, how can required services be delivered in a high quality and timely manner so that DRG target days are met, physicians and patients are satisfied, labor costs are minimized, and the hospital remains financially solvent?

When a patient is admitted to the hospital, it is either known ahead of time what resources will be required

(elective surgical patients), or it is not known with any degree of certainty, as with the patient admitted with an undetermined diagnosis. In the latter case, it can only be anticipated that demand will be placed on those departments whose services will be required to establish a diagnosis.

The object is to develop a treatment plan (routing) that details the services and procedures required by each patient. In the case of the elective surgery patient, this is fairly straightforward. The physician can supply this information prior to the time of admission. Where a patient is admitted through the emergency department, and a diagnosis is made immediately, a treatment plan can be readily established. In this type of admission, treatment plans serve as input to the capacity planning and control system.

The patient who is admitted for purposes of determining a diagnosis places the greatest unknown demand on the hospital's resources. For this patient, the physician's initial plan is to order those services required to provide information for establishing the diagnosis. These diagnostic orders will serve as input to the capacity planning and control system until the diagnosis is made. Once the diagnosis is made, a treatment plan is developed and loaded into the system database.

The next task is to assign due dates for completing the treatment plan and discharging the patient. Once the diagnosis is known, a DRG can be assigned. The assigned DRG with its reimbursable length of stay (LOS) determines due dates. In turn, the assigned due date determines the relative priority of the various services to be provided at each work center.

It is difficult to determine how to actually use the available resources, given the fact that a considerable portion of demand is unknown until patients are admitted to the hospital.

Before the services required for a particular patient can be scheduled through the various work centers, the standard time for each service or procedure plus interoperation times (transit plus queue times) must be known. Queue is a characteristic of any interrupted flow process. The process of patient treatment can be described as an interrupted flow process, because the treatment process is not one smooth continuous path from one test or procedure to the next. Consequently, the work centers providing procedures, tests, or services exhibit a work-in-process characteristic known as a queue. A queue is defined as the work in standard hours at a given work center waiting to be processed. As demonstrated in other waiting line situations, as the queues increase so does the average queue time and the quantity of work in process. Figure 4 illustrates this phenomenon.

As shown in the figure, as long as the hours loaded into Work Center A are equivalent to the capacity available, the work queue will remain constant. However, if more standard hours are loaded into the work center in a fixed period of time than the center can accommodate, the queue size and the work in process will increase. Consequently, total lead time will increase due to delays in providing the required procedures.

As soon as a patient is admitted to a hospital, in essence, the work in process is increased and consumption of capacity begins. In order to minimize excessive queues and to ease the flow of a given patient from the time of admission to discharge, scheduling and work center loading must be performed. Scheduling may be defined as the assignment of desired starting dates and times for the tests, services, or procedures that are anticipated for a typical patient in a specified DRG. Work center loading is defined as the determination of the total standard hours of labor required for each procedure for all patients in each work center by date and time. These activities are related in that scheduling provides the basis for following the progress of required procedures through the various departments, while loading is a priority control technique that highlights bottlenecks and underloads resulting from attempts to meet the schedules.

The capacity planning and control system performs both of these functions in a two-step process. First, each treatment plan containing the required services and corresponding processing and interoperation times, plus the due date, is loaded using finite capacity assumptions. This will reveal which patients are likely to miss the assigned due date for the DRG provided. When this occurs, the scheduler establishes higher priorities for those patients anticipated to be late or to expand work center capacity through scheduled overtime. The second step is to rerun the load with the reassigned priorities or additional work center capacity to complete the required services on time. The result of these iterations is a daily dispatch list for each work center

FIGURE 4

CAPACITY CONSTRAINT ON WORK CENTER A

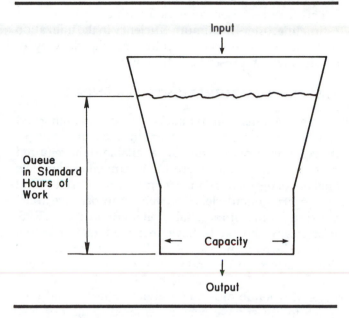

that will list in priority sequence those services and procedures to be performed each day. Each work center reports the completion of the required services so that the system is updated and remaining work can be tracked.

Hospitals will never be able to completely schedule the workload so that all the peaks and valleys over time are eliminated. However, the HCRPS will minimize the variances through efficient capacity management. For example, scheduling the admission of elective patients on the basis of available capacity in the various nursing units rather than infinitely loading will decrease the queue size and work in process. The capacity of the nursing units would be in units of hours of nursing care available during a given period. The underlying assumption here is that by managing the queue of the primary work center (i.e., the first major work center providing services), work required of the secondary work centers (e.g., ancillary departments) will tend to be properly balanced.

This feature is particularly valuable because not all tests and procedures must follow a given sequence, especially when a patient is admitted with an undifferentiated diagnosis. To develop a diagnosis, the attending physician may order a number of different tests and procedures involving more than one work center. Efficiency could be vastly increased if the specified tests or procedures could be routed among the work centers so as not to unnecessarily increase the workload at work centers already loaded to capacity.

This feature, when combined with completion time estimating, offers maximum efficiency in the utilization of finite resources while optimizing the delivery of services within prescribed DRG limits.

MATERIAL REQUIREMENTS PLANNING

An activity that runs parallel to capacity planning and control is required to ensure that the right quantities of the right types of materials are available at the required time to support patient care and treatment. A complete analysis of the material management function is beyond the intent of this article. However, it is imperative to cite the significance of material availability in the HCRPS. Historically, hospitals have managed their material inventories by using a set of stock replenishment procedures, decision rules, and records to ensure continuous physical availability of all items. The three crucial questions of when to order, how much to order, and how much to invest have been considered in light of cost, lead time, and past usage. A more fundamental attribute of the hospital's material inventory management system might be the nature of demand. Orlicky states that "demand for a given inventory item is termed *independent* when such demand is unrelated to demand for other items—when it is not a *function* of demand for some other inventory item."[6] Demand of this type must be forecasted.

In contrast, demand is considered dependent when it is directly related to or derived from the demand for another inventory item or product. In most manufacturing firms this approach of inventory management aptly fits. For example, in manufacturing garden tractors a requirement for engines, wheels, and paint will occur only when there is a demand for garden tractors. Carrying wheels or engines in inventory when there is no demand represents potential needless capital and space investment.

Independent demand that is managed by use of order quantity, reorder point, service level, and safety stock procedures focuses on the individual item. Conversely, material management from a dependent demand perspective focuses on the end-product requirements (demand) over time. Steinberg, Khumawala, and Scamell have presented a system that illustrates the

applicability of dependent demand logic and a corresponding material requirements schedule for a surgery suite. Based on the time horizon of a week the scheduled surgeries by type and by physician generate a dependent material requirements listing. The components of each surgery come from the surgery requirements file, which is equivalent to a single item bill of materials.[7] This rationale can be expanded to the point that a bill of resources required for each DRG could be identified and utilized to determine material requirements in forthcoming time periods.

In light of intensified competition and the need to minimize costs while providing quality care, the need is critical to evaluate the material management portion of the overall HCRPS. A recent study by Showalter, Forseth, and Maxwell focuses specifically on the hospital food service delivery system.[8] Numerous production concepts, information system requirements, and delivery components of the food service operation have parallels in the manufacturing environment. Concepts such as dependent demand material management can be applied to hospitals without having to reinvent the wheel. It appears that some inventory reduction and material availability improvement can occur when overall demand is viewed from an end-item (DRG), time-phased requirement perspective. The essence of the material requirements planning module of the HCRPS is that material in sufficient quantities must be on hand when needed so that care and treatment can proceed as scheduled or required.

•   •   •

The health care industry is facing a new era of cost control, stiff competition, fixed government reimbursement, and a rapidly changing product offering. The operation of not-for-profit hospitals may soon be a memory. The need exists for a system to tie together the key functions of a hospital and at the same time be workable for top and middle management. The HCRPS provides such an integrative, closed-loop system. The strategic planning, marketing, operations, master scheduling of anticipated demand, capacity planning, and material requirements planning functions of a hospital or health care facility must interrelate so that the system is balanced properly, the customers are satisfied, and the organizational objectives are achieved.

It is important to recognize that the HCRPS will require significant changes in the modus operandi of most physicians and administrators. Overcoming resistant attitudes and behaviors of key personnel will most likely be the major obstacle to successful implementation and execution of such a closed-loop system. It is encouraging to note the earlier successful adoption and adaptation of concepts and programs such as standard costing, productivity, quality control, and others to health care management. Just as these new ways of operating required adjustments and change, so will the total system management approach require some, but the system technology and the supporting computer hardware and software requirements have been available for some time. A fairly steep learning curve confronts health care managers, but the eventual payoff in profitable use of resources will be worth the effort.

REFERENCES

1. Mazziotti, D.F. Remarks to the Berks County of Pennsylvania Manufacturers Association, May 24, 1985.
2. McSpadden, B. "MRP II, Fact or Fiction." *Systems User* 6 (July 1985): 32-35.
3. Drucker, P.F. *Management*. New York: Harper & Row, 1974, p. 99.
4. Ibid.
5. Clark, J.T. "Capacity Management—Part Two." In APICS *23rd Annual Conference Proceeding*. Falls Church, Va.: American Production and Inventory Control Society, October 1980.
6. Orlicky, J. *Material Requirements Planning*. New York: McGraw-Hill, 1975, p. 22.
7. Steinberg, E., Khumawala, B., and Scamell, R. "Requirements Planning Systems in the Health Care Environment." *Journal of Operations Management* 2, no. 4 (1982): 251-59.
8. Showalter, M.J., Forseth, M.S., and Maxwell, M.J. "Production-Inventory Control Systems Design for Hospital Food Service Operations." *Production and Inventory Management* 25, no. 2 (1984): 67-83.

Planning evolution in hospital management

Gilbert D. Harrell
and
Matthew F. Fors

In today's competitive health care market, hospitals are adopting more sophisticated and aggressive planning systems. The development of hospital planning can be visualized as an evolutionary progression from financially based systems to advanced systems of strategic analysis. This article offers a prescriptive model that hospital administrators can use to assess their organization's planning capabilities and move along the path to more effective planning.

Health Care Manage Rev, 1987, 12(1), 9–22
© 1987 Aspen Publishers, Inc.

During the past decade, hospitals have found themselves in a markedly more hostile environment. Competition in the health care market has increased rapidly and in many areas the very structure of health care delivery has changed with the introduction of health maintenance organizations (HMOs), preferred provider organizations (PPOs), urgent care centers, and other new forms of patient contact. In addition, recent changes in hospital reimbursement from third party payers may reduce the cash inflow for typical inpatient hospital care. Faced with new competitors, rising costs, and lower reimbursement, hospitals have begun to look closely at alternative care delivery mechanisms to achieve new growth. Many have undertaken extensive organizational restructuring and have launched major new ventures in search of competitive success.

The challenges in today's health care market have placed great pressure on hospitals to develop more sophisticated and aggressive planning systems. Yet, many hospitals continue to rely on traditional forms of planning that focus on the internal factors of administration. These approaches prove to be weak support systems for hospital management in a dynamic market. One survey suggests that few hospitals currently have a market-based strategic plan in place.[1] During the past three to four years, some hospitals have adopted planning systems that took nearly 20 years to evolve in other industries. While these institutions use more advanced systems, they are still on the steep side of the learning curve in marketing and strategic planning.

To understand the move to sophisticated planning approaches, one can visualize hospitals progressing through a series of distinct planning stages. This "evolution" offers a prescriptive model for advancement of hospital planning. By viewing the development of strategic planning as a series of stages, hospitals can assess their capabilities and prepare to move

Gilbert D. Harrell, *Ph.D., is Professor of Marketing and Transportation Administration, Michigan State University, East Lansing. His research, consulting, and teaching focus on strategic planning, marketing and sales management, and marketing research and buyer behavior.*

Matthew F. Fors, *M.B.A., is a consultant specializing in hospital and medical marketing and business strategy. His consulting and research experience includes work with hospitals, physicians, and medical suppliers.*

on to the next level of planning sophistication. At the very least, hospitals should seek to move to the next level, with the ultimate goal of reaching more advanced stages. In addition, new strategic planning systems may be forthcoming to accommodate the unique aspects of the hospital environment. This article presents an evolutionary path for hospital planning, illustrates how current strategic thinking can be applied, and raises the challenges that future hospital planning systems must address.

FIVE PLANNING PHASES

The concept of evolutionary phases in formal planning has been examined in work with industrial goods manufacturers.[2] The findings support the idea that planning does evolve along typical paths as organizations gradually increase their planning capabilities. For hospitals, five distinct planning phases can be identified. Each phase represents a major step in the evolution from elementary planning methods to more advanced strategic planning systems. The five phases are

1. financial planning and control systems;
2. environment-based planning;
3. project market planning;
4. strategic business unit (SBU) portfolio development; and
5. strategic portfolio application.

First, the characteristics of each planning phase and its implications for hospital management are discussed. Then a summary is given of current trends that foreshadow future planning systems.

Phase 1: financial planning and control systems—an internal focus

Prior to the 1980s, the health care field was growing in quantum leaps. Health care expenditures more than tripled from 1970 to 1980, reaching 9.5% of the GNP by the end of the decade.[3] This growth was stimulated by expanding government-subsidized health care programs, increased population, and a proliferation of new health care services due to technological advancements. In the 1960s and 1970s, when construction costs were relatively low and the need for increased hospital beds was forecast, facilities planning occupied a good deal of the hospital staff's planning effort. At that time, the health care delivery system consisted primarily of private practicing physicians and affiliated hospitals. A major challenge was to acquire funds for expansion at low rates

and subsequently apply those funds to build capital structures. Much of the competitive focus of hospital administrators was directed at building market share by adding beds with proper local approval. Hospitals were clearly in the growth stage of their life cycles.

Compounding the picture was the dramatic increase in third party pay and government financing. This required internal structures to shuffle large amounts of data and paperwork. Additionally, the availability of more sophisticated, and consequently more expensive, medical apparatus placed a high premium on administrators' efforts to acquire funds at a reasonable rate. A natural outgrowth was the introduction of financial accounting systems to guide cost control and cash flow management. High speed computers, spawned in the previous decade, provided the hardware to get the job done. Financial accounting systems were supported by software that could accommodate the required high volume and perform fairly elementary financial analysis. As inflation became an important variable, hospitals continued to emphasize the importance of financial planning and record keeping to slow rising costs.

During this period, accurate financial planning was possible because forecasting was relatively easy. Although environmental factors were changing, the direction of change was consistently upward with predictable rises in demand for many of the hospital's services. The financial control systems produced fairly accurate documentation of administrative actions. The greatest concern was the ability to get information quickly and project further into the future.

Financially based planning systems lack a major ingredient that is required in today's environment. They are unable to effectively analyze and interpret the market impact of environmental and competitive changes. Many hospitals have failed to move from internally focused financial planning systems, and these organizations have suffered competitively because of it. Other hospitals that are somewhat isolated from competition in smaller communities and remote areas have managed to survive despite this internal focus.

Phase 2: environment-based planning—orientation to marketing

The environment-based planning approach is a necessary phase in moving from an ethnocentric perspective to an external perspective. The ethnocentric perspective is characterized by great reliance on the views of technicians and medical practitioners within the hospital hierarchy. The environmental-based perspective, by contrast, is outwardly focused and directed toward the hospital publics.[4]

During the mid-1970s, many organizations discovered the importance of broad, basic, innovative, and futuristic goals.[5] These corporations benefited by developing mission statements that placed them in line to take advantage of growth opportunities. Thus firms were prompted to shift from looking only at the internal resources of the organization to applying greater attention to opportunities in the marketplace.

During the mid-1970s, many organizations discovered the importance of broad, basic, innovative, and futuristic goals.

As with other industries, most hospitals appear to have moved into or through the environment-based planning phase. At this stage, hospitals examine market opportunities on a nonquantitative, "visionary" basis. Some hospitals created mission statements that focused more on the treatment of diseases rather than the care of patients. Others with a more progressive attitude began to look at patients as health care consumers in a broader sense, rather than simply treatment seekers. These hospitals found it valuable to conduct studies of patients to determine the requirements of positive health care. Thus, at this time, marketing research was added to most planning groups as a major function. The studies helped to describe the potential roles of the hospital as well as to evaluate the hospitals' performance as perceived by patients.

During this phase, many hospitals identified several constituents other than patients that should be addressed in searching for their particular niche in the community. These included physicians, community organizations, business enterprises, and labor groups. Perhaps the most important public to be identified by hospitals was the private practicing physician who had found increased leverage through multiple hospital affiliations. Many hospitals and physician populations have had a long history of antagonism. A good deal of it can be traced to the dependence each party has on the other and the lack of power either group has to accomplish its unique

goals. Yet, by looking outward, many hospitals quickly recognized the tremendous importance of physicians not only in serving patients, but also in generating demand for hospital services. Studies support this role and have indicated that most patients are heavily influenced by their physicians in their choice of hospital care.[6]

The transition from internal financially based systems to market-oriented planning philosophies represents a major shift in strategic thinking for hospitals. However, in order to have a positive impact, these mission statements and philosophies have to be translated into actual hospital strategies and programs.

Phase 3: project market planning—the search for structure

The project market planning phase is characterized by attempts to apply market-oriented philosophies to hospital opportunities in an organized fashion. This phase extends the environment-based planning systems by focusing more on the actual activities to accomplish project goals. Its strength is in providing very systematic guidance for individual hospital projects. The market planning phase of the planning evolution can be recognized by use of detailed outlines that are often referred to as "planning guides." The outlines typically specify great amounts of information that must be documented. Consequently, a bulk of the planning effort usually revolves around a situation analysis of the hospital's market position. This stimulates the expansion of marketing research activities by the hospital. Many top administrators receive a continual flood of offers by research companies and associations to perform marketing surveys and to supply general market information to support this type of planning system.

Unfortunately, project market planning is really a "snapshot" approach to planning. At given points in time, a relatively accurate record of the market conditions can be ascertained and specific hospital objectives and action plans can be devised. However, in a rapidly changing environment, the system is too stagnant and limited in scope. Little consideration is given to the total framework under which the hospital operates. For example, a hospital might have one project for an oncology unit, another one for the cardiovascular unit, and a third for the birthing unit. In many cases, a scattering of individual projects will occur that lack the systematic integration needed to move forward with total programs and major operational commitments. Additionally, this planning approach requires a great deal of marketing attention to individual programs. Such time and expertise may not be available to some hospitals given the limited number of marketing personnel who are knowledgeable in the health care field.

Phase 4: SBU portfolio development—a step toward integration

Portfolio planning has now become a standard approach for strategic thinking in many businesses. This approach was popularized by Boston Consulting Group as a means to graphically depict a firm's opportunities in the market. The use of portfolios is appealing to planners because it recognizes distinctions among different product or service areas of the firm, supports the development of unique strategies for each area, and uses a straightforward graphic format to communicate strategic thinking. A variety of different methods for constructing portfolios have been developed and in certain cases tailor-made portfolios are advocated to meet a company's unique needs.[7]

During the past three to four years, the portfolio approach has been applied to the planning practices of some hospitals. As in other industries strategic business units provide a means to categorize the hospital's activities for planning purposes. Each unit is based on a composite of products, technologies, functions, and specific markets served by the hospital. By carefully defining each unit, hospital planners are able to identify separate entities that could be operated as quasi-independent businesses. A subtle paradox is that by defining the hospital as a set of SBUs that could operate independently, hospitals are actually better able to coordinate the activities of the entire hospital.

Using this approach, one major hospital identified the following strategic business units:
- newborn and maternal care;
- child and adolescent care;
- adult medical care;
- surgical care;
- mental health care;
- ambulatory/primary and outpatient care; and
- clinical support services.

The SBUs are then placed on a portfolio grid that positions them according to the hospital's strength in the unit and the amount of opportunity represented by the particular unit. Figure 1 shows an example of the basic grid that is used and how the SBUs were positioned by the sample hospital. The SBU positions are established through a combined assessment of secondary market data, community market research, and administrative business judgment.

The portfolio planning concept recognizes that different businesses are in varying phases of the life cycle and therefore will produce or use cash in varying degrees. Category A is represented by strategic planning units of low hospital resource strength and high market opportunity. These particular units offer the greatest amount of growth potential, but also are likely to require large amounts of cash flow and hospital resources to move them into Category B. As shown, surgical care represents an attractive hospital opportunity but one that will probably entail high investments in equipment and medical staffing to expand.

Category B represents those units in which the hospital has a great amount of resource strength and that also offer high opportunity. Here, the cash flow could be positive or possibly break-even. These are SBUs where the hospital has the greatest excellence and uniqueness (in this case, mental health services). Thus, the hospital should continue to support this area and will probably accrue long-term value from its operation.

Category C is represented by those units that are in the mature phase of their life cycle and thus offer low growth opportunity even though the hospital is particularly strong there. In most cases, these SBUs should still generate a good deal of capital. If they do not, it is usually due to one of three factors. First, it could be that this part of the hospital is being mismanaged and economies of scale are not being properly utilized to generate cash flow. Second, it is possible that a very strong regional health care competitor has kept prices down, thereby hindering profitability. Third, government intervention, which mandates reduced fees, could be preventing cash from flowing out of this area. An example is the case of adult inpatient care. Although aging of the general population has provided the hospital with continued patient volume and a dominant share has been maintained, a major proportion of patients rely on Medicare reimbursement. Medicare limits potential revenues and suggests that new forms of care should be explored, such as outpatient or home health care alternatives.

FIGURE 1

SBU PORTFOLIO

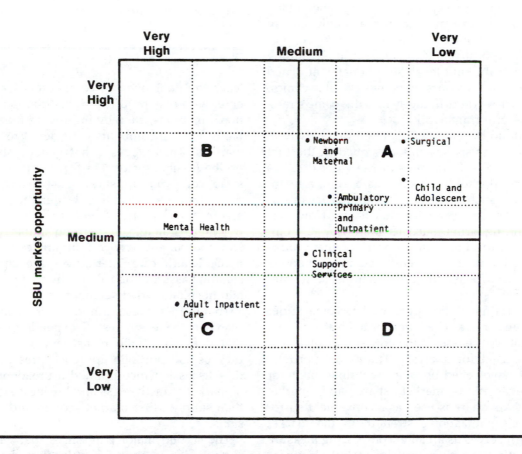

Category D is represented by those businesses that offer only limited or negative growth opportunities and in which the hospital is not very strong. Obviously, these particular SBUs are unlikely to warrant extensive future investment.

SBU portfolio development represents a very important stage in planning evolution. It offers a means to systematically divide the hospital into operational units and evaluate the cash flow implications of each unit. For each hospital, the picture will differ even within the same market area. For example, in a major metropolitan area, mental health programs represent major growth opportunities for one hospital because

of its unique resources and experience. Consequently, those programs are classified in Category B. Yet, another hospital in the same city might classify those programs in Category D because it has different resources and a different perception of what represents an attractive market opportunity. Although different, both assessments are realistic.

Hospitals that have used the portfolio approach have benefited from careful analysis regarding the competitive position of the hospital, as well as the opportunities for each of its strategic planning units. The system also provides graphic representations that make it easier to communicate with hospital board members and other administrators. Furthermore, by visualizing the business according to a series of strategic planning units, alternative forms of management organization become apparent. For example, some hospitals have developed planning teams to represent each unit. These teams are made up of hospital administrators, physicians, nursing staff, and other representative parties. Since many hospitals already operate through a multiplicity of management committees, this team structure provides a logical focal point for much of the planning that is done at the unit level. Additionally, affiliated organizations such as nursing homes, satellite clinics, and urgent care centers fit nicely into this same strategic business unit framework.

SBU portfolio development is often tied closely to the financial analysis systems described in the first planning phase. In fact, much of the work that has been done on portfolio analysis has been of a financial nature. As such, even the SBU approach can suffer from too much of an internal focus. However, some consulting firms, such as McKinsey & Company, which introduced the concept to many business organizations, have carefully maintained an external market focus in unit identification and planning.

Recently, the portfolio approach has come under attack by some critics. There appear to be at least two fundamental weaknesses. One criticism involves the dimensions used for analysis. Traditional portfolio approaches have relied on only two dimensions for business evaluation—market share and market growth. Market share is used as a convenient surrogate for an organization's strength in the market while growth serves as an all-encompassing measure of a market's attractiveness. In reality, business strength consists of a complex arrangement of the resources that an organization can bring to bear, including technological advantages, personnel knowledge and experience, client and supplier relationships, and research and development capabilities. Similarly, market attractiveness cannot be understood by examining only growth rates. Instead, management must consider total market volume, profit potential, competitive pressure, and many other aspects in deciding where to invest company resources.

Reliance on share-growth matrices as a basis for harvesting certain businesses has resulted in near catastrophes for a number of major manufacturers.[8] Market leaders may decide to comfortably harvest high share-low growth markets and inadvertently

Business strength consists of a complex arrangement of the resources that an organization can bring to bear, including technological advantages, personnel knowledge and experience, client and supplier relationships, and research and development capabilities.

leave the door open to competitors who selectively enter with new production, distribution, and promotional methods, thereby improving the profit potential of what incumbents considered to be lackluster markets. This suggests that generic strategies may not be feasible for certain firms and conditions.[9] Instead, companies must cautiously watch for competitive entry even where their leadership position seems secure. Parallels are evident in the health care industry where dramatic distribution shifts are under way. New outpatient services, urgent care centers, and home health care alternatives are changing long-standing assumptions about the true potential of certain hospital market segments.

To address these inherent problems, some researchers have suggested expanding the elements that define portfolio measurement.[10,11] Notice that the hospital portfolio approach presented earlier in this discussion incorporated a broadened definition of market attractiveness and business strength rather than simply using market growth and share dimensions.

The second major criticism is that while portfolio analysis does a good job of labeling the positions of various strategic planning units for comparison, it is incomplete because it does not specify the actual activities that should be undertaken within each unit and subsequently for the hospital as a whole. For example, what strategies should be used to strengthen the hospital resources in SBUs that offer high opportunity? The analysis is largely descriptive rather than prescriptive. The key to effective use of portfolio planning is in moving beyond the analytical stage to implementation. Many companies have encountered difficulty in connecting portfolio theory to practice because they fail to allocate resources or to build strategies based on portfolio positions.[12] Similarly, many hospitals also stop short after simply identifying circumstances and positioning SBUs.

FIGURE 2

PHYSICIAN PORTFOLIO

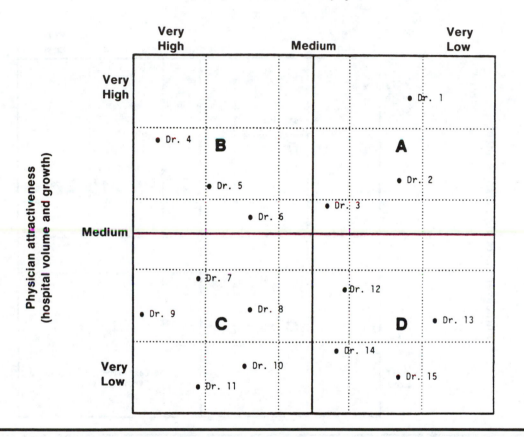

Hospital penetration within physician's business

They fail to move to the next stage to develop actual hospital strategies.

Phase 5: strategic portfolio application—blueprints for action

After identifying strategic planning units, hospital administrators must come to grips with key organizational and management decisions. In the strategic portfolio application phase, the administrator's effort extends beyond building an appropriate planning structure to include developing procedures for actual strategy formulation. This will involve strategies directed at patients, physicians, referral agencies, support groups, and competitors. As an example, let us examine how the strategic portfolio planning system might be used to design strategies for physicians.

As noted, physicians should properly be viewed as both a potential resource and as a customer of the hospital. Looking at physicians in this way, it is useful to analyze a portfolio of physicians in the relevant health care community. A hospital's physician may be positioned according to two portfolio dimensions: physician attractiveness (defined as the physician's current volume of hospital work and projected growth); and hospital penetration (defined as the share of physician's business currently received by the hospital). Figure 2 provides an example of how this type of analysis might appear for a given hospital.

FIGURE 3

PHYSICIAN SEGMENT PORTFOLIO

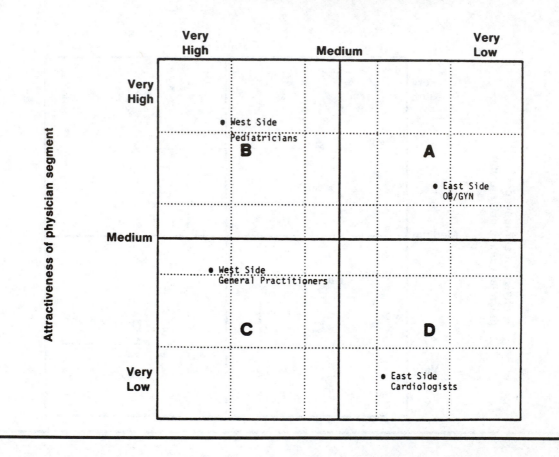

Hospitals with a great number of physicians in Category A are in an attractive medical community; however, they lack strength within the community, as measured by low physician support. Hospitals with a great number of physicians in Category B are in an attractive market and have a great deal of strength. Hospitals with a great number of physicians in Category C are probably in a very mature medical community and may experience growth problems in the future. Hospitals that may have most of their business coming from physicians in Category D are in a dangerous strategic position and must alter their approach or they will fail. The most healthy hospitals will probably have a mixture of physicians in Categories A, B, and C.

As a second step, it is a relatively simple but important matter to group the physicians by segment using geographical location, physician specialty, and other descriptors. Once these segments are identified, they should also be placed on a portfolio to summarize the categories of physicians to which the hospital is directing its appeals. Figure 3 is an example of how four such segments might be positioned.

The third step is to build strategies for each segment. This is accomplished by identifying those strategic variables that can be controlled by the hospital

FIGURE 4

STRATEGIES FOR PHYSICIAN SEGMENTS*

	A	B	C	D
	East Side OB/GYN's	West Side Pediatricians	West Side General Practitioners	East Side Cardiologist
Allocation of Time Contact Frequency	Moderate Extensive	Heavy Extensive	Moderate Periodic	Low Limited
Administrator Involvement	Top administrator involvement	Regular inclusion of senior people	As necessary but handle at lower echelons wherever possible	Avoid top involvement unless unusual situation
Type of Contact	Concentrated personal communication	Personal contact and groups	Group contact and mailings	Limited group contact
Competitive Focus	Challenge competitors' providers by aggressively seeking to build new relationships with this physician group	Solidify and maintain existing relationships. Defend against competitive hospitals	Preserve current physician relationships. Watch for competitor thrusts	Satisfy problems or concerns do not invest heavy time/effort
Message	Stress unique benefits of affiliation vs. competitive hospitals (i.e., special programs and support services)	Emphasize long term cooperation and value of affiliation to physician	Reinforce commitment to physician but underscore importance of increasing contribution	Stress need to boost contribution where appropriate
Objectives	Obtain____ # new physicians and staff, increase share with existing physicians	Hold all current physicians, maintain or increase their contribution level	Retain physicians and current volume	Take what is contributed. Do not attempt to increase hospital's share of this segment

* Letters A, B, C, D refer to the blocks in the grid shown in Figures 1, 2, and 3.

administration. These could include such elements as administrator involvement, type of contact, message to be communicated, and so on. Appropriate strategies can then be developed based upon the portfolio position of each physician segment, as illustrated in Figure 4.

The same strategic portfolio planning system can be used on a number of critical levels for strategy

FIGURE 5

COMPETITOR PORTFOLIO

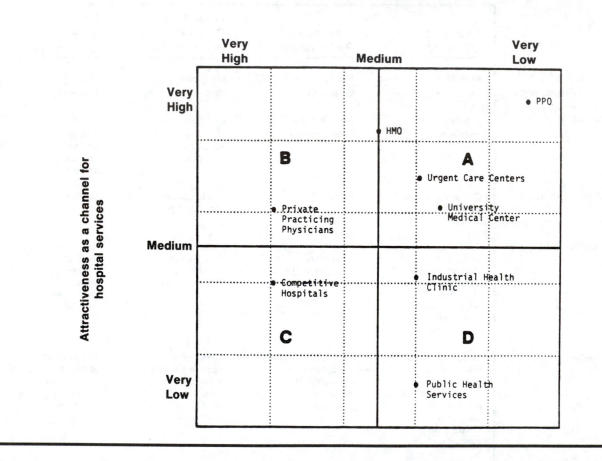

development. Earlier, it was noted that an important aspect of strategy is to understand the competitors' positions. Aggressive hospitals are not only monitoring their own situations, they are also carefully looking at the situations of other hospitals and other forms of health care delivery. One hospital has been successful in charting the positions of local distribution channels for health care, as illustrated in Figure 5. The portfolio shows competitive hospitals as well as other types of delivery systems. It is also possible to show individual competitors within each type. In this hospital community, the HMO is in Category A but possibly moving quickly into Category B. Thus, the hospital must be careful to monitor the progress of HMOs to ensure that a good deal of hospital volume is not lost. Furthermore, the hospital may wish to look at the HMO not only as a competitor, but also as a possible customer of the hospital's services. That is, through cooperative relationships or shared services, the HMO may actually prove to be a key source of hospital referrals and business building. Figure 6 describes some of the ways that alternative health care delivery systems might be addressed with different strategic approaches.

FIGURE 6

COMPETITIVE CHANNEL STRATEGIES*

	A	B	C	D
Strategic Elements	HMO	Private Practicing Physicians	Competitive Hospitals	Public Health Services
Hospital Channel Emphasis	High	High	Medium	Low
Amount of Resources	Moderate	High	Low	Very Low
Administrative Organizational Posture	Initiate personal one-to-one contact between top administrator and competitor leaders	Develop task teams with possible medical staff involvements	Continue current contact structure unless problems arise	Rely on existing interface systems and contacts
Activities	Explore cooperative relationships to enter new market segments and add new services	Determine how existing base can be strengthened to expand patient sourcing. Focus on combined efforts	Welcome referrals but remain separate	Only limited effort to hold present volume. Give in to competitors if necessary
Competitive Thrust	New ventures, mergers, or shared services	Cooperate for mutual benefit	Maintain aggressively competitive posture	Accept referrals to hold community relations and fulfill hospital mission where appropriate
Objective	Expand volume by____%	Maintain or increase volume	Hold current volume	Accept____%. Decline

* Letters A, B, C, D refer to the blocks in the grid shown in Figures 1, 2, 3, and 5.

ADVANCED HOSPITAL PLANNING SYSTEMS: CHALLENGE FOR THE FUTURE

Thus far, the series of planning phases that hospitals pass through as they move from elementary to sophisticated planning systems have been described. Few hospitals currently use highly sophisticated systems, but more are moving in that direction. Portfolio planning has proven quite valuable in its application to hospital strategy formulation. However, the process for developing and implementing strategic plans encounters a severe test in the hospital setting. Certain peculiarities in the decision-making environment of hospitals suggest that a special approach to strategic planning is required to fully address their unique needs. Future hospital planning systems must accommodate and exploit these structural differences to maximize the effectiveness of strategic planning efforts.

Unlike most corporate organizations, hospitals function through a highly complex arrangement of committees, task forces, and ad hoc planning groups. These planning subsets exist at all levels of the hospital, from staff groups within individual departments up to advisory committees of the hospital board. While the presence of planning groups is not totally foreign to companies in other industries, only in hospitals does this structure have such a pervasive and ongoing impact on the decision-making process. Moreover, participation on hospital planning groups typically includes individuals from inside as well as outside the hospital. For example, it is common to find a balanced mix of representatives from hospital administration, the medical staff, the hospital board, and possibly an external community representative.

Such groups may be charged with developing standards, monitoring performance, and assessing programs. In addition, they often have responsibility for outlining objectives and formulating strategies for recommendation to the president, chief executive officer, and full hospital board. In short, these committee structures play a crucial role in determining hospital objectives and defining strategic alternatives.

This decision-making structure has developed for good reasons. It is based on the hospital's need to accommodate the divergent goals of several constituencies and enlist their cooperation and support in order to accomplish hospital objectives. In most situations, it is vital that the hospital administration garner the backing of physicians, the board, and perhaps local community groups or industries for a given program to succeed. Conversely, the medical staff is aware that it too lacks sufficient power to carry out its desired goals without support from the other sectors. As a result, consensus is achieved through personal interaction in small planning groups that provide the mechanism to raise the concerns and motivations of each sector, resolve potential conflicts, and move forward with plans that incorporate these divergent perspectives.

Advanced hospital planning systems must utilize highly participatory and interactive methods to accommodate the decentralized group decision processes used in the hospital environment. One can imagine that such systems would include iterative planning stages in which strategic options are drafted, revised, and refined in an organized fashion in order to achieve maximum support from administrators, physicians, the board, and other key groups. Still, it will be necessary to maintain personal contact between representatives of each group since negotiation and persuasion are fundamental in arriving at decisions in the hospital planning environment. The important goals of the system must be to raise viable and creative approaches, facilitate decision making, and integrate these decisions into a cohesive hospital plan of action.

While future hospital planning systems must be participatory and integrative, these are necessary but not sufficient qualifications. In a dynamic health care market, the system must also permit rapid decision making in response to sudden market shifts in customers, competitors, and legislation. This is the essence of the challenge for hospital strategic planning.

In a dynamic health care market, the system must also permit rapid decision making in response to sudden market shifts in customers, competitors, and legislation.

A participatory and integrative system must be designed that also provides rapid identification of strategic responses and moves the hospital to action in the marketplace.

An important key to reconciling these conflicting planning requirements will involve the methods for gathering strategic information. In truly strategic organizations, planning is actually a decision-making mechanism and plays a fundamental role in executive actions. Ultimately, the need for elaborate written procedures, planning books, and the like will be dispensed with as planning is translated directly into action. For hospitals, the ability to provide up-to-date and usable input to strategic planning will facilitate longer lead time for decisions and allow the participatory decision process to move more rapidly. Sophisticated information systems will be designed to operate across hospital functional areas and provide a full range of computer tools to record, analyze, and interpret information. For example, computer graphics may be used to model alternative scenarios and predict the likely outcome of various actions. Such "what if" types of planning activities will open new doors for effective management and present realistic ways of assessing the impact of strategic decisions. At the same time, this information can give hospital planning groups the added insights to avoid the lengthy, detailed study now required to assess health care needs and develop program choices.

RECENT TRENDS IN CORPORATE PLANNING

It would be remiss to conclude this discussion without noting several important trends within corporate planning today. Together these interrelated trends suggest that a new step in planning evolution is taking shape.

"Back to basics"

Since the mid-1970s, the focus of corporate planning has undergone a significant shift. Earlier planning approaches emphasized the process of strategic planning at the expense of strategy implementation. This preoccupation with the mechanics of planning was perhaps a natural outcome of the popularization of portfolio concepts. Today, many leading firms are placing greater emphasis on strategy application and less on the planning process itself. In view of the economic recession in the early 1980s, and increasing competition in low-growth conditions, managers must respond quickly to rapid shifts in competitive pressure. Thus, planning is being realigned to get "back to basics" in many companies. This means focusing squarely on obtaining and maintaining a competitive advantage.[13,14] This new posture also has heightened the importance of good market research about current market conditions. An increasing number of firms are finding a need to better understand customer needs and attitudes toward competitors in order to secure a superior image in the marketplace.

Greater line management responsibility

A second trend is evident in the type of personnel involved in planning. The responsibility for strategy development, which was relinquished to "corporate strategists" in the 1970s, is being returned to line management in many organizations. There is greater hands-on involvement of managers in strategy formulation and a coincident downsizing of formal strategic planning departments. This move is designed to obtain maximum benefit of management's knowledge about markets, customers, and competitors, as well as to strengthen their commitment in carrying out strategies. Resultant strategies are based on a better understanding of market dynamics and managers obtain a sense of ownership in shaping the destiny of their business unit or department. Involvement of line managers may also help them acquire greater appreciation for a long-term perspective in planning. Day-to-day actions take on a new meaning if they are steps to a self-ascribed goal.

Entrepreneurial new venture teams

The third major trend is reflected in a new form of organizational structure. Certain large organizations such as General Motors, Kodak, and 3M have established independent teams for new ventures. These entrepreneurial teams often consist of managers, technicians, and salespeople who are charged with developing and marketing a new product or service entirely outside the traditional organizational structure. The goal is to bypass the typical roadblocks and red tape that can stifle creativity and delay response within the traditional corporate channels. As yet, the results are not all in, but this new entrepreneurial approach may hold great promise for revitalizing innovation.

In moving to more sophisticated planning approaches, hospitals should take note of these recent trends and incorporate them into their planning where possible. Administrators will want to avoid getting lost in the mechanism of the planning process and maintain the focus on implementation of competitive strategies. Basic marketing research should be emphasized to build understanding of health care customers, competitors, and market conditions. How is the hospital perceived relative to competitors in key market segments? What criteria do these customers use in selecting a hospital? What can the hospital do to enhance its standing on characteristics customers use to select a hospital among alternatives? These are fundamental questions that warrant research into consumer attitudes and the development of strategies for attitude change.

While a formal planning group may offer a comfortable feeling that "someone is doing something" about the hospital's future, department managers and other personnel (nurses, physicians, technicians) should be brought into the planning activity to share their experiences and insights. The process may not be as "neat" or convenient as a centralized group of designated planners, but the rewards of management involvement may pay off in commitment and follow-through.

Finally, progressive hospitals may wish to experiment with entrepreneurial venture teams to facilitate the development and launch of new health care services. Such teams can move important projects ahead with the speed and concentration needed for success in an increasingly competitive marketplace.

● ● ●

Today, most of the literature regarding hospital marketing and strategic planning focuses on the need for planning and particularly underscores the importance of a philosophy of customer orientation. Unfortunately, little of the literature is analytical or prescriptive in nature. It does not fully describe the approaches that can be used to develop aggressive strategies. The concept of evolutionary planning phases should encourage administrators to push beyond descriptive marketing literature to develop and apply creative strategies for planning units, patient segments, physician segments, and competitors. By recognizing the unique advantages and disadvantages at each stage, hospitals can benefit from the experiences of firms inside and outside the health care industry.

REFERENCES

1. Kropf, R., and Goldsmith, S.B. "Innovation in Hospital Plans." *Health Care Management Review* 8, no. 2 (1983): 7–16.
2. Bluck, F.W., Kaufman, S.P., and Walleck, A.S. "Strategic Management for Competitive Advantage." *Harvard Business Review* 58 (July–August 1980): 154–161.
3. News release by Health Care Financing Administration. Washington, D.C.: HCFA, October 10, 1984. Statistics cited in *Health Care Financing Review*, Fall 1985.
4. Kotler, P. *Marketing for Non Profit Organizations.* Englewood Cliffs, N.J.: Prentice-Hall, 1975.
5. Levitt, T. "Marketing Myopia." *Harvard Business Review* 38 (July–August 1960): 46–56. Reprinted as *Harvard Business Review Classic* 53 (September–October 1975): 26–48.
6. Boscarino, J., and Steiber, S.R. "Hospital Shopping and Consumer Choice." *Journal of Health Care Marketing* 2, no. 2 (1982): 15–23.
7. Wind, Y., Mahajan, V., and Swise, D.J. "Designing Product and Business Portfolios." *Harvard Business Review* 59 (January–February 1981): 155–65.
8. James, B.G. "SMR Forum: Strategic Planning under Fire." *Sloan Management Review* 25 (Summer 1984): 57–61.
9. Day, G.S. "Diagnosing the Product Portfolio." *Journal of Marketing* 41 (April 1977): 29–38.
10. Wind, Y., Mahajan, V., and Swise, D.J. "An Empirical Comparison of Standardized Portfolio Models." *Journal of Marketing* 47 (Spring 1983): 89–99.
11. Wensley, R. "Strategic Marketing: Betas, Boxes, or Basics." *Journal of Marketing* 45 (Summer 1981): 173–83.
12. Haspeslagh, P. "Portfolio Planning: Uses and Limits." *Harvard Business Review* 60 (January–February 1982): 58–73.
13. James, "SMR Forum: Strategic Planning under Fire."
14. Hussey, D.E. "Brief Case: A Portfolio of Commentary and Opinion." *Long Range Planning* 18, no. 2 (1985): 107–108.

An empirical investigation of the nature of hospital mission statements

C. Kendrick Gibson,
David J. Newton,
and
Daniel S. Cochran

An exploratory study of hospital planners was completed to determine if there was agreement between theory and practice concerning mission statement components and development. Results showed that mission statements have received little attention as part of the overall strategic planning process.

Health Care Manage Rev, 1990, 15(3), 35-45

Interest in strategic planning and how it should be performed is capturing the attention of the hospital industry as it has other sectors of the economy. Several authors have discussed strategic planning as it relates to the hospital industry. This particular article focuses on an important part of the planning process: developing effective mission statements for guiding hospitals.

The mission statement gets little recognition in most strategy applications. Perhaps this is due to lack of understanding of the importance of the mission statement: The importance of developing the mission, however, cannot be overstated. In fact, many believe that the development of the mission should supersede everything else in strategic planning. Leontiades, in an early article, proposed that the proper relationship of planning activities is (1) developing the overall mission, (2) developing strategies, and (3) formulating specific plans and programs.[1]

Snow and Hambrick, among others, have pointed out that there is a distinct difference between the process of developing the strategy and the actual implementation of the plan.[2,3] In addition, measurement of results is difficult when there is no standard. The mission statement can be the document that helps clarify issues and guides middle managers as they make decisions that affect the organization.

Even so, there has been little guidance for hospital managers in developing an effective mission statement. The purpose of this article is to present some of the literature concerning what should be included in a mission statement and to present the findings of an exploratory study concerning mission statements in the hospital industry.

WHAT IS A MISSION STATEMENT AND WHAT DOES IT DO?

Lazer and Culley have defined the mission statement as the fundamental reason the organization exists. This is determined by asking "What business is the organization in?" and "What is its basic purpose?"[4(p.130)]

C. Kendrick Gibson, *Ph.D., is a Professor in the Department of Economics and Business Administration and Director of Strategic Planning at Hope College in Holland, Michigan.*

David J. Newton, *M.H.A., is Vice-President for Planning at Butterworth Hospital in Grand Rapids, Michigan.*

Daniel S. Cochran, *Ph.D., is an Associate Professor in the Management Department at Mississippi State University in Starkville, Mississippi.*

Drucker stated that these questions may be obsolete in a fast-changing environment, and the appropriate questions are "What will our business be?" and "What should our business be?"[5] Ackoff has supported these ideas by stating that a mission statement should commit the organization not to what it must do in order to survive, but to what it chooses to do in order to thrive.[6]

Focusing on mission statements does not diminish the importance of a vision statement. Block has stated that a vision statement is an expression of optimism or a statement related to greatness and hope for an organization. He believed that what some organizations have called credos or core principles were, in fact, vision statements. A vision statement comes from the heart of the leadership group and is radical and compelling.[7] As such, it lays the groundwork for a mission statement, which then adds meaning to the vision by helping to clarify what is to be done.

A frequently quoted definition of a mission statement is that it "is a broadly defined but enduring statement of purpose that distinguishes the organization from others of its type and identifies the scope of its operations in product (service) and market terms."[8] The mission statement is of value in helping an organization to focus its resources to accomplish specific things. The mission statement should at least help distinguish one hospital from another.[9] Ackoff supports this idea by stating that the mission should establish the individuality, if not the uniqueness, of an organization.[6] Quinn writes that a mission statement should attempt to create élan or an identity larger than the limits placed on the firm by the individuals themselves.[10] Byars and Neil stated that the mission defines the current and future business activities that will be pursued by an organization; it becomes a unifying force, providing a sense of direction and a guide to decision making for all levels of management.[11] The mission offers this distinctiveness by clarifying the role and purpose of the organization.[12]

The second attribute or characteristic of a mission statement is that, ideally, it should be exciting and inspiring.[6] Zaleznik found that effective missions help satisfy people's needs to produce something worthwhile, to gain recognition, to help others, to beat opponents, or to gain respect.[13] Employees of hospitals want to believe that they are engaged in something important as much as employees in other organizations. Ackoff believed the mission should play the same role in an organization that the Holy Grail did in the crusades.[6]

Third, the mission should facilitate a change in the behavior of the organization.[6] The mission is the first step in the development of goals and objectives that stretch and focus the organization. McMillan believed that most hospital missions are too general and useless in that they do not prompt any actions.[14] Unless mission statements facilitate the development of objectives and measures toward attainment, then the mission is of no value.[6]

Knowing what a mission statement is and generally what it can do for an organization is of little value if managers have no knowledge about what should be contained in the statement itself. The components of mission statements are an important part of any discussion about missions in hospitals.

MISSION STATEMENT COMPONENTS

Research concerning what should be in a complete mission statement has progressed slowly and has focused primarily on business organizations outside the health care industry. In one concept article by Pearce, the mission is described as the statement that presents the basic goals, characteristics, and philosophies that shape the strategic posture of a firm. As such, the statement should identify the scope of the firm's operations in product and market terms.[8]

Several component parts of an effective mission statement were suggested by Pearce. Without going into each in detail, these components were

- the basic product or service, primary market, and technology to be used in delivering the product or service;
- organizational goals stated in a strategic sense—such as growth, profitability, stability, or survival;
- organizational philosophy—the code of behavior that guides the operations of the organization;
- organizational self-concept—a self-evaluation and self-concept based on a realistic evaluation of its strengths and weaknesses; and
- public image—how those outside the organization should or do view the particular entity.[8]

These components were used to create a practical framework for developing an effective mission statement by Cochran et al.,[15] who contrasted examples of various components from corporate and university missions. In addition, they discussed how organizations could evaluate the quality and usefulness of a statement.

David et al. later completed an empirical study of Fortune 500 companies and accredited business schools in an attempt to determine how useful these components were. They found that these components were exhibited in more than half of all statements from both groups. They concluded that the content was indeed important to mission statements, and that higher-performing firms had more comprehensive statements. On the other hand, many of the responding organizations did not have a written mission statement.[16] Pearce and David used the same data to complete a slightly more detailed analysis to explain why this was so. Attention was drawn to the lack of a mission statement by the fact that many corporate leaders asked for help in statement development. At that time it was believed that lack of knowledge about the components of an effective statement hampered, if not prevented, mission development.[17]

Others have shed light on the relevant pieces of a mission statement. Carl Sloane, a management consultant, believed that a mission statement should be built around a clear definition of the business management wants to be in and should include guidelines for what the organization would be in that business. It was also important that the mission statement include enough information to make it useful to operating managers, in order to gain commitment.[18] Want believed the proper components were purpose, principal business aim, corporate identity, policies of the organization, and values.[19] These are very similar to the components proposed by Pearce.

MISSION STATEMENTS IN THE HOSPITAL SETTING

In spite of interest in mission statement development in the business setting, few have attempted to specify what should be in the mission statement for a hospital organization. Two efforts are reviewed here. McMillan believed that an effective statement should at least deal with the following list of variables.[14] A comparable variable suggested by Pearce is indicated by parentheses.

- hospital location and geographic area of service (market);
- description or identification of the hospital (self-concept, product definition);

In spite of interest in mission statement development in the business setting, few have attempted to specify what should be in the mission statement for a hospital organization.

- specialty departments to be established, educational needs to be met, research pursuits (service, technology);
- technological level of medicine to be delivered (technology);
- role of the hospital in its local health care environment (strategic goals, self-image);
- particular philosophies and attributions (values); and
- cost and size (strategic goals).

Ainsworth's ideas related to the value and usefulness of a mission statement for hospitals and offered a few general guidelines. The components he believed important were

- statement of the reason for the existence of the institution (strategic goals, product or service);
- commitment of the institution to a specific purpose (goals, product or service); and
- inclusion of restrictions, if any, concerning services that would not be provided[20] (product or service).

RESEARCH OBJECTIVE AND METHODOLOGY

The literature concerning hospital mission statement components was found to offer little empirical evidence for hospital managers concerning how mission statements were viewed by managers and what components are important. This exploratory project was done to offer insight into these issues and to provide a basis for further research.

Using a survey questionnaire, the authors sampled members of the Society for Hospital Planning and Marketing of the American Hospital Association. A systematic sample of 700 people was selected from the membership. The responses used in the analysis were limited to individuals who were personally involved in the strategic planning process in their organizations. Only those organizations that had mission statements at the time of the survey were included. These criteria were established to help ensure that the responses were based on personal experience with and knowledge about hospital mission statements.

Survey materials included a cover letter, brief definitions of strategy, a mission to help clarify what the survey was about, and the questionnaire itself. The questionnaire consisted of the following four parts:

1. information about the organization for categorizing responses according to factors such as bed size;

2. general information about planning and mission statements in the particular organization;
3. twelve Likert-scaled questions concerning the use of mission statements in the organization; and
4. a section concerning mission statement components using Pearce's components list as a guide. This section asked respondents to evaluate the description of each component as offered by Pearce and to improve on it from their points of view. In addition, respondents were to indicate whether or not they believed the component was relevant for their organizations and whether or not their mission statements included the component.

The survey was pretested with five hospital planners selected from the list. Suggestions for improvement were incorporated into the final survey prior to mailing.

Usable responses were received from 176 individuals representing slightly over 25% of the sample population. These individuals served in hospitals of all different sizes and tended to categorize themselves into small, medium, or large hospital organizations. Thirty-five (20.1%) could be considered small in size, with 200 or fewer beds. There were 70 (40.2%) in the medium category, with 201 to 400 beds, and 69 (39.7%) in the large category, with more than 400 beds. Ninety-five percent of the respondents characterized their hospital organizations as either not-for-profit (67.8%, $n = 118$) or religious not-for-profit (27.1%, $n = 47$).

DISCUSSION AND RESULTS

Competitive situation

Organizations represented in this survey tended to reflect the widespread concern over competition and its effect on hospital futures. Over half of these respondents (61.8%, $n = 107$) reported that they faced strong competition in their environments. Only seven institutions (4.0%) reported low competition, and the remainder reported average competitive environments ($n = 59$, 34.2%).

Trends in occupancy seemed to reflect this environment. Nine organizations (5.2%) reported very low occupancy rates of less than 50%, while 73 organizations (41.8%) stated that occupancy was between 50% and 69%. The largest group reported occupancy levels between 70% and 100% ($n = 82$, 52.6%). Of this category, 25% of the respondents were at 80% occupancy or above, but only 8 organizations (4.6%) were between 90% and 100% occupancy.

Only a few organizations reported facing significant increases in occupancy trends ($n = 10$, 5.8%). On the other hand, many more stated that they were experiencing a significant decline in occupancy ($n = 30$, 17.5%). Combining those with significant declines and those with slight declines in occupancy showed that 59.1% ($n = 101$) of the respondents were facing a decline in occupancy of some type.

These occupancy characteristics and the respondents' perceptions of their competitive environments seem to support the need for mission statement development and careful thought about the future of each organization. Average managers who have experienced good years of expansion and success will find it more difficult to adjust in hard times without an agreed-on mission. More direction and thought about the purpose and capabilities of the organization would seem to be necessary for continued success.

Mission statement use in respondent organizations

The organizations in this sample tended to use and view mission statement development and use in much the same way as their counterparts in the business community. Tables 1 through 4 summarize the level of agreement expressed by respondents about 12 aspects of mission statement development and use. Table 1 presents the overall responses. The reader will note that respondents recognize the importance of mission statements and generally feel positive about each of the survey statements evaluated. In addition, 84.2% ($n = 144$) stated that their organizations had mission statements.

Table 2 separates respondents into groups according to whether they reported low, average, or highly competitive environments and presents the mean scores for each of the statements. Generally, those organizations facing high levels of competition agreed more than other groups that their planning was more operational than that of others, and they were slightly more tentative than other groups concerning agreement about several of the areas. Presenting the data this way, however, overlooks the number of respondents that may have disagreed, especially those facing high competition. Within this high competition category, several organizations are not similar to most of the other organizations. For instance, of the 107 institutions reporting a highly competitive situation, 15 (14%) indicated that they believed a mission statement was not an important aspect of planning by either disagreeing strongly or disagreeing with the first statement. In

---

TABLE 1

LEVEL OF AGREEMENT CONCERNING VARIOUS ASPECTS OF PLANNING

		Level of agreement* (*n* = 173)					Mean value
		1	**2**	**3**	**4**	**5**	
1. The development of a mission statement has been and is an important aspect of our planning.	Frequency %†	3 1.7	18 10.4	29 16.8	57 32.9	66 38.2	3.954
2. Developing mission statements is a top management function and involves few individuals within the organization.	Frequency %	16 9.2	45 26.1	19 11.0	62 35.8	31 17.9	3.272
3. The board of trustees is instrumental in the development of the mission of the organization.	Frequency %	10 5.8	12 7.0	23 13.4	57 33.1	70 40.7	3.959
4. A planning committee/team is responsible for the development of the mission statement and the strategic plan.	Frequency %	13 7.5	17 9.8	15 8.7	72 41.6	56 32.4	3.815
5. The mission statement is used as a guide for gaining commitment to organizational values and goals.	Frequency %	5 2.9	5 2.9	31 17.9	51 29.5	81 46.8	4.145
6. Our mission statement is clear and helps middle level managers make more effective and relevant decisions.	Frequency %	8 4.6	32 18.5	60 34.7	53 30.6	20 11.6	3.260
7. The development of a mission statement involves several levels of managers including the board of trustees, medical staff, and both senior and middle management.	Frequency %	18 10.4	49 28.3	20 11.6	41 23.7	45 26.0	3.266
8. We have found that a mission statement is too difficult and time consuming to develop.	Frequency %	110 64.7	32 18.8	18 10.6	6 3.5	4 2.4	1.600
9. Our planning is more operational than strategic.	Frequency %	37 21.5	56 32.6	30 17.4	41 23.8	8 4.7	2.576
10. A consultant has been used to help develop a mission for our organization.	Frequency %	87 51.7	29 17.1	16 9.5	26 15.4	11 6.5	2.083
11. We do not have a mission statement as an inherent part of our strategic plan.	Frequency %	128 74.9	16 9.3	10 5.8	7 4.1	10 5.8	1.567
12. The mission statement of our organization has a high degree of shared commitment. We can see how our individual actions affect each other and our overall goals.	Frequency %	11 6.4	30 17.6	46 26.9	60 35.1	24 14	3.327

* 1 = Strongly disagree, 2 = Disagree, 3 = Neutral, 4 = Agree, 5 = Strongly agree.

† Row percentages may not total 100% due to rounding.

TABLE 2

MEAN LEVELS OF AGREEMENT CONCERNING PLANNING ACCORDING TO LEVELS OF COMPETITION

	Low competition (n = 7)	Average competition (n = 59)	High competition (n = 106)
1. The development of a mission statement has been and is an important aspect of our planning.	4.429	3.966	3.916
2. Developing mission statements is a top management function and involves few individuals within the organization.	2.714	3.475	3.196
3. The board of trustees is instrumental in the development of the mission of the organization.	4.429	4.051	3.877
4. A planning committee/team is responsible for the development of the mission statement and the strategic plan.	4.286	3.729	3.832
5. The mission statement is used as a guide for gaining commitment to organizational values and goals.	4.000	4.153	4.150
6. Our mission statement is clear and helps middle level managers make more effective and relevant decisions.	3.143	3.220	3.290
7. The development of a mission statement involves several levels of managers including the board of trustees, medical staff, and both senior and middle management.	4.143	3.288	3.196
8. We have found that a mission statement is too difficult and time consuming to develop.	1.143	1.655	1.600
9. Our planning is more operational than strategic.	1.857	1.163	2.623
10. A consultant has been used to help develop a mission for our organization.	1.714	2.293	1.990
11. We do not have a mission statement as an inherent part of our strategic plan.	1.000	1.483	1.651
12. The mission statement of our organization has a high degree of shared commitment. We can see how our individual actions affect each other and our overall goals.	3.857	3.263	3.327

addition, 45 of these respondents (51.4%) believed that statement development was not a top management responsibility.

Fifty-six respondents (55.1%) in the highly competitive situation were neutral toward their mission statements or thought them unclear and unhelpful to middle managers. Perhaps that was because 50.5% (n = 54) felt that few levels were involved in statement development. Nineteen (17.9%) either did not know if their organizations had statements of mission or believed that they did not. Finally, 51.4% (n = 55) did not believe there was a high degree of shared commitment.

Of those organizations facing high competition, many need to develop a more concentrated focus about how they will respond to their environment in order to get everyone to work toward the same objectives.

Low occupancy has been a primary factor in motivating organizations to plan. While only nine organiza- tions reported extremely low occupancy rates (0–49% of occupancy), these were apparently heavily involved in analysis and planning for the future. The strength of their responses compared to those of other groups was quite high. Table 3 presents those results. As before, frequencies within categories yield valuable informa-

TABLE 3

MEAN LEVELS OF AGREEMENT CONCERNING VARIOUS ASPECTS OF PLANNING ACCORDING TO OCCUPANCY

	Low occupancy 0%–49%) ($n = 9$)	Medium occupancy 50%–69% ($n = 73$)	High occupancy 70%–100% ($n = 91$)
1. The development of a mission statement has been and is an important aspect of our planning.	4.333	4.027	3.857
2. Developing mission statements is a top management function and involves few individuals within the organiza- tion.	2.444	3.192	3.418
3. The board of trustees is instrumental in the development of the mission of the organization.	4.778	3.904	3.922
4. A planning committee/team is responsible for the develop- ment of the mission statement and the strategic plan.	3.778	3.973	3.692
5. The mission statement is used as a guide for gaining commitment to organizational values and goals.	4.333	4.137	4.132
6. Our mission statement is clear and helps middle level managers make more effective and relevant decisions.	3.667	3.315	3.176
7. The development of a mission statement involves several levels of managers including the board of trustees, medical staff, and both senior and middle management.	4.111	3.438	3.044
8. We have found that a mission statement is too difficult and time consuming to develop.	1.111	1.630	1.625
9. Our planning is more operational than strategic.	2.222	2.597	2.593
10. A consultant has been used to help develop a mission for our organization.	2.111	2.042	2.114
11. We do not have a mission statement as an inherent part of our strategic plan.	1.000	1.556	1.633
12. The mission statement of our organization has a high degree of shared commitment. We can see how our individual actions affect each other and our overall goals.	3.778	3.315	3.292

TABLE 4

MEAN LEVELS OF AGREEMENT CONCERNING VARIOUS ASPECTS OF PLANNING ACCORDING TO
TRENDS OF OCCUPANCY

	Significant decline (*n* = 30)	Slight decline (*n* = 70)	Slight and significant increase (*n* = 69)
1. The development of a mission statement has been and is an important aspect of our planning.	4.000	3.859	4.029
2. Developing mission statements is a top management function and involves few individuals within the organization.	3.067	3.254	3.420
3. The board of trustees is instrumental in the development of the mission of the organization.	3.900	3.873	4.088
4. A planning committee/team is responsible for the development of the mission statement and the strategic plan.	3.867	3.775	3.870
5. The mission statement is used as a guide for gaining commitment to organizational values and goals.	4.200	4.070	4.188
6. Our mission statement is clear and helps middle level managers make more effective and relevant decisions.	3.367	3.197	3.246
7. The development of a mission statement involves several levels of managers including the board of trustees, medical staff, and both senior and middle management.	3.600	3.113	3.217
8. We have found that a mission statement is too difficult and time consuming to develop.	1.667	1.652	1.500
9. Our planning is more operational than strategic.	2.467	2.746	2.435
10. A consultant has been used to help develop a mission for our organization.	2.467	2.029	1.925
11. We do not have a mission statement as an inherent part of our strategic plan.	1.467	1.557	1.588
12. The mission statement of our organization has a high degree of shared commitment. We can see how our individual actions affect each other and our overall goals.	3.333	3.271	3.353

---

tion. Within the medium-occupancy group, for instance, 52.1% (*n* = 38) did not believe their mission statements were clear and useful to middle managers. Similarly, 45.2% (*n* = 33) did not believe that several levels of management were involved in statement development, and 36 (49.3%) did not agree that shared commitment was high.

Disagreements existed among those with high occupancy rates as well. However, the implications may be less evident, given the stronger performance of their

TABLE 5

MISSION STATEMENT COMPONENTS' RELEVANCY VERSUS IRRELEVANCY AND WHETHER INCLUDED OR NOT IN RESPONDENT MISSION STATEMENT

Component	Relevant		Irrelevant		Included		Not included	
	n	%	n	%	n	%	n	%
1. Customer or primary market	154	(95.7)	7	(4.3)	130	(88.4)	17	(11.6)
2. Products or service	136	(86.1)	22	(13.9)	99	(66.9)	49	(33.1)
3. Technology	110	(71.9)	43	(28.1)	67	(45.9)	79	(54.1)
4. Organizational goals	130	(82.8)	27	(17.2)	79	(53.0)	70	(47.0)
5. Organizational philosophy	150	(94.3)	9	(5.7)	124	(83.8)	24	(16.2)
6. Self-concept	89	(57.8)	65	(42.2)	39	(27.1)	105	(72.9)
7. Public image	135	(84.4)	25	(15.6)	97	(65.5)	51	(34.5)

particular organizations. Ninety-one organizations reported high occupancy levels, but of these, 31.9% (n = 29) were neutral toward or believed that mission statements were not important. In fact, 63.7% (n = 58) either did not know what their missions meant or were unclear about how to use them. These hospitals did not involve several levels of the organization in discussions, since 58.2% (n = 53) either disagreed with or were neutral to the statement related to involvement. Finally, 29.7% (n = 28) believed that their planning was more operational than strategic. This may be expected, given strong demand.

Occupancy trends have affected the type of planning done by some organizations, too. Sixteen of 30 in the group facing significant declines (53.3%) were involving more levels of the firm than just top management in mission development. Even so, 15 (50%) did not think their mission statements were clear enough or provided enough guidance to middle managers, and the same proportion did not believe a shared commitment had been developed. Table 4 presents the mean results for occupancy levels, whether low, medium, or high occupancy existed. On the average, the three groups were quite similar in the views toward the 12 statements, even if there were several who were not in the mainstream of opinion.

Mission statement components

Even though most of these respondents agreed that mission statements are important and were in general agreement concerning use, they were less alike in their evaluations of what should be included in a mission statement. Table 5 summarizes whether respondents believed certain components were relevant and whether their own statements included the components listed.

Most respondents believed that the components presented were relevant. For only one component, self-concept, was there a large number of respondents who did not see the value of stating or explicitly defining the component. Sixty-five (42.2%) of those responding to that question believed self-concept to be irrelevant. Technology was also believed by many to be relatively unimportant to the hospital mission statement. Forty-three (28.1%) believed this aspect to be irrelevant.

Although most individuals thought the listed components relevant, several components were often not included in the mission statements of the individuals' hospitals (see Table 5). These frequently omitted components and their proportions of omission were

- self-concept (72.9%),
- technology (54.1%),
- organizational goals (47.0%),
- public image (34.5%), and
- product or service (33.1%).

Those most often included in mission statements were the customer or primary markets to be served and an organizational philosophy. This may be due to the experience hospitals have with developing written statements about these areas, to affiliations with religious groups, or to traditions and values commonly associated with medical institutions.

These findings may also reflect that respondents had not previously considered mission statements to the extent that was required in the survey. This could account for the fact that many components believed relevant were not included in mission statements.

• • •

The results of the survey seem to support several conclusions. First, that a dialogue is needed within the health care industry concerning which components should be in a mission statement and how such a statement should be developed. Written comments as well as marked responses to questionnaire items indicate considerable diversity in opinions about whether missions should be expanded and shared with many individuals or few. With the exception of this study, the literature related to the development of missions in the hospital industry offers little guidance to practicing managers.

Second, many organizations have statements of philosophy or value but have not developed a strategic focus to their mission statements. This should be of particular importance to those institutions reporting declines in occupancy and highly competitive environments.

Third, commitment to the strategic direction of the organization can be improved by increased efforts to involve more levels of management in development and by more frequent communication about what actions are necessary to achieve the mission of the organization. This is particularly so in organizations facing stiff competition and declining occupancy.

Several respondents sent copies of their mission statements for review and offered comments beyond the items included in the questionnaire. A brief analysis of these revealed two ideas that seemed to guide most responding organizations in their work concerning mission statement development. First, respondents seemed overly concerned with brevity. A statement that is too brief becomes a motto only, offering little guidance. Brevity could also be a mistake for such a challenging environment. Although the environment changes rapidly, the mission statement is the cornerstone of the hospital strategic plan. As such, considerable thought and effort must be applied to its development if strategic and implementation plans are to be relevant. Second, fear of disclosure seemed to keep some information out of mission statements. Careful dissemination of complete statements is vital to proper implementation. Perhaps there should be two statements: one for internal use and one, similar to a vision statement, for release to the public. The published version could offer the general framework to be followed by the institution, while the internal statement could include confidential or more complete information.

Finally, strategic management is often defined in terms of a stream of decisions leading to the development of strategies to accomplish specific objectives.[21] These decisions are effective only in light of the mission of the organization. The understanding of what a mission should be has progressed beyond answering the questions "What businesses are we in?" or "What businesses should we be in?" Hospitals should consider whether they have gone far enough in recognizing the centrality of mission statements to effective strategic planning.

REFERENCES

1. Leontiades, M. "The Confusing Words of Business Policy." *Academy of Management Review* 7, no. 1 (1982): 45–48.
2. Files, L.A. "Strategy Formulation in Hospitals." *Health Care Management Review* 13, no. 1 (1988): 9–16.
3. Snow, C.C., and Hambrick, D.C. "Measuring Organization Strategies, Some Theoretical and Methodological Problems." *Academy of Management Review* 5, no. 4 (1980): 527–38.
4. Lazer, W., and Culley, J.D. *Marketing Management, Foundations and Practices.* Boston, Mass.: Houghton Mifflin, 1983.
5. Drucker, P.F. *Management: Tasks, Responsibilities, Practices.* New York, N.Y.: Harper & Row, 1974.
6. Ackoff, R.L. "Mission Statements." *Planning Review* 15, no. 4 (1987): 30–31.
7. Block, P. *The Empowered Manager: Positive Political Skills at Work.* San Francisco, Calif.: Jossey-Bass, 1988.
8. Pearce, J.A., II. "The Company Mission as a Strategic Tool." *Sloan Management Review* 23, no. 3 (1982): 15–24.
9. Griffith, J.R. "The Mission of the Well-Managed Community Hospital." *Michigan Hospitals* 24, no. 7 (1988): 43–46.
10. Quinn, J.B. *Strategies for Change: Logical Incrementalism.* Homewood, Ill.: Irwin, 1980.
11. Byars, L.L., and Neil, T.C. "Organizational Philosophy and Mission Statements." *Planning Review* 15, no. 4 (1987): 32–35.
12. Thieme, C.W., Wilson, T.E., and Long, D.M. "Strategic Planning for Hospitals Under Regulations." *Health Care Management Review* 6, no. 2 (1981): 35–43.
13. Zaleznik, A. "Power and Politics in Organizational Life." *Harvard Business Review* 48, no. 3 (1970): 47–60.
14. McMillan, N.H. "The Mission Statement: Where It All Begins." In *Planning for Survival, A Handbook for Hospital Trustees.* 2d ed. Chicago, Ill.: American Hospital Association, 1985.

15. Cochran, D.S., David, F.R., and Gibson, C.K. "A Framework for Developing an Effective Mission Statement." *Journal of Business Strategies* 2, no. 2 (1985): 4–17.

16. David, F.R., et al. "An Empirical Investigation of Mission Statements." In *Proceedings*, edited by D.F. Ray. Mississippi State, Miss.: Southern Management Association, 1985.

17. Pearce, J.A., II, and David, F. "Corporate Mission Statements: The Bottom Line." *Academy of Management Executive* 1, no. 2 (1987): 109–16.

18. Pascarella, P. "Is Your Mission Clear." *Industry Week* 219, no. 4 (1983): 75–77.

19. Want, J.H. "Corporate Mission." *Management Review* 75 (August 1986): 46–50.

20. Ainsworth, T.H., Jr. "The Mission Statement: Essential Ingredient in Planning." *Trustee* 29, no. 9 (1976): 34–36.

21. Jauch, L.R., and Glueck, W.F. *Business Policy and Strategic Management*. 5th ed. New York, N.Y.: McGraw-Hill, 1988.

Patrolling the turbulent borderland: Managerial strategies for a changing health care environment

Mark Burns
and
Alfred R. Mauet

Contemporary health services administrators face tasks of complex decision making. One approach is to identify the dominant problem, then respond. An inventory of such problems and responses can play a vital role in organizational survival.

Administrators of health services organizations have always had to face problems of information gathering, decision making, and implementation. Yet, the targeting of appropriate problems (for attention and action) has often been shaped by factors in the health care environment that often are beyond the managers' control—developments in technology, management methods, and governmental intervention. Today, the rate of change in these outside forces has become so rapid that this organizational environment itself must be regarded as unstable, even turbulent.[1] Federally sponsored health planning has come and gone; diagnosis related groups (DRGs) are "in." Insurance-oriented business conglomerates are exerting unprecedented pressure on the health care industry. Competitors for market share are multiplying in both number and variety.[2,3]

This instability of the health care environment has almost become a truism. Most contemporary managers of health services organizations are well aware that they must deal with other organizational actors—allies, competitors, regulators, suppliers, community groups—and that these organizational actors are themselves changing constantly, often at an almost dizzying pace. The critical question for managers is how to adapt to these continual shifts and changes. Ideal paper solutions all too often collapse upon collision with the uncertainties of the real world of health care. Furthermore, dealing with a turbulent organizational environment demands something better than the inertia of knee-jerk traditionalism. For example, no longer can managers assume federal tolerance for escalating health care costs—not to mention ready availability of federal funding for pilot programs.[4-6]

One practical approach to the problem of rapid change is to consider what appears to be the dominant

Mark Burns, *Ph.D., is an Associate Professor of Political Science and Director of the Health Administration Program, Auburn University, Auburn, Alabama. He has published in the areas of health planning, interorganizational behavior, and organizational innovation.*

Alfred R. Mauet, *M.P.A., is a graduate student and research assistant in the doctoral program in the Department of Science and Technology Studies at Rensselaer Polytechnic Institute, Troy, New York.*

The authors thank Camilla Stivers for raising several issues crucial in the development of this article.

problem in the interorganizational environment of a health services organization. That is, the health services manager must analyze the primary concern posed by the complex external interrelationships of his or her organization with other relevant organizations, then act accordingly. Drawing on earlier research in the theory of organizations by Burns and Mauet,[7] the authors suggest that at least five major types of problems exist in the interorganizational environments of health services organizations, each of which should be met by a specific strategic focus for managerial action.

Once an administrator has identified the most crucial interorganizational problem facing his or her organization, a strategic focus for action becomes evident, along with its associated objective. The next step is a choice of tactics. In only a few cases will the health care manager be able to implement all the potential tactics at once or with equal vigor. While these choices will be partly constrained by managerial and organizational style, the authors suggest a few cautionary guidelines for each strategic focus that may aid the decision process.

RESOURCE DEPENDENCY

"Why don't we ever have enough...?" "Enough" in this case could be enough money, clients, legal authority, or whatever resource seems to be in critically short supply. Resources are mainly obtained from the organization's surrounding environment; therefore, a useful initial tactic is an internal needs assessment.[8,9] Specifically, the administrator will need to address such questions as what do departments, divisions, and offices most require to do their jobs? What element is most lacking?

The mirror image of an internal needs assessment is the development of inventories of external resources. One question that could be asked is, what is available in the surrounding environment that might be used to meet a facility's needs? Marketing surveys can be one useful source of information to obtain such data.

Once internal needs are compared to available external resources, actual resource gathering can begin. For example, although lobbying is a term usually associated with government agencies, in actuality all health care organizations engage in some lobbying for resources. A hospital administrator who appears before a certificate of need (CON) review board in order to seek a legal mandate for construction is lobbying; a clinic administrator who appears before a local Rotary club to better inform its members about clinic physicians' services is lobbying. Lobbying is simply a plea—blatant or subtle—for what an individual or institution does not have, directed toward "those who do."

Increasingly, resource sharing arrangements are proving to be another popular approach in the health care industry. Whether full mergers, shared services, or any of the numerous possibilities in between, resource sharing can often reduce acquisition costs for expensive equipment as well as produce benefits from economies of scale.

The manager who finds resource dependency to be the dominant problem of the organization will need to beware of some of the associated pitfalls of coping with it. For example, needs assessments and resource inventories can be over emphasized to the neglect of careful analyses of longer-term problems. Obtaining short-term "soft" funding for a community wellness program may be less crucial over the long-term than a plan to deal with the effects of a declining physical plant. Also, lobbying and resource sharing may result in compromises with fundamental organizational mission and commitments that prove embarrassing or destructive at some later point. For example, resource sharing may acquire a momentum of its own and result in an organization being absorbed by a larger "helper" in a corporate merger to an extent far beyond the original intentions of the management of the smaller facility.

CONTINGENCY

"Does anyone know what's going on around here?" When a health services organization seems to be bewildered by the dizzying pace of externally induced change (i.e., competition from other organizations, multiplicity of federal regulations, shifting community needs), it may be time to take steps to more effectively map its environment. Any organization must be somewhat responsive to its environment, but those that wish to stay on top of the competition must try to not merely react to change but to anticipate it and plan for it *before* its impact becomes critical.

In this regard, a major tactic of value is staff capability building. No matter how small the organization, some portion of its human capabilities needs to be devoted to scanning the environment for signs of relevant change. For example, some health services administrators were aware of DRGs when they were a mere experiment in New Jersey; their institutions reaped a corresponding benefit when DRGs became a major national policy.

Training staff in the scanning or mapping process

may necessitate some reorientations. Because a criticism of American business administration in general tends to be its short-time horizon and preference for quick fixes,[10,11] some retraining or development of longer horizons may be necessary. In particular, the importance of leading indicators, even hunches, may have to be stressed.[12]

No matter how small the organization, some portion of its human capabilities needs to be devoted to scanning the environment for signs of relevant change.

When retraining is less feasible, importing longer horizons may be possible; for example, hiring new, more future-oriented staff. Looking for new suppliers, market entrants, and organizational forms and alternative services more amenable to long-range planning may be another defensive move.[13] For example, faced with investor pressure to devote undue attention to matters of short-term profits rather than development of longer-range strategic policies, an investor-owned health services organization may seek to "go private" via leveraged buyout. Similarly, a shift to bond financing rather than equity financing may facilitate lengthening organizational time horizons.

The number of staff that can be devoted to scanning the environment will of course depend on the size of the institution. In a major hospital, such a duty may fall to a planning division. However, even smaller facilities can take advantage of what staff they have. An administrator of a smaller hospital, for example, may have a clerical employee who spends a portion of work time scanning professional journals for articles in key areas of interest and then prepares brief summaries for the administrator's attention. Monitoring developments at professional conferences can also be a useful tactic. Plugging into a contact network may be another—a phone call or an informal lunch meeting may often be sufficient for an administrator to obtain some basic hints as to what's happening in a crucial area of concern.

Depending on the rate of apparent change in the role of the organization, long-range forecasting may be important. This is particularly true at the corporate level, where sweeping strategies of market infiltration and development may take years, even decades, to evolve.

Although the contingency strategy tends to be more inherently appealing than resource dependency, to administrators with an activist orientation, it, too, has potential problems. Less reactive than the previously discussed strategy, contingency strategy nonetheless can lead to obsession with "fighting fires" rather than to engagement in long-range planning. In particular, many organizations will choose to sacrifice long-range planning in favor of quick peeks at the horizon of next year or possibly next quarter. The quick fix of adapting to transient environmental shocks may override long-range opportunities to actually exploit or shape the environment. An attempt to co-opt a small market segment of current interest may preclude longer-term development of more extensive segments. For example, a mid-size hospital in a northeastern state turned its attention to the creation of an outpatient care facility while ignoring the more involved but potentially more lucrative development of a competitive health benefit plan or health maintenance organization (HMO) for marketing to the public.

ORGANIZATIONAL MYTH MAKING

"Who are we?" Although the concept of an organization having central goals or values is not new,[14] in recent years numerous additional studies have sought to explore the relevance of organizational culture (a pervasive set of internal organizational myths affecting performance) for health services organizations and other enterprises.[15-19] In particular, Ouchi's persuasive study would seem to suggest that organizations in which employees have a clear sense of mission are more effective. In part such effectiveness stems from enhanced morale of employees but, more importantly for purposes of this article, the effectiveness stems from perceptions of other organizational actors in the organization's environment that it is mission oriented, that its employees "stand for something."

Thus, administrators whose health services organizations seem to be burdened by a mythology that is vague or ineffective need to frankly evaluate what can be done to convince not only their own employees, but also their public, of their positive characteristics. For example, at one small southeastern hospital located in a foothill region, a number of malpractice suits were brought against its medical staff. When an anonymous local humorist labelled it "Blood Valley General," the nickname quickly attained popularity in the area, giving the facility a definite *negative* mythology to grapple with.

A major first step for many organizations will be to trace the traditions of the facility. Are its historical orientations those of public charity, religious service, an intense profit motive? Were there particular administrators, trustees, or staff whose image shaped impressions of the institution, both internal and external? In the case of older organizations, this step may involve discussions with older or retired staff members for their observations as well as interviews with current staff to determine current perceptions. Gradually, even a negative culture can be changed through a sustained educational effort[20] in which strenuous efforts to activate dormant positive traditions—or implant new ones—can lead to renewal of the provider as community support returns. Once a general sense of tradition has been obtained, closer analysis may have to follow. What legacy of values was left in a hospital by a beloved, but slightly eccentric, director of nursing who served for 15 years? Did the director leave an impression of the importance of the serving ethic or memories of toleration for less-than-competent administration? Or both?

In some cases, a subtle or not-so-subtle process of value oriented linguistic negotiation may have to occur. A more progressive incoming director of a large long-term-care center for the elderly may have to persuade, cajole, and otherwise reorient the perceptions, values, and even language of staff members steeped in traditions of custodially oriented care promoted by a previous administrator. To be effective, such a process would have to be somewhat mutual at the very least.

In choosing to concentrate on a strategic focus of organizational myth making, the manager should keep several precautions in mind. In exploring an organization's traditions, it may be tempting to enshrine them rather than modify them to fit current circumstances ("Father O'Riley always intended this to be a charity hospital, and that's how it's going to stay"). On the other hand, management may lose sight of the value of organizational culture as a unique commodity with its own inherent value, viewing it merely as a tool for the amoral manipulation of employees ("Father O'Riley is dead. We're going to become profit oriented and anyone who doesn't like it can leave").[21] Instead of either extreme, a subtle reweaving of culture to suit both tradition and current needs may be the best alternative ("To carry on Father O'Riley's tradition of service, we have to break even").

DOMAIN CONSENSUS

"Why don't they understand us?" The major problem related to domain consensus is the creation of agreement on the activities of the health services organization in the collective consciousness of its community, particularly in the minds of key figures in other organizations (e.g., clients, consumers, and politicians). Management that emphasizes domain consensus seeks not only to project the self-understanding of self-image of its organization onto the minds of significant actors in the environment of the health services organization, but also to promote and negotiate a common understanding of its task domains. The manager asks, "Do they agree with our goals? Do they agree with our methods?" and acts accordingly.[22]

Part of domain consensus may involve transmitting better information to the general public about the methods and goals of the organization. How many people in the community know that a particular hospital has a drug rehabilitation program? Do most of the residents of a small community realize that the local health care center for the elderly provides other types of long-term-care services as well? Do they understand the long term goals of these facilities, and do they agree with them?

However, the manager employing a domain consensus strategy goes considerably beyond simply seeking to foster an essentially favorable public impression of the organization. So-called "community influentials" may also be of importance. While formal government officials (mayors, council members, or state senators) are of concern, less obvious figures such as religious leaders and officers of civic clubs should also be considered.

Suppliers, allies, and competitors may all be participants in shaping or reshaping a consensus about the goals of the organization.

Finally, other organizations within the environment of the health services organization will need to be taken into account. Suppliers, allies, and competitors may all be participants in shaping or reshaping a consensus about the goals of the organization and how it plans to attain them. Specifically, the emphasis needs to be not so much on the organization per se as on influentials *within* the organization such as corporate presidents and agency heads.[23]

Whether created informally or by such formal mechanisms as service agreements or contracts, a successful domain consensus strategy should have the effect of reducing interorganizational conflict over goals and actions. The corresponding increase in mutual trust should allow greater freedom of action for the organization in the future.

On the other hand, an overemphasis on negotiation as a process may undercut substantive concerns.[24,25] In their eagerness to achieve consensus, organizational managers may sacrifice substantively useful programs or goals. Furthermore, the structures created through domain consensus should also be viewed as potentially fragile, and as entities that may not necessarily survive their creators. Finally, there is no guarantee that agreements negotiated among one group of actors (e.g., hospital suppliers) may not provoke hostility from others (e.g., federal regulatory officials). Indeed, as the health services industry matures, less formal networking arrangements may well be a preferred domain management strategy for the formalization of multi-actor consensus.[26]

ORGANIZATIONAL DESIGN

"Can't we do anything right?" If a health services organization seems to be experiencing repeated difficulties in its response to shifts in the environment in which it operates, it may be necessary to invoke an organizational design strategy. To be successful in a continuously shifting environment, such an approach necessitates continuous adjustments.[27]

Fits between internal design and external reality must be carefully examined. For example, is information about certain external developments simply not reaching key decision makers rapidly enough? If so, perhaps a more sophisticated management information system should be installed. Perhaps tasks should be more carefully developed along more rigorously functional lines. Goals of the organization may then require more careful specification than in the past. Alternately, a radical decentralization to move decision making closer to the point of action may be desired. For example, one medium-sized northeastern hospital set up a series of satellite operations; considerable independence was allowed to the managers of the individual enterprises. Serving as both profit centers and feeders, these units were deliberately granted this degree of

independence to allow them maximum latitude to adapt to local circumstances.

An organizational design strategy may provide the best opportunity to shape the environment of a health services organization rather than a mere response to change by restructuring the organization to anticipate environmental needs before they materialize. Refinements can bring this goal closer and closer, for example, by continually improving outpatient services that are useful.

On the other hand, a few cautionary notes are in order: Overemphasis on organizational design may lead to obsession with formal analyses ("The numbers say so"), to the neglect of intuitive approaches.[28] Similarly, a rigid, vertically oriented command structure may displace the use of informal but necessary lateral flows of information. (Even the hospital "rumor mill" may have its value.) Finally, design strategies may lead to overemphasis on the design process itself, rather than on the substantive goals of the organization. In "outwitting" its environment, an organization may neglect its substantive identity.[29]

• • •

In this article the authors have offered an inventory of interorganizational problems facing contemporary health services administrators, suggested some appropriate strategies and tactics, and examined some of the most serious pitfalls associated with these approaches. Not every health services organization will encounter these problems at the same phase of its history.[30] Similarly, given differing perceptions, not all managers will accurately perceive the existence of such problems. Nonetheless, the certainty of rapid change in the contemporary health services environment makes the effective consideration of such issues a major challenge for administrators at every level of service and in every type of health services organization.

REFERENCES

1. Terreberry, S. "The Evolution of Organizational Environments." *In Readings in Organization Theory: Open-System Approaches*, edited by J.G. Maurer. New York: Random House, 1971.

2. Brown, M. "From the Editor." *Health Care Management Review* 11, no. 2 (1986): 5–6.

3. Brown, M. "From the Editor." *Health Care Management Review* 9, no. 3 (1984): 5–6.

4. Levine, C. *Managing Fiscal Stress: The Crisis in the Public Sector.* Chatham, N.J.: Chatham House, 1980.

5. Hirschhorn, L., and Associates. *Cutting Back: Retrenchment and Redevelopment in Human and Community Services.* San Francisco: Jossey-Bass, 1983.

6. Whetten, D.A. "Organizational Decline: A Neglected Topic in Organizational Science." In *New Directions in Public Administration,* edited by B. Bozeman, and J. Straussman. Monterey, Calif.: Brooks/Cole, 1984.

7. Burns, M., and Mauet, A. "Administrative Freedom for Interorganizational Action: A Life-Cycle Interpretation." *Administration and Society* 16 (1984): 289–305.

8. Aldrich, H. "Resource Dependence and Interorganizational Relations; Local Employment Service Offices and Social Service Sector Organizations." *Administration and Society* 7 (1976): 419–54.

9. Yuchtman, E., and Seashore, S. "A Systems Resource Approach to Organizational Effectiveness." *American Sociological Review* 32 (December 1967): 891–903.

10. Hayes, R., and Abernathy, W. "Managing Our Way to Economic Decline." *Harvard Business Review* 58 (July/August, 1980): 67–77.

11. Ouchi, W. Theory Z. New York: Addison-Wesley, 1981.

12. Peters, T.J., and Waterman, R.H. *In Search of Excellence: Lessons from America's Best-Run Companies.* New York: Warner Books, 1982.

13. Autry, P., and Thomas, D. "Competitive Strategy in the Hospital Industry. *Health Care Management Review* 11, no. 1 (1986): 7–14.

14. Barnard, C.I. *The Functions of the Executive.* 30th anniv. ed. Cambridge, Mass.: Harvard University Press, 1968.

15. Goldsmith, S.B. *Theory Z Hospital Management: Lessons from Japan.* Rockville, Md.: Aspen Publishers, 1983.

16. Ouchi, Theory Z.

17. Peters and Waterman, *In Search of Excellence.*

18. Denhardt, R.B. In the Shadow of Organization. Lawrence, Kans.: Regents Press of Kansas, 1981.

19. Mitroff, I., and Kilman, R. "On Organization Stories: An Approach to the Design and Analysis of Organizations through Myths and Stories." In *The Management of Organization Design, Vol. I: Strategies and Implementation,* edited by R. Kilman, et al. New York: North Holland, 1976.

20. Goldsmith, M., and Leebow, W. "Strengthening the Hospital's Marketing Position." *Health Care Management Review* 11, no. 2 (1986): 83–93.

21. Smircich, L. "Concepts of Culture and Organizational Analysis." *Administrative Science Quarterly* 28 (September 1983): 339–58.

22. Ford, D., and Burns, M. "The Politics of Domain Consensus: Applications to Long-Term Care." *Journal of Health and Human Resources Administration* 9 (Spring 1987): 423–47.

23. Kronenberg, P.S. "Interorganizational Politics and National Security: An Approach to Inquiry." In *National Security and American Society,* edited by F.N. Traeger, and P.S. Kronenberg. Lawrence, Kans.: University of Kansas Press, 1973.

24. Thompson, J.D., and McEwen, W. (1958). "Organizational Goals and Environment: Goal-Setting as an Interaction Process." *American Sociological Review* 23 (February 1958): 23–31.

25. Selznick, P. *TVA and the Grass Roots.* Berkeley: University of California, 1949.

26. D'Aunno, T.A., and Zuckerman, H.S. "A Life-Cycle Model of Organizational Federations: The Case of Hospitals." *The Academy of Management Review* 12 (1987): 534–45.

27. Galbraith, J. *Organization Design.* Reading, Mass.: Addison-Wesley, 1977.

28. Peters and Waterman, *In Search of Excellence.*

29. Thompson, J.D. *Organizations in Action.* New York: McGraw-Hill, 1967.

30. Burns and Mauet, "Administrative Freedom for Interorganizational Action."

PART II

STRUCTURE

Vertical integration: exploration of a popular strategic concept

Montague Brown
and
Barbara P. McCool

News headlines continue to proclaim the virtues of vertical integration, networking, regionalization, cluster markets, and other methods of organizing health care.[1] With insurers entering major joint ventures with providers (Aetna with Voluntary Hospitals of America [VHA]; Provident and Transamerica Occidental with American Healthcare Systems [AHS]; Equitable with Hospital Corporation of America [HCA]), it would seem that something fundamental is occurring that might presage a more vertically integrated health care delivery system.

The idea of vertical integration in health care easily stirs the imagination and holds the attention of policy makers, health administrators, and, increasingly, entrepreneurs. Those seeking to regulate expenditures want vertical integration to avoid duplication of services. Those seeking to ensure quality and efficiency attempt to own or control whatever resources a patient might need within an episode of illness or even a lifetime. More pragmatic people seek to bring downstream services and upstream services under their wings for many reasons: to stabilize markets, to use excess capacity, to secure profits from related services, and, from time to time, to capitalize on the prestige one hopes will enhance an entire line of services.

The concept of regionalization of health care services for a particular population, territory, or trade area has a long history: the Lord Dawson Report in England in 1920[2]; the Committee on the Cost of Medical Care in the United States in 1932[3]; the Commission on Hospital Care in 1956[4]; the Regional Medical Program in 1966[5]; and AHA's Ameriplan proposal,[6] which sought some form of integrated care for a geopolitical region.[7-10] Since these ideas seem to surface frequently, one can reasonably question whether the current enthusiasm will lead to major change or whether it merely represents another fad.

One should remember that earlier calls for regionalization and vertical integration came during times of physician and hospital shortage. Access and comprehensiveness were big issues. Today, there is a sur-

Montague Brown, *M.B.A., Dr.P.H., J.D., is Chairman and CEO of Strategic Management Services, Inc., in Shawnee Mission, Kansas, and Editor of* Health Care Management Review.

Barbara P. McCool, *R.N., M.H.A., Ph.D., is President of Strategic Management Services, Inc., in Shawnee Mission, and Associate Editor of* Health Care Management Review.

Health Care Manage Rev, 1986, 11(4), 7–19
© 1986 Aspen Publishers, Inc.

plus of hospitals, beds, and physicians, coupled with high cost and overuse. If these old ideas fit today, it will have to be for different reasons than those cited in earlier days.

The literature on the regionalization of health services discusses many, if not all, of the underlying reasons for vertical integration. However, the literature and rationale for regionalization go beyond the ideas of economy and medical efficiency to endorse political governance.

Many proponents of regionalization basically are seeking a way to govern. For those who prefer governance within the framework of the political system, regional health care systems can be directed by elected and appointed government officials and institutions. For others who prefer private, voluntary institutions, regional systems can work under a governmental charter or framework, but can be essentially self-directed by their own voluntary governing bodies. Those who sit at the supposed apex of a vertically integrated system seem to think it equally natural and desirable to have such a system governed and controlled by the medical elite at the academic health science center. In a pluralistic system such as the United States, regionalization represents a move toward greater vertical integration and centralization of control.

Whatever the motive, proponents of vertical integration generally share the arguments of economy, efficiency, quality, and access associated with the concept.

WHAT IS VERTICAL INTEGRATION?

Vertical integration is a term used in marketing and economics to describe complex systems that link resource development, manufacturing, distribution, and consumption. For example, food chains, when linked vertically, own and operate the farms, processing plants, and distribution systems, and provide food to their customer base in a variety of forms, including meal service. Their integration may also involve them in energy production for their farms, factories, and transportation systems.

In health care, vertical integration commonly refers to the ability of one provider system (i.e., owner or controlling entity) to provide all levels and intensities of service to patients and health care consumers from a geographically contiguous region when these clients present themselves to that system. Primary, sec-

In health care, vertical integration commonly refers to the ability of one provider system to provide all levels and intensities of service to patients and health care consumers.

ondary, tertiary, rehabilitative, custodial, and other care modalities are available within one system. In contrast, mere ownership of a variety of different service modalities in separate areas of the country should be analyzed as a form of diversification, perhaps, but not as vertical integration of service from a consumer's perspective.

In a system of vertically integrated services, a patient presents himself or herself for primary care and moves from one level to another as is medically appropriate, using the most economical and best service necessary and remaining within the ambit of the same provider. One can argue that the greater the extent that all problems are met by one provider, the greater is the vertical integration of that provider. A fully integrated system is capable of providing all services to all patients who present themselves for care.

In addition, since medical care has long been treated by consumers as a service for which one needs to purchase risk protection, a vertically integrated system will provide financial services, much as General Motors provides financial services such as loans to assist in buying a car so that consumers can use its products. Traditionally Blue Cross/Blue Shield provided such services independently of provider. Now providers are adding financial risk services to their portfolios to augment traditional financial risk services.

History of vertical integration

Hospitals and hospital chains were first attracted to vertical integration because of economies of scale and increase in market share. Economies of scale (quality, cost, production efficiency, profit potential, access to supply of inputs, and access and control of customer markets) relate to decisions about when to own, operate, control, or make an element or service versus contracting for, entering a joint venture, or buying it in the open market. These decisions are made with due consideration for quality of medical care, access for consumers, and competitive factors in the market.

Motivated by economy of scale issues and competitive concerns, the prudent strategist in previous times operated, merged, networked, or otherwise linked with as many elements of a vertically integrated system of hospitals and services as possible. This same strategist also sought to attract independent primary care physicians, who were often in short supply. The strategist sought to network with these physicians for referrals, education, and the economic opportunity brought about by their endorsement of the brand name (most prestigious, biggest, or best) of the system and its secondary and tertiary services.

Two-stage process

The strategist developed a two-stage process of vertical integration. In the first stage, he or she took advantage of the many economies of operation for hospitals and related services that were available, especially when there were units in contiguous geographic areas. For example, one top-notch management group with specialists could handle 10 or 20 hospitals rather well. Laundries, mobile diagnostic technology, educational systems, representation to government, access to capital, and the like provided attractive opportunities for systems of hospitals with a scale of approximately $300 million to $900 million in revenues.

The greatest opportunity to achieve economies of scale resided in a second stage of integration—control over medical referral patterns. This second stage depended more heavily on physician market competitive factors than on the known economies of scale in hospital operations. In other words, vertical integration had to overcome the resistance (i.e., the refusal to refer patients) of individual practitioners ready to attack any upstream competitor (hospital or specialist) that threatened their opportunities and their freedom to control their own patients.

Indeed, the experiences of voluntary multihospital systems in the late 1960s and 1970s show that integration of medical referrals is easier to attempt than to accomplish. These hospital systems set out to build regionally integrated cluster-type systems that would offer all levels of medical care: treatment in primary settings by independent practitioners; first-level hospital care; specialist care; and, ultimately, subspecialist care. What they found was that physicians insisted on vertical levels of care at one site, their primary site, and not someone else's primary base. Few, if any, voluntary systems achieved very good results in trying to influence referrals to the other geographically contiguous hospitals they owned. The system's ownership or management of additional hospitals simply did not overcome traditional physician referral patterns. Thus, voluntary hospital systems were able to achieve some degree of vertical integration of hotel-type support services (e.g., bed and board), management services, and capital economies, but not vertical integration of patient care.

Investor-owned chains

Investor-owned chains also have a history of showing supply-side gains but no real vertical integration. During the 1970s these chains, with their capital advantage, rushed into the most readily penetrable market areas that appeared to have been abandoned by privately owned hospitals: growth areas needing new capacity and overflow areas with breakaway physicians who, for their own competitive reasons, wanted another hospital.

As growth occurred in such investor-owned, horizontally integrated, single-site, and single-purpose hospitals, management specialization developed around organization building, reimbursement, and regulatory process. Shared purchasing, dedicated suppliers, and proprietary interest in manufacturing and distribution were always potential ways to gain additional revenue, but these options were not used much as long as no pressure existed on the pricing side, which controls utilization. Today, with more consumer sensitivity to the price of services, any savings in supply costs go directly to the bottom line, so the scramble for economies in hotel services makes much more sense. Any savings on cost in a price-oriented system benefit the provider's bottom line directly. Of course, the provider may lower prices, thus passing savings to buyers. Again, these economies of operation do not reflect real vertical integration.

Multihospital systems

A number of multihospital systems have owned and operated prepaid plans, rehabilitation centers, nursing homes, and home care programs, and have offered many subspecialty medical services at one location or another. Such services offered in diverse locations represent a form of diversification but do not address the issues of integrated services for a defined population. Having such experiences and capabilities does, however, aid in positioning such firms for ultimately bringing their other resources into systems of vertically integrated services.

Current interest in vertical integration

Since investor-owned systems historically have ignored the opportunities for integration upward into tertiary services and downward into risk services (e.g., ambulatory care, diagnostics), ventures such as Wesley Medical Center in Wichita, Kansas, Lovelace Clinic in Albuquerque, New Mexico, St. Joseph Hospital in Omaha, Nebraska, Humana's Louisville, Kentucky, operations, and similar deals came as a shock to the voluntary and university communities. Corporations thought to be interested only in the simple primary care hospitals in single-hospital or overflow-hospital markets were suddenly interested in hospitals with the potential for becoming the linchpin in a vertically integrated system. The more skeptical observers, of course, seemed to think that such ventures were merely window dressing engaged in for prestige and for marketing purposes, not serious business ventures with their own merits. Less attention seemed to be given at the time to the inherent potential in aggressively seeking preferred provider status with multiple managed care systems or in building or buying such systems to complement the provider capacity in place.

Increasing profitability

This new interest in vertical integration in markets where excess capacity exists is understandable as chains such as HCA, American Medical International (AMI), and others announce lower earnings from operations. Having maximized their economies of operations, these chains are now turning to vertical integration to increase their profitability from underutilized assets.

To achieve this goal, the chains must have a solid base of primary physicians, tertiary capacity, and as many ties as possible with insurance companies and managed care systems. Three tasks comprise the real competitive challenge to the chains and regional systems: (1) backward integration to risk services, (2) joint ventures with physicians, and (3) forward integration into referral services. Unless mastered, these tasks represent the Achilles' heel of the for-profit and not-for-profit regional systems.

Changing competitors

Vertical integration may also play an increasing role among some hospitals in areas sparsely populated by chain operations. In fact, some observers have said that these hospitals may drop out of the national voluntary alliances, realizing that their biggest competitive threat stems from the potential vertical integration of other systems in their own regions, not from hospital chains.

Now, with the major move by investor-owned chains and voluntary alliances to join with insurance firms to vertically integrate backward into risk services, and with risk service firms striving to move subscribers into managed care systems in order to meet customer demand for more cost control, the entire range of assumptions about who is competing with whom is open for serious examination.

Management and governance

In summary, the traditional development of voluntary regional systems, as well as national chains, is built on management, supply, and related economies, not true vertical integration of medical care. Until last year, the voluntary national alliances followed the pattern of the national chains by buttressing their potential advantages in operating costs and ignoring the development of an integrated system of medical referrals.

Even without full vertical integration, voluntary alliances and investor-owned chains can gain much from rebuilding horizontal, somewhat integrated, systems to take advantage of buying power, regional management system sharing, and intramarket program sharing. The biggest roadblock to this process is the notion of local prerogative and discretion. Hospital administrators, especially those who run the larger voluntary and investor-owned chains, have maintained and reinforced the notion that the local administrator has control and autonomy. But these concepts retard movement toward the greater efficiency that national buying and program (product) development afford.

ENVIRONMENTAL FACTORS SUPPORTING VERTICAL INTEGRATION

Four key factors tend to support vertical integration. First, the distribution of disease in populations dictates vertical integration. Most illnesses are common problems that can be treated by primary practitioners. Because of the relative frequency of these illnesses, primary practitioners can be supported by a relatively small population base. Secondary and tertiary practitioners deal with less frequent problems and thus need a population catchment area of much greater size. A population base in excess of a million may be required for some subspecialty practices, while a family physician can fill a practice in an area that has a few thousand families.

Secondary and tertiary practitioners must depend on the vigilance of the primary care physician to identify those problems requiring specialized care and then to refer the patient to a specialist when more complex diagnostic and therapeutic services are needed. Thus, it is the nature of complicated diseases and complex, expensive technology and specialized treatment to require some form of regionalization or, as has happened most often, a network of referral relationships that move patients to the specialist and then back to the primary practitioner.

Secondary and tertiary practitioners must depend on the vigilance of the primary care physician to identify those problems requiring specialized care and to refer the patient to a specialist.

Second, quality of care by secondary and tertiary practitioners can be ensured only when these physicians continue to develop their skills by serving large population groups. This is a quality of scale issue. It is also an economic value issue, since offering a service without maintaining quality will ultimately cost the practitioner business from sophisticated buyer groups.

Third, there is an efficiency issue involved. Volume helps decrease production cost (at least over some theoretical range of size), and in medical specialties it also increases quality (again, over some theoretical range of activity). Superior value can be produced if there exist the scale and market share to support those specialty services that work efficiently. A comprehensive system has the potential to attract a large volume of patients, thereby lowering the unit cost of services and specialized technology.

Fourth, there is an inherent appeal to the idea that wherever a person comes in contact with a system of care, there exists an incentive within that system that encourages quality performance and economic treatment, smooth and timely movement among services, and easy communication among caregivers. A good example of this is the perceived quality image of the Kaiser Permanente system.

ENVIRONMENTAL FACTORS INHIBITING VERTICAL INTEGRATION

There are several key reasons the health care field has not moved toward the concepts of regional and vertical integration.

Physician autonomy

First, physicians enjoy their independence as economic and medical practitioners. Physicians have always had a keen sense of the potential for hospitals to influence their practice patterns. This potential power and a potential counterweight to it are well known to any physician soon after he or she enters the profession. The question is how to control big, strong, financially well-heeled hospitals. Such hospitals can be controlled by keeping two hospitals viable and using both for patients and referrals. Patient referrals and hospital use patterns are potent tools of control, especially for the primary care physicians who are at the entry level of the medical system. Therefore, some physician groups would resist any movement by hospitals toward scale and increased leverage.

Of the many potential threats to physician autonomy, a hospital's dominance over specialty practices is the oldest and greatest. Physicians truly fear the potential of a dominant institution that fully controls their access to hospital and related services. Regional or vertically integrated systems greatly increase the potential for institutions to control physicians through their ability to shift referrals among competing physician specialists and among competing hospitals. If any geopolitical region had only one vertically integrated set of services, physician power to shift referrals and maintain power or leverage over hospitals would be lost or at least severely diminished. Whether the system is government owned, voluntary, or investor owned makes little difference.

Physicians appear to like the notion of vertical integration of their practices, within their practices, and for their practices where opportunities exist to achieve revenue, profit, quality, and efficiency. In theory, all the ideas that make vertical integration attractive to hospitals (and increasingly attractive to insurance companies) make vertical integration attractive to the practitioner, as long as it is under his or her control.

When there were not enough specialty physicians, there was no incentive for specialists to vertically integrate in order to pressure the primary care physicians for referrals. They did not need more patients. As long as this traditional referral pattern existed, specialists kept their autonomy and so did primary physicians. Perhaps even more important, any moves by secondary and tertiary physicians to invade the primary territory were, and still are, punished by the primary physicians whose referrals control the system of secondary and, especially, tertiary medicine. However, with the current surplus of specialits, increased vertical integration becomes an option.

Pluralistic system

The second, and supporting, set of reasons for the lack of any serious movement toward regionalization or vertical integration involves the history and underlying motives for societal support for a system of private and public hospitals. For many reasons, the United States has developed a pluralistic system (a variety of owners) of hospitals. This approach is supported by underlying beliefs about religion, ethnicity, and politics. It also suits the intensely competitive nature of medical practice. In the past, competing physicians could almost always find a religious group, a public body, or more recently an investor group to build a hospital for their use, as long as there was some assurance of getting a sufficient number of patients to fill the hospital, carry the debt burden, and secure profits for the equity investment required.

In the past, hospital owners took advantage of the cost-plus reimbursement system. When physicians wanted their own shop to free themselves from outside restrictions or the weight of colleagues more senior or more in control in existing institutions, hospitals made it easy for them to move. When growth occurred, all benefited. One could put a service in place and charge what one needed for a good return, so both physicians and hospitals profited.

Support of status quo

Another reason for the lack of vertical integration is the fact that the prepayment systems (basically Blue Cross and Blue Shield) were constructed to reinforce those existing arrangements, not undercut them. Insurance was cost, place, physician, and hospital neu-

tral. More recently, with the advent of managed care programs, physicians and hospitals are under intense pressure to sign up with plans that force them to share economic risk for the care of patient groups.

Support of multiple delivery sites

A fourth reason is that cost-based reimbursement, with its neutral stance toward organization and integration of services, basically supported the development of multiple delivery sites, various degrees of aggregation desired by the provider of service, and competition among all arrangements for the patronage of the individual patient. Under the cost-based system, professional desires regarding technology, place, and service configuration were paramount decision factors. There was no incentive to integrate services.

Now this approach faces rapid obsolescence because of buyer pressure, competitive prices for services, strict utilization review, increasingly fearful insurers who want to get ahead of the game in cost-effective managed care systems, and a real glut of hospitals, beds, services, and physicians. Faced with this obsolescence, many groups are now considering vertical integration.

IMPLEMENTING VERTICAL INTEGRATION

What are the options for hospitals and multihospital systems to improve performance in multifacility markets, in areas with substantial concentration, and in thinly serviced markets? Before moving to find answers to this question, one should consider how justified the new-found and widely spread belief in vertically integrated systems really is. After all, vertical systems consistently have failed to materialize almost every time they have been attempted in this century.

Access to physicians who control referrals

The first factor in achieving a measured level of vertical integration is access to the full range of physicians who control referrals. This acknowledges that the vast majority of people are not in managed care programs. Thus, as utilization rates go down, physicians will seek to move their patients to the hospital most likely to offer the broadest service array for their patients. They will enter joint ventures for economic gain, but not if such ventures threaten to tie them up with organizations that lack services their patients may need, i.e., those systems that are not vertically integrated.

For example, in Houston, Texas, both HCA and AMI need access to the kinds of services available at tertiary hospitals like the Texas Medical Center, a large biomedical complex with multiple tertiary facilities. By contrast, in Wichita and in Denver, Colorado, those firms can provide internally almost all the care patients might require in a managed care system. Humana has a similar capacity in Louisville.

Availability of managed care programs

The second factor in achieving a measured level of vertical integration is preferred access to and availability of health maintenance organizations (HMOs), preferred provider organizations (PPOs), traditional insurance, and other more directly managed care programs. The chains and voluntary alliances are moving to cover this area. Both have made attempts to enter the risk services business.

Any major move by VHA, HCA, or Humana into the full range of risk service products makes that organization's members major competitors with all other systems—hospitals, networks, and insurance. Up to this point, these organizations have been primarily competitors in the market for hospital services. By vertically integrating, they may become formidable in all levels of care and a real competitive threat to any providers that are not vertically integrated. As many of these systems form local alliances, they force others to form counterweight alliances to compete with them. Many older coalitions and status quo arrangements crumble under this pressure.

With alliances and chains bringing the kind of capital needed to capture managed care opportunities, all providers will begin to understand the ultimate power of a new strategy of vertical integration.

With alliances and chains bringing the kind of capital needed to capture managed care opportunities, all providers will begin to understand the ultimate power of a new strategy of vertical integration. Patients are the coin of the realm for physicians. Hospitals need them. Universities need them. Tertiary care systems need them. By vertically integrating, chains and alliances can have a stake in every market, and they will discover that having a stake in bringing patients to providers makes all other economic joint ventures with physicians seem insignificant by comparison.

VERTICAL INTEGRATION IN DIFFERENT ENVIRONMENTS

Actually achieving economic advantages of scale in a horizontally integrated firm makes it possible to add all savings to the bottom line in a product priced or managed care environment. Thus shared and centralized services should be developed within cluster and concentrated markets, to the extent that they make economic sense. Even selective backward integration into supply areas, where the firm could benefit from any excess profits being generated by suppliers, can be lucrative in some areas.

Many economies of operation can be achieved by consolidating and centralizing business service functions of existing units. Ensuing economies of scale on purchasing, supplies, standardization of equipment, and the like can and should be done as soon as possible, after a thorough analysis of gain, line by line, area by area. Moves of this type are already under way by most alliances and firms. For each product, the unit of analysis may be as large as the company or as small as two units. For some lines of business, the proper unit for economies and competitive advantage may be larger than the parent firm itself. Risk service may well fall here. In essence, vertical integration takes on the persona of the environment in which it is developed. Several examples follow.

Concentrated markets with tertiary capacity

In concentrated markets the major gain, beyond shared service economies, stems from the potential for moving patients among programs through physician referral. This is the key to vertical integration. Most approaches to influencing physician referral patterns have involved buying or entering joint ventures with primary care hospitals, or entering joint ventures for diagnostics, ambulatory care centers, managed care programs, PPOs, and other such risk products that can be used to direct patients. But for the near term (three to five years, and possibly longer), winning primary physician loyalty to referral physicians and referral hospitals is the key to achieving vertical integration of medical care capacity in markets where firms own or operate tertiary capacity. In such markets additional equity investments in all levels of services that can utilize existing assets (space and services) also may be attractive.

These concentrated markets should be organized around such concepts as medical care markets and major trade areas, areas within which the population normally seeks and receives 80 to 90 percent of its medical care. Management for the entire market should be under one manager. Such managers might report to a strategic business unit that has overall regional responsibilities for marketing, strategic analysis, investment, and general management of all company activity in the region.

Markets in which firms have several primary hospitals

In markets with limited tertiary capacity within the owned and managed system, it will be necessary for primary hospitals to create substantial joint ventures to link with tertiary programs. Only in this way can an organization gain the greatest returns from the care needed by patients who are initially attracted to primary care physicians and primary care treatment in dispersed hospital systems.

This is true for several reasons. First, any managed care, PPO, or HMO insurer wants to contract with the most complete network of providers. If significant types of referral care are not in one's own facilities, then the next best option is to enter a joint venture, network, or independently build and offer such services. In this way, hospitals can become attractive to managed care programs.

Second, under contracting market conditions that necessitate a choice of which hospital to save, physicians typically abandon the overflow or primary care facility in favor of the full-service facility or system. Physicians consider full-service facilities as the best alternative for serving their patients. Not coincidentally, these systems also help physicians maintain their own practice viability. Ironically, when one does not have major referrals for tertiary services, it is not as necessary to seek physician loyalty on referrals. Unlike the markets with tertiary care programs, in primary care markets there is less likelihood that physicians will want or need to move their patients from

one hospital to another. However, as managed care continues to gain ground, those hospitals without the more complex tertiary abilities will lose business as physicians choose to save the more complex facilities needed for their patients. Thus, hospitals must band together with tertiary care systems in order to survive. Fortunately for those with primary care facilities, tertiary facilities are also in oversupply and need alliances for referrals, just as primary hospitals need their referral backup to make their linkage with managed care firms effective.

Third, the supplier with the greatest control over referrals will have the most capital available to offer the next level of technology for medical care and the most advanced systems will become more attractive to upscale consumers, a lucrative target market. For these three reasons, it is essential that primary hospitals link with one or more tertiary care facilities.

Independent hospitals in markets with several hospitals

The solo hospital in a market with several hospitals will need to pursue a niche strategy designed to hold what business it can while fending off competitors seeking additional patient days.

Several basic approaches can be developed to support a solo strategy. First, the hospital can link or network with a referral center and try to maintain utilization of primary care services. Second, it can seek to become a primary provider for all managed care plans as they develop. Under this scenario, the hospital must try to keep one plan from becoming dominant in the marketplace. Third, the hospital can try to become the primary provider for at least one managed care plan. When possible, securing an equity position in one or more managed care plans will aid in keeping the directed patient flow from becoming too narrow, or, if it does become narrow, this position will help the hospital to benefit from that flow.

Specialty hospitals will need to find ways to secure the specialty business from all managed care plans or link closely with the general provider most likely to deliver the largest part of the specialty referral market segment to them. Many specialty hospitals depend heavily on the routine work they receive to maintain their more esoteric services, so any strategy that cuts heavily into their overall business may threaten their ability to maintain these referral services.

Teaching hospitals

Teaching hospitals basically fall into two categories: (1) the major university health science centers where much of the basic health science research is conducted. These centers have a teaching mission, with the hospitals devoted principally to research and education, and (2) the teaching hospitals that offer three or more major residency programs. These hospitals put more focus on patient service, with teaching and research being less primary activities.

Health science centers

The health science center is likely to have substantial financial support for both its research and its educational role, in addition to the support that is derived from providing patient services. To the extent that these outside support systems can be maintained and enhanced, the health science center will need and be able to compete in the marketplace for referrals from the sophisticated managed care programs. This assumes, however, that the health science centers can and do control their service cost and maintain relatively unique program offerings. Having a research base will continue to make such institutions attractive for the more difficult cases; managed care systems such as Kaiser Permanente, Health America, Maxicare, and others will always need help with their more complex cases. For such firms to try to keep their patients out of these centers of excellence will ultimately test their credibility as major suppliers. Barring a large market share for one firm, they will need to contract for such services for the foreseeable future. This represents a major opportunity for tertiary care suppliers. In fact, health science center and teaching hospitals might aggressively seek contracts to take on the management of the more complex cases before the insurance programs of such managed care companies decide to take responsibility for them.

Competitors for the more complex and specialized cases will come not from the managed care companies but from those tertiary and teaching centers that do not have major investment in and responsibility for research and teaching of medical students. Additional competition will come from those regional hospital systems and national hospital management companies that have strong regional networks and can offer tertiary services from within their systems.

At this time, it would appear that health science centers can compete effectively, provided they aggressively manage their costs (seek efficiencies) and are careful to seek the role of tertiary supplier for managed care systems early in their development. In other words, the game is just beginning. Many options remain open to those who see change coming, are open to meeting the challenge, and are aggressively examining their markets to determine when to join others, contract, or remain outside the competitive arena when appropriate.

Other institutions

Those teaching institutions that depend heavily on patient revenues to support their teaching role are at greatest risk of losing some of their preeminence and their roles as centers of excellence. They are faced with the difficult situation of using price discounts to get volume, while simultaneously finding it increasingly difficult to support the residency programs that make it possible to maintain their center of excellence strategy. Ultimately, those who deal with this issue should survive. But they, unlike the academic health science center, will need to network with a large number of providers, managed care firms, and national alliances to secure aggregate volumes of patients necessary for their tertiary programs to maintain quality while performing efficiently.

Since state and federal supporters of academic health science centers are likely to aid their clients in maintaining their viability over the intermediate term of competitive developments, most teaching hospitals will not receive such support. For this reason, some will undoubtedly fail as major tertiary centers of excellence for some services. Maintaining costly specialized programs can be an unbearable burden in a price-sensitive market, especially when buyers seek lower cost.

It is likely that the teaching and tertiary care centers outside of health science complexes will have the greatest need to build regional networks, to link formally and informally with all possible referral sources, and to build as many managed care connections as possible. This expectation seems to be borne out by the large numbers of such institutions that have made up the initial membership of VHA, AHS, and Sun Alliance. Teaching hospitals also seem natural partners for investor-owned firms and managed care firms. The number of joint ventures between these hospitals and investor-owned firms indicates that teaching hospitals are aware that they have a stronger need for multiple alliances than do academic health science centers.

Alliances between health science centers and management chains

The alliance strategy is relatively new and none of the major linkages to date seem to preclude new initiatives to form alliances between the stronger academic health science centers and hospital management chains. Managed care companies also seem to want strong alliances with primary care providers and referral agreements with those tertiary care providers who wish to maintain their research and teaching capacity but who do not need to subsidize teaching and research programs. In other words, while teaching and tertiary hospitals would like to play a major role in primary care, both hospital chains and managed care companies want to retain this role for their own operations. Thus, it is likely that chains and managed care programs will be selective in seeking out tertiary referral lines with the major academic health science centers. They will reserve the primary and secondary care roles for themselves. In the process, they will bypass their close competitor, the teaching hospital, which has more limited tertiary capacity.

Managed care companies

Managed care companies are in the business of providing or negotiating for the provision of health care services purchased by employers or other groups. They are required to provide such services within the limits of a contract they make with these employers and groups. At one extreme is the owned and operated health service, such as Kaiser Permanente, which packages physician, hospital, and risk management services within its own family of companies. At the other end of the spectrum is the insurance firm, which contracts for risk and limits liability by specifying the range within which it will cover services or the amount of total payment. In other cases, employers may manage their own risk, specify eligible providers, contract for administration, and use excess insurance coverage to avoid large losses.

Competition among managed care firms is increasing, putting pressure on premium price and thus pushing all suppliers in the direction of more tightly managed utilization and cost controls.

Increased competition

Competition among managed care firms is increasing, putting pressure on premium price and thus pushing all suppliers in the direction of more tightly managed utilization and cost controls. As these firms compete for the buyers' attention, they will need to control utilization more and more and seek low prices from suppliers of services not offered directly by the managed care firm itself.

Probably the lowest-cost producers of primary care are family physicians. Some of the early HMO service suppliers sought out family physicians, general internists, and similar primary care providers as the core of their original network. Low-cost or low-price hospital providers and willing specialists have been secondary priorities. As patient volume has grown, specialists have been asked to take greater risks and hospitals have been asked to offer greater discounts in order to get the volume business offered by managed care firms that can select the provider for their clients.

Under conditions such as these, physician and hospital providers are under tremendous pressure to take the risk and start their own managed care firms. But in doing so, they must delicately balance their own risk management offerings so that they can gain market share while maintaining business and referrals from competing managed care firms.

Put another way, as providers develop their abilities to offer managed care services directly to employers and groups, they must do so in a fashion that does not simultaneously drive away business from other managed care firms (now competing firms) and from referring physicians whose practices are tied more directly to other managed care firms and hospitals.

If hospital and physician provider groups initiate their own risk services and managed care programs, they may lose referrals from these competing groups.

On the other hand, if they have not positioned themselves to be the provider of choice in such groups, they run the risk of eventually being left out of more tightly managed groups.

Role of insurance companies

Managed care firms are, with a few exceptions, relatively new. Some have developed with little regard for utilization control and have depended heavily on the lack of tightly managed control for their profitability. As competition builds for the managed care premium dollar, the more loosely managed firms will lose out to more tightly managed groups. But as managed care firms succeed as a sector of the health care industry, it becomes more important than ever for any insurance firm wishing to compete for the full service benefit dollar to offer managed care. Therefore, health care managers now see, and can expect to see, many more insurance firms seeking managed care business, buying up established managed care firms, merging traditional benefit companies into managed care firms, and entering joint ventures between big benefits firms and provider networks and firms.

In short, the strategies of insurance and benefits firms are so new in their adoption and so tentative in their execution that it seems safe to conclude that the industry is only beginning to discover and answer many of the questions posed and implied here. Few of the strategies that have unfolded so far appear to be clear-cut winners. Few of the players seem secure in the belief that they have the answers. The only thing that seems certain is that change is here. For those who like the excitement of a game in its early stages, this is a great opportunity to participate in the definition of a new health care provider. For those who see only insurmountable problems, retiring to the sidelines or merging with someone more comfortable with the risk seems a more likely strategy.

For those who think that vertical integration is the right way to go, there is plenty of room to maneuver. They can mold the health care system into a more efficient and probably more vertically integrated mode of care. Who will do this is an open question. Where it can be done is similarly open. But since vertical integration runs counter to so many interests, it will remain a high-risk strategy, however it is implemented.

ASSESSMENT OF FORCES IN THE HEALTH CARE FIELD

Powerful forces are active in the health care field. Voluntary hospital alliances are flourishing as providers seek refuge in networks that will allow independent hospitals and independent physicians to retain control over their destinies in the face of impending radical changes in reimbursement that favor competitive pricing and full-service arrays.

Assumptions underlying the fears of independent hospitals and physicians

Several assumptions are currently causing great anxiety among independent institutions and practitioners. One assumption is that the powerful hospital chains will use their ability to get market equity to buy up the good business opportunities to the exclusion of the voluntary hospitals. Just how such chains could come up with the new equity to perform this miracle is unclear. (It would probably require in the neighborhood of $50 billion in equity and a similar amount of debt to accomplish this feat.) Given the beating the chains have taken recently in the stock market, this scenario seems improbable. Therefore, the implication that the powerful companies will take over the field seems to be basically a fear tactic to encourage the forging of more horizontal and vertical voluntary alliances.

Another fear is that the powerful insurance and managed care systems will take over control of patients and usurp the role of providers in the system. This argument also assumes that only a few firms will dominate the industry. For this to happen, hundreds of benefits insurers would need to abandon the field; the full-service firms (HMOs) would have to become the sole, or at least dominant, model of delivery; and traditional providers would need to insist on high utilization under traditional methods of payment. Just the opposite seems to be occurring. Utilization is decreasing dramatically. Employers are managing their own care and benefits in a much more effective manner. Traditional providers are adjusting to this new approach, cost is coming down, and providers are accepting PPOs and other price-sensitive approaches fairly well. Also, more and more benefits companies are developing a wide range of approaches to ensure their survival in the marketplace. The world may be changing but it appears that many traditional owners (hospitals and physicians) are responding well to market forces. As a result, they are not losing their control over their hospitals and practices.

A third assumption is that businesses and personal consumers are ready and willing to make changes in how they consume health care services in order to secure a better price and value relationship. This assumption appears to be true. It is unlikely that the industry has fully explored consumers' willingness to change. However, this change is occurring incrementally. Many of the firms that moved first and fastest have experienced difficulty with their model approaches. As consumer groups move inexorably toward tighter controls of their own utilization, providers increasingly respond, albeit reluctantly.

Just how much of the market share will go to tightly managed care firms before traditional suppliers offer equally attractive utilization rates and prices, with greater freedom for consumers to choose physicians? Surely a 5 percent or 10 percent shift to HMOs is too little; but at 20 percent or 30 percent penetration, can traditional suppliers fail to respond? When the responses come, should there not be counter responses? The game has begun, but surely it is not yet decided.

Current situation

As these fundamental changes occur, providers are indeed finding that circumstances can make for strange bedfellows. Disbelief that change will come has given way to fear that all is lost, only to be replaced by confidence in all-purpose alliances to fight the change. As the battle lines are drawn and readiness to do battle pervades, tenable options emerge with new lines of alliance, vertical and horizontal integration occur, and new partnerships begin to develop.

New alliances

Vertical integration itself is beginning to emerge as an idea whose time has come. In the early stages many parties saw themselves at the core of such a system. They began the process hoping to solidify this coveted position. Some weaker, more timid players immediately threw in the towel and merged with the stronger partners. Others hedged and joined alliances to wait, see, and sample. A lot of money has been invested in these exercises but for the most part they were exercises, not the consummation of a vertical system.

Perhaps it is in these alliances that some of the potential for building vertical systems exists. Given the many different services offered for the total health care dollar, it may be that any given provider not only will be a strong part of one alliance, but will play an important role in many alliances. The United States is, after all, a pluralistic society. Many vendors, physicians, and hospitals are interdependent on the unique economies of specialized sectors of the health care economy.

Significance of new delivery systems

The HMO represents a particular subset of integration. The shared purchasing program represents another subset, and it is unlike the first, though important for its own merit. Maybe the health care industry is moving toward many different types of vertical integration. If new delivery systems do represent subsets of vertical integration, perhaps what is beginning will lead to a more vertically integrated system of services. But it is unlikely to lead to one or two or even a hundred or more super systems. It is more likely that the traditional mode of physician and medical care in general will evolve toward more efficient patterns. Pattern is the key term. In a pattern or set of relationships, more vertically related activities can evolve if and when they provide efficiency or provide a competitive or marketing opportunity for gains in terms of economy, medical care, or access.

Positive economic and medical care gains from joint ventures, networks, and diversification may occur without the parties involved giving up their control in these new negotiated relationships. Gains for consumers can occur without providers totally abandoning their traditional roles and missions. However, these roles will need to be redefined and renegotiated within the context of the larger societal goal of efficiency and access.

Total integration unlikely

It is unlikely, however, that health care will ever become fully integrated. It is possible, if not probable, that a totally owned and operated vertically integrated system would look and act much like a state owned and operated system, with all the barriers to innovation and change that this might represent. That is, the traditional notion of vertical integration

It is unlikely that health care will ever become fully integrated.

may well be a bigger blunder in design than going along with the old cost-plus system despite that system's history of duplication and overuse.

If this is the case, total integration, vertical or horizontal, is undesirable. What is needed are the creativity and innovation that come from highly pluralistic approaches and the energy that comes from competitive behaviors within a pluralistic system that forces change, growth, or failure.

Rational approach to vertical integration

As today's strategist explores vertical integration, he or she must look for an underlying rationale at each step. Is it for medical quality, efficiency, consumer acceptance, competitive advantage, or some related criterion? In analyzing the alternatives, issues of vertical integration and horizontal integration, corporate restructuring, diversification, merger, and alliance are great starting points, but as goals they fall short. They should be viewed as means or mechanisms for progress, not as goals or outcome measures. Indeed, there is a move toward greater vertical integration not because it represents an unalloyed virtue but because more general risk taking by larger groups of providers stimulates most cost-effective methods of care.

Totally owned and operated vertically integrated systems are not likely to occur as a result of market competitive forces unless all programs, resource requirements, and abilities can be brought to operate at the optimal level of utility simultaneously. This type of situation has never existed in any kind of organization. It certainly does not exist in medical care as it currently operates. Lumping everything into one organization would create a lump, not a set of orderly programs in harmony with one another and collectively meeting consumer needs.

● ● ●

Health care managers can and probably will network, enter joint ventures, and build and operate in a much more rational fashion—meaning more vertical

and horizontal relationships. But these efforts will not result in a neat textbook example of what a vertical system might represent. The system will be pluralistic. It will meld together and it will break apart whenever the parts do not fit. It will have control and coordination between individuals, groups, and corporations with many voices being heard. The 1990s will not look like the 1970s, but many of the same owners and physicians will be doing many of the things they did in the 1970s with greater efficiency and sound value to consumers, and in competition with others seeking to serve similar markets. In addition, they will be doing things with more and different partners than would have been envisioned in the last decade, or even today.

REFERENCES

1. *Hospital Literature Index* 40 (1984): 207–8.
2. United Kingdom. Parliament. Consultative Council on Medical and Allied Services, Ministry of Health of Great Britain. *Interim Report on the Future Provision of Medical and Allied Services.* Cmd. 693. 1920.
3. Committee on the Cost of Medical Care. *Medical Care for the American People: The Final Report of the Committee.* Committee Pub. No. 28. Chicago: University of Chicago Press, November 1932.
4. Rosenfeld, L.S., and Makover, H.B. *The Rochester Regional Hospital Council.* Cambridge, Mass.: Harvard University Press, 1956.
5. Clark, H.T. "The Challenge of the Regional Medical Programs Legislation." *Journal of Medical Education* 41 (1966): 71–74.
6. American Hospital Association Special Committee on the Provision of Health Services. *Ameriplan: A Proposal for the Delivery and Financing of Health Services in the United States: Report of the Special Committee on Health Service.* Chicago: AHA, 1970.
7. Brown, M., and Money, W.H. "Promise of Multihospital Management." *Hospital Progress* 56, no. 8 (1975): 36–42.
8. Brown, M., et al. "Trends in Multihospital Systems: A Multiyear Comparison." *Health Care Management Review* 5, no. 4 (Fall 1980): 9–22.
9. Brown, M. "Multihospital Systems in the 80s–The New Shape of the Health Care Industry." *Hospitals* 56 (March 1, 1982): 344–61.
10. Brown, M. "Community Hospitals: Caring, Curing, Commerce. Systems Commerce and the Caring Tradition." *Hospital Progress* 64 (May 1983): 37–44, 62.

Vertical integration in health services: Theory and managerial implications

Douglas A. Conrad
and
William L. Dowling

A vertically integrated health care system is an arrangement whereby a health care organization offers, either directly or through others, a broad range of patient care and support services. This article discusses the market forces and strategic considerations driving the recent trend toward vertical linkages in health care markets and examines some of the managerial implications and issues associated with this vertical restructuring trend.

Health Care Manage Rev, 1990, 15(4), 9–22
© 1990 Aspen Publishers, Inc.

The health services market is undergoing radical transformation, a transformation that began with extensive horizontal integration and multisystem formulation in the 1970s and has been followed more recently by extensive vertical integration and diversification in the 1980s. We believe that these recent trends in vertical linkages in health care markets will continue throughout the foreseeable future. There are definite economic and clinical benefits associated with such vertical structuring. Our goal is to try and understand the market forces and strategic considerations that are driving the vertical reorganization of the health care system and to present some of the managerial implications and issues associated with this vertical restructuring.

The article proceeds in 4 parts:
1. definition of vertical integration,
2. presentation of a theoretical framework that sets out the underlying determinants of vertical integration and its associated benefits and costs,
3. examination of inter- and intraorganizational forms responding to those underlying determinants of vertical integration, and
4. managerial implications and issues associated with development of vertically integrated health care systems.

We draw on microeconomic theory, particularly the literature on transaction costs and competitive strategy that emerged in the late 1970s and early 1980s, as well as on empirical evidence and insights concerning practical managerial and organizational issues. Those managerial and organizational issues translate into agenda for future research and investigation by both the academic community and the fields of practice. This research needs to be informed by collaboration among management practitioners, clinicians, and academics working within the frameworks of their basic scientific disciplines.

DEFINITIONS

A vertically integrated health care system is an arrangement whereby a health care organization (or

Douglas A. Conrad, *Ph.D., is a Professor in the Department of Health Services, University of Washington in Seattle. He also serves as Director of the University of Washington's Graduate Program in Health Services Administration in Seattle.*

William L. Dowling, *Ph.D., is Vice President for Planning and Policy Development at Sisters of Providence health system. He is also a Clinical Professor in the University of Washington's graduate program in Health Services Administration in Seattle.*

closely related group of organizations) offers, either directly or through others, a broad range of patient care and support services operated in a functionally unified manner. The range of services offered may include preacute, acute, and postacute care organized around an acute hospital. Alternatively, a delivery system might specialize in offering a range of services related solely to long-term care, mental health care, or some other specialized area.

Full functional integration requires both administrative and clinical integration. As a corollary, the management and operation of vertically integrated services will tend to be closely coordinated or centralized. The major purpose of such integration is to enhance the system's overall effectiveness or profitability, not necessarily the effectiveness or profitability of each individual service line.

Clinical integration of the health care services provided to individual patients implies geographic proximity, since both the delivery of patient care and, consequently, the geographic boundaries of a vertically integrated delivery system are generally local or regional. These boundaries conform to natural patient care service areas or markets.

The importance of particular health care services being coordinated within a local or somewhat larger regional market—as opposed to a national or large regional area—will depend on the geographic scope of the market for the relevant services. For example, an individual receiving specialized cancer care might well be served by a tertiary referral hospital far from his or her residence. The tertiary hospital care could be augmented by home health care and long-term care for the cancer patient in his or her local market. If the various elements of the individual's care were integrated within a single health care system, organizational and clinical integration could still exist even though the various levels of the patient's care were delivered in physically distinct settings. This highlights the need to define the geographic nature of the market for a given service before judging whether the patient care functions are integrated.

Put simply, vertical integration is the coordination or linkage of businesses (service lines) that are at different stages in the production process of health care. For example, an acute care hospital vertically integrates when it acquires or establishes different levels or types of care such as ambulatory care, long-term care, or home care. The principal aims of vertical integration are to enhance coordination among the elements or stages of the production process (Porter[1] has called this proc-

> *The primary purposes of vertical integration in health care are to enhance the comprehensiveness and continuity of patient care and to control the sources of patients or other users of a delivery system's services.*

ess "the value chain") and to control the channels of demand for, or distribution of, a firm's core services. In the case of the hospital, the core service is acute inpatient care. Control and coordination of ambulatory care, long-term care, home care, medical products supply, and even wellness and health-promotion activities serve either to promote referrals to the hospital's core (inpatient) service line or to improve its distribution (as in the example of postdischarge care).

In short, the primary purposes of vertical integration in health care are to enhance the comprehensiveness and continuity of patient care and to control the sources of patients or other users of a delivery system's services. In the past, vertical integration in health care focused on closing gaps in the availability of services and improving the continuity of patient care. In today's competitive and reimbursement-constrained environment, controlling the flow of patients to an institution is often the key to maintaining market share. The emphasis on controlling demand and/or channels of distribution has increased as competition has intensified.

DIMENSIONS OF VERTICAL CONTROL

In defining vertical integration in general, one can distinguish four dimensions of the vertical control continuum, which is a more general way of describing vertical integration.[2] These four dimensions are

1. the breadth of the integration; for example, the range of diagnosis related groups (DRGs) cared for by the vertically integrated system;
2. the degree of within-firm purchases and internal sales of vertically related services, as contrasted with the use of external sources ("outsourcing") for inputs and sales to other firms of one's service outputs;
3. the number of stages in the vertically related value chain integrated or explicitly coordinated by a single organization; for example, the health maintenance organization (HMO) that provides a wellness program, ambulatory care, acute inpa-

tient care, long-term care, and home health care, as well as the full continuum of primary and specialty care for given clinical conditions, would be integrated at many stages in the value chain; and

4. the form of integration, that is, the nature of the coordination or ownership arrangements that link related services.

The breadth of vertical integration is a strategic decision for the firm, one that balances the firm's efficiency and effectiveness in delivering services among different product (e.g., DRG) types. For example, the firm that chooses to offer a wide array of service types—for instance, from comprehensive mental health services all the way through specialized cancer care and sophisticated trauma services—has presumably made a conscious decision that it can function efficiently and effectively across that wide array of services. An organization can vertically integrate in one product stream (e.g., cancer care) without necessarily integrating vertically or even offering significant services in other areas.

The decisions about breadth depend on synergies across service types, just as decisions about "depth" turn on the efficiency and effectiveness of an organization across different levels of a vertical value chain. For instance, there are cross-benefits between offering general medical-surgical services and possessing a trauma care capacity. Similarly, the chemotherapy and radiological services required in a comprehensive oncology program also serve to support the delivery of general medical-surgical care.

The degree to which a single level of a vertically integrated firm purchases all of its inputs from internal sources and provides the outputs of its level exclusively to other divisions or levels within the firm also involves a strategic balance. The use of external sources in addition to internal sources for inputs stimulates competition within the firm as to the source of supply of drugs, laboratory tests, and other inputs to the delivery of services. Outsourcing also maintains strategic flexibility in the event that the firm's own capacity is compromised by external events, such as staffing shortages or declines in demand for the organization's primary output.

The business knowledge gained through provision of one level's service to another level within the same organization can be used to develop outside markets for the organization's services. For example, the in-house pharmacy or laboratory that supplies the needs of a hospital could also arrange the sale of those products to other organizations such as physician practices.

This strategy serves to enhance the prospects for internal vertical integration by raising the scale of output at any one stage (through enhanced numbers of markets for that stage of production), and thus may justify the integration by creating gains through economies of scale.

The number of stages in the value chain that a single firm decides to control—so as to better coordinate its contracts and other arrangements—will be driven by consideration of the cost savings from coordinating input and output flows as well as of gains in the continuity and quality of patient care derived from more closely controlling the different stages of service. For instance, the provision of health promotion and disease prevention services within a health services organization that also operates a hospital provides a base for the hospital's activities in acute patient care, either by generating referrals or by providing advance information regarding patient needs that aids in coordinating these patients' later care. A key to the decision to vertically integrate a series of related stages is an organization's conscious commitment to serve a population base. The depth of integration is thus driven both by the ability to share information, physical capital, and patient care human resources across different levels of health services activity and by the gains to continuity of care that result from doing so.

The organization can add or gain control of a product or service line through many different means:

- internal development of new services
- acquisition of another organization or service
- formal merger
- lease or sale/lease-back arrangement
- franchise
- joint venture
- contractual agreement
- loan guarantee
- informal agreement or affiliation

Each of these different forms of vertical control has different risks, costs, and benefits. An organization's decision to vertically integrate is not a simple zero-to-one choice, but rather, involves a continuous balancing act among these different forms of vertical control.[3]

In addition to the four generic dimensions of vertical control discussed above, a unique "fifth dimension" in health care exists—the potential integration of health insurance with health services delivery.

At one level of analysis, the linkage of the source of health care payment with the source of health care delivery simply seems to represent decisions along each of the four dimensions already discussed:

1. It represents the addition of a new stage in the production of process—backward integration into delivery from the viewpoint of the third party payer, or forward integration into payment for its own services by the health care delivery organization.

2. A third party payer who hired or purchased its own physician services network would be choosing the "common ownership" form of backward integration into delivery, whereas the payer who signed a long-term arrangement for physician services with a single multispecialty group practice would be integrating by contract.

3. Given the decision to integrate backward by contract, the third party payer increases its degree of vertical integration by forming exclusive contracts with physicians rather than preferred provider contracts.

4. Similarly, a local multihospital system with a broad service line (e.g., mental health, cancer care, cardiac specialty care) might sign an exclusive contract with a third party payer to deliver service to that payer's enrollees. If the payer previously offered only psychiatric coverage, such a move would increase the breadth of the insurer's integration with delivery.

Insurance/delivery system integration involves a fifth dimension in that the fundamental "ethos" of the business is changed. The insurer now manages the care process directly rather than just paying the bills. On the flip side, the delivery system changes its perspective from a "revenue center" for itself to that of a "cost center" to the integrated health delivery and financing system. The integrated delivery and financing system both manages the economic risk of health care and assumes that risk.

Accordingly, integration of financing and delivery calls for new management expertise. This movement into previously "foreign territory" by both payers and providers requires different competitive strategies than those of providers. The competition between integrated financing and delivery systems is over premium dollars, not prices; that is, the control of utilization, not the maximization of volume, becomes crucial to success. Prepaid health plans compete for persons, not procedures.

THEORETICAL FRAMEWORK

The box entitled "Determinants of Vertical Integration" summarizes what we believe to be the fundamen-

---

Determinants of Vertical Integration

Production cost savings
  Shared fixed inputs
  Synergies between vertical stages
Transaction cost savings and service coordination benefits
  Information economies
  Savings on costs of negotiating and administering contracts
  Coordination of services among related stages (continuity of care)
Overcoming market imperfections
  Regulatory constraints
  Monopoly power on buyer or seller side
Management and internal organization factors
  New organizational forms
  Organizational "culture"
Environmental conditions

---

tal determinants of, and benefits sought by, vertical integration. Since there exists little empirical research that assesses the costs, risks, and benefits of vertical integration under different conditions, these determinants are justified conceptually rather than empirically. The major drivers of vertical integration are

- production cost savings;
- transaction cost savings and improved coordination of services (i.e., continuity of care);
- overcoming market imperfections;
- responding to management and internal factors; and
- responding to environmental changes that alter market conditions, production technologies, and transactional relationships.

Environmental forces

We begin with observations about some of the environmental conditions influencing vertical integration. In our judgment, the two critical environmental forces behind the rapid evolution of vertically linked systems are (1) new prospective payment arrangements that significantly alter the interdependencies between economic agents at different levels in health care delivery—hospitals and physicians, payers and providers (both institutional and individuals)—and between informational intermediaries and those parties responsible for paying for and providing health care services; and (2) dramatically increased cost and price sensitivity by purchasers of health care services, which has given rise to a demand for increased organizational efficiencies and price reductions.

The increased price sensitivity of purchasers has tightened the interdependencies among hospitals and their physicians, physicians and their support professionals, medical products and informational technology suppliers, service providers themselves, and among third party payers and individual and institutional providers. Backward integration by employer groups and insurance companies into the delivery of care is just one symptom and response to these increased interorganizational interdependencies.

Prospective payment is perhaps the single most important contemporary example of an environmental shift that alters the interdependencies among stages in the health services value chain. Movements to more closely integrate hospitals and their medical staffs through employment relationships, strict probationary periods prior to the granting of full admitting privi-

---

Prospective payment is perhaps the single most important contemporary example of an environmental shift that alters the interdependencies among stages in the health services value chain.

---

leges, and preferred provider contracting between insurers and providers and between institutional and individual providers, each respond to the increased interdependencies forced by prospective payment. Hospitals are also moving to coordinate their relationships with their physicians and to structure enhanced predischarge care and referral relationships, together with better postdischarge care, by employing or exclusively contracting with groups of physicians to provide the full range of inpatient and outpatient services. This form of vertical integration is increasingly being forced on the delivery system by the payer side.

Another factor fostering vertically integrated arrangements is the aging of the population. Heightened attention to the treatment of chronic diseases encourages organizations, particularly hospitals, to develop pre- and postacute care arrangements for facilitating the care of a given person over time. Chronic disease involves long-term care and long-term rehabilitation, which requires coordination of many different services. A key decision for many organizations will be how to structure enhanced continuity of care between different

levels in the process of caring for individual patients. The increased prevalence of chronic disease, brought about by the aging of the population, reinforces the need for an integrated delivery system.

At the same time, the aging of the population has increased the relative importance of the Medicare program to the overall delivery system. Both the nature of chronic disease and the growing significance of the Medicare population, already under a per case form of prospective inpatient payment, are pushing the system toward capitated payment structures. Within capitated structures, the providers quickly learn to reduce transaction costs among different parties in the system by entering into contractual arrangements or by devising closely coordinated networks. These moves bring about integration in one form or another at both the clinical and the administrative levels of the organization.

Efficiency and effectiveness "drivers"

The key to production cost savings does not seem to be at the unit-cost level, but rather in relation to the utilization of inputs between different stages in health care delivery. If HMOs have shown us one thing, it is that the principal gain from vertically structured arrangements flows from substituting the use of less-expensive treatment modalities for acute inpatient care. Organizations increasingly will need to focus on finding synergies between different levels of the care process, and these will depend on using the talent in one part of the business, for example, ambulatory care or prevention/wellness, to economize on utilization at other stages in delivery (most typically, the hospital or nursing home levels).

Transaction cost savings center on economies in the transfer and use of information between different levels of care. For example, the nursing home that coordinates its admissions with an integrated hospital and physician clinic system can design supportive acute inpatient care arrangements for those episodes that require hospitalization within the context of a single linked system. A common organization may save on the cost of entering into and enforcing contracts between different care providers as it substitutes internal management and organizational culture for pricing incentives as mechanisms for organizing services at different levels in the care process.

Tighter linkages between different levels of care (e.g., through combining skilled nursing home care with hospital acute inpatient care in a common organization) not only save transaction costs, but also should yield improved coordination and continuity of care. Systematic preadmission and postdischarge planning save on the transaction costs of "errors" between steps in the value chain while also improving the quality of services delivered at each point in the process.

Regulatory constraints and market imperfections

In addition, vertical integration can be a means to work around regulatory constraints or market power on the buyer or seller side. For example, a hospital might form its own HMO, along with a physician group, as one means to avoid hospital rate-setting restrictions in a particular state. By doing this, the hospital substitutes disclosure and regulation of its HMO premiums by the state insurance department for control over its rates as an acute hospital by a state rate-regulation agency. The regulatory control in this case is moved up from an intermediate stage (the hospital rates) to the final stage of production (total premiums to the buyer), thus potentially economizing on the costs of regulatory compliance. Vertically integrated systems are also one means of exerting countervailing power against groups (such as organized physicians in a local area) that charge above-cost prices to hospital producers. Similarly, the physician group that integrates forward into its own preferred provider organization (PPO) arrangement through coordination with other physician groups can overcome strong market power exerted on the buying side by a sole community hospital or other monopoly provider of hospital services. In both cases, whether the monopoly is on the buyer or seller side, the integration serves to eliminate the social inefficiencies that result when any one player in the marketplace can control the transaction prices for health services.

INTEGRATIVE MECHANISMS

A key to the success of vertical integration rests with the nature of the coordinative mechanisms crafted to support that integration. These mechanisms merit emphasis in this article, and we now turn to a discussion of integrative instrumentalities, which fundamentally determine the success of vertically linked strategies.

Administrative coordination mechanisms

The first step in developing a vertically integrated delivery system is the building of administrative mechanisms to coordinate and integrate services. We focus first on administrative mechanisms at the interorganizational level. The box entitled "Administrative Coordination/Integration: Interorganization or System Level" illustrates the variety of these interorganizational mechanisms, which range from tapping the benefits of single ownership to utilizing the advantages of proximity among different organizational units.

Given the different mechanisms for achieving interorganizational coordination, an integrated delivery system does not have to own or even provide every service itself; it may enter into cooperative relationships with other entities to achieve the desired degree of coordination among services. An example of such a cooperative relationship would be the use of a transfer agreement between a hospital and a nursing home that specifies incentives for bringing nursing home patients back to the hospital for subacute care. Through the use of such innovative contracting arrangements, the organization can manage other elements of the delivery system without accepting the final business risk for its operation. An HMO or a PPO that contracts with providers of all the different levels and types of care illustrates an extreme example of this coordinative mechanism.

Intraorganizational administrative coordination

Administrative mechanisms are also required within the organization (intraorganizational) to more closely link different stages in the production process of health services. The box entitled "Administrative Coordination/Integration: Intraorganization or Program Level"

Administrative Coordination/Integration: Interorganization or System Level

Single ownership	Informal agreement
Internal development	Coordinating/steering
Acquisition/merger	committee
Lease	Planning
Franchise	Budget and operations
Shared ownership	Marketing
Joint venture	Shared coordinator/manager
Partnership	ager
Management contract	Governing board participation
Contractual agreement	pation
External party (e.g., HMO)	Management participation
Interorganizational	Proximity
Affiliation agreement	

> **Administrative Coordination/Integration: Intraorganization or Program Level**
>
> Program/product line form of organization
> Matrix organization
> Program coordinator/manager
>   Extent of authority?
>   Physician, nurse, manager head?
>   Single individual, team?
> Liaison roles to link departments
> Program steering committee/team
>   Authority?
>   Membership?
> Program planning committee/task force
> Program budgeting
> Program data
>   Integration of financial and patient data around programs
> Administrative policies and procedures
> "Culture"
>   Encourage direct communication/problem solving across departments

displays a spectrum of these linking methodologies. We pinpoint a few examples here for further discussion. These internal administrative integrating processes may take the form of assigning the responsibility for coordinating different components to a program manager, using program planning task forces, and integrating clinical and financial information around specific clinical programs or services.

A study of Japanese management in the last several years (e.g., in the works of Ouchi[4])has revealed the importance of multidimensional and multidivisional organizations in responding to the changing health care market place. The matrix organization illustrates one such innovation, wherein a manager is alternately responsible to both a functional manager (e.g., marketing, finance) and a product-line manager (e.g., surgical services).

Some of the most important vertical linkages in health services will not involve the integration of the entire organization's complete product line or service mix, but rather the design and implementation of vertically integrated programs (e.g., a heart center organizing the comprehensive spectrum of primary, secondar, and tertiary cardiovascular services for a defined patient population). A new set of administrative coordination "technologies" may need to be established to make these programs work. The vertical integration of

programs raises questions not only concerning product management and matrix organization models, but also regarding

- the appropriate mix and locus of function and program authority and accountability;
- the nature and composition of steering committees and program planning task forces;
- the integration of clinical, financial, and sociodemographic information; and
- the crafting and nurturing of new organizational "cultures" and the administrative policies and procedures that support "vertically linked," direct communication and problem solving across interrelated subunits of the organization.

Patient care coordination

Although such administrative mechanisms are necessary conditions for cost-effective vertical integration, they are hardly sufficient. For a system to be fully integrated, patient care itself must be coordinated and its continuity assured. Sample approaches to this critical step are outlined in the box entitled "Clinical Mechanisms for Patient Care Integration."

The common thread running through these different mechanisms for patient care coordination and integration is their emphasis on connecting patient services at different stages in the care process. The managed care plan does this by developing HMO and PPO products, using exclusive or preferred contracting with a defined set of providers as the means for linking different levels of patient care, as well as their financing. Case management—whether directed by a primary care physician, nurse specialist, or interdisciplinary team—integrates

> **Clinical Mechanisms for Patient Care Integration**
>
> Managed care plan
> Case management
> Case manager (e.g., physician, nurse)
> Interdisciplinary team
> Primary care "gatekeeper"/case manager
> Medical director
> Clinical coordinator/clinical nurse specialist
> Single medical record
> Discharge planning
> Program-oriented quality assurance activity
> Continuing medical education and in-service training
> Consumer information and referral program

The managed care plan develops HMO and PPO products, using exclusive or preferred contracting with a defined set of providers as the means for linking different levels of patient care.

by explicitly managing and assuming responsibility for the care of individual patients and by coordinating patient care with the various social and financial support resources needed over the course of an individual's illness. Case management models hold particular promise for integrating the care of chronically ill persons, for whom the case management team functions much like a "personalized HMO."

To elaborate on just one other example, the single (integrated) medical record that would follow the patient over time and across delivery settings offers an important opportunity for coordinating patient care. The integrated record would serve three critical functions; it would

1. link information on illness episodes over time;
2. capture diagnostic, treatment, and health status information sufficient to provide an intertemporal health assessment for the patient; and
3. record outcomes of the nursing and medical interventions applied to the patient.

These different coordinative mechanisms serve to reinforce a variety of intra- and interorganizational forms, each of which is adapted to fit a particular set of environmental, market, and organizational managerial circumstances. Our next task is to examine these organizational forms under the terms of our conceptual framework.

A MATRIX OF ORGANIZATIONAL FORMS

Table 1 matches the determinants of vertical integration (as suggested by our conceptual framework) with different intra- and interorganizational forms of vertical integration observed in the marketplace. This is by no means an exhaustive list of integrated arrangements, nor does it represent an ordered (i.e., from more to less integrated) continuum of vertical structures. Instead, Table 1 gives a series of examples that are meant

to provide a "reality test" of the relevance of our conceptual framework.

We discuss each of the examples in Table 1 briefly and only to emphasize key insights, since the detailed analysis is contained within the table itself. First, the development of the closed-staff-model HMO has been a response to the environmental pressures of cost sensitivity on the part of health care purchasers and to the supply and mix of physicians in local markets. The production and transaction cost benefits of the closed-staff-model HMO are driven by strong internal utilization management and organizational integration of hospitals, ambulatory care facilities, and physicians.

Individual practice associations (IPAs) and PPOs are somewhat newer organizational forms, created primarily to balance the tradeoffs between purchasers' access to a broad range of providers and the production cost and transaction cost efficiencies that result from tighter integration. These more "loosely coupled" arrangements are capturing increased market share relative to closed-staff HMOs (although both are gaining relative to "unmanaged" fee-for-service arrangements) because consumers are attracted by the large numbers of participating providers they offer.[5] It remains to be seen whether the utilization controls of IPAs and PPOs will be as effective as the more tightly structured closed-staff HMOs.[6]

The integrated hospital-multispecialty physician group practice model, which predates the HMO and PPO models, developed in a market context different from that of managed care plans. In Seattle, a multispecialty physician group practice is one of four core organizations making up the vertically linked Virginia Mason Medical Center: the physician group practice partnership, the hospital, the fund development foundation, and a research center.[7] The hospital–clinic integration was in place even before Medicare and Medicaid ushered in retrospective cost-based reimbursement in 1965. The primary "drivers" behind this organizational form appear to be the desire for closer coordination of referral and patient care relationships between specialty and primary care physicians and the benefits of convenience to physicians and continuity of care to patients from the integration of ambulatory and inpatient care. The internal management culture promotes this integration through several mechanisms, such as

- a single set of written objectives relating to patient care, education, and research for all the core organizations;

- maintenance of "medical center discipline" by top managers; and
- overlapping management responsibilities for organizational components (e.g., the executive administrator of the Mason Clinic is also vice president of the hospital).

The hospital-based, primary care group practice is described by Shortell and Zajac as a "hybrid" organizational form, one that combines features of a joint venture (i.e., a shared equity investment by initially autonomous physicians and a hospital) with those of an internal corporate venture (i.e., the closer linkage of a hospital with the primary care physicians who admit patients there).[8] In this case, the venture is knitted together by a joint equity investment of physicians and the hospital and by internal staffing of a semiautonomous unit (i.e., the group practice itself). Consistent with our conceptual framework, Shortell and Zajac posit that resource scarcity (prospective and restricted payment to doctors and hospitals) and competition (e.g., due to the increasing supply of physicians and to excess hospital bed capacity) are the primary environmental stimuli for these ventures. Their survival and success in the marketplace will be determined by their ability to craft performance-based incentives, overcome medical staff resistance to new referral and admitting practice patterns, and structure sufficient operating autonomy for the group practice, while at the same time maintaining both the strategic importance of the group practice and its integration with the hospital's and the physician members' core services.

The managed care product is an innovation of the 1980s that reflects the competing pressures for autonomy and control experienced by today's health care organizations.[5] The example, Pointer, Begun and Luke (referred to in Table 1) comprises four hypothetical organizations operating in the same local market. These organizations form a "strategic alliance" to offer a managed care insurance product that covers physician services, hospital care, and skilled nursing services.[9] Depending on the circumstances of a particular market environment, these organizations would use a combination of arms-length contracting and joint ownership to design, deliver, and market the managed care product. The members of the alliance come together for a specific strategic purpose, but remain parallel and, in some cases, competing organizations in other local markets and other service lines.

Finally, the McKesson Corporation, a large distributor of drugs, health care products, and other consumer goods illustrates the notion of a value-adding partnership (VAP).[10] All five determinants of vertical integration are germane to this example, as shown in Table 1. While the primary technologic innovation behind the VAP between McKesson and the independent drugstores it serves is a computer information system, the key to McKesson's success in prescription drug services is its management's commitment to monitoring and strengthening each link in the value chain from product supplier, to distributor (McKesson itself), to drug store, to final consumer. The history of this VAP illustrates that such partnerships develop first between adjacent stages in the value chain (e.g., distributor and independent drug store), but are then reinforced at stages close to the final consumer (e.g., in the form of computerized information on the effects of different drug combinations).

MANAGEMENT ISSUES

We close with a series of questions for those who do, and those who would, manage vertically integrated health care systems. Although we do not know the answers to all of these questions, we believe that they must be addressed if vertical integration is to be pursued efficiently and effectively in specific situations. The issues raised by these questions fall into five categories:

1. The fit of the vertical integration strategy with the core mission of the organizations involved.
2. Capital requirements and capital financing approaches.
3. The design of organizational processes, incentives, and responsibility/accountability mechanisms in support of vertical integration.
4. The amounts, types, and sequencing of the expertise and resources required to effectively carry out vertical integration.
5. The need to broaden both clinical and managerial perspectives on case-mix management and quality assurance.

Fit and mission

1. What can an organization do to ensure that diversification into areas other than traditional patient care services does not threaten its basic character, identity, and values?

This question emerges with particular force as the organization seeks to integrate different levels of patient care and "population-based services" (e.g., home

TABLE 1

THE "INTEGRATIVE BALANCE": INTRA- AND INTERORGANIZATIONAL FORMS

Form of vertical integration	Determinants Production cost savings	Transaction cost savings
1. Closed-staff-model HMO (common ownership, fully integrated value chain)	Primarily through utilization management of inpatient care	Continuity of care through integration of facilities and medical staff
2. IPA-model HMO (separate ownership; contracting between the "plan" and physicians, hospitals; contract-based integration of value chain)	Utilization management; less-rigorous utilization management incentives than in closed-staff HMO	Still essentially market in contracting between plan and physicians, hospitals
3. Insurer-sponsored PPO (separate ownership; contracting on preferred vs. closed-panel or exclusive basis; contract-based integration)	Minimal; achieved primarily through unit cost reductions stimulated by price discounting	Replaces repeated contracting with one-time costs of establishing preferred provider network
4. Integrated hospital-multispecialty physician group practice (shared governance of the hospital and clinic; partially integrated value chain)	Not a prominent factor	Continuity of care benefits; referral and practice network; increased congruence of hospital and physician goals
5. Hospital-based ambulatory primary care group practice (shared-equity investment by hospital and physician group; internal staffing of semi-autonomous unit; partially integrated value chain)	Minimal factor	Some continuity of care gains due to tightened referral network between the hospital and primary care physicians (PCPs)
6. Local-market-based managed care product (formation of "quasi-firm" by short-term general hospital, multispecialty physician group, skilled nursing facility, and insurance carrier; partially integrated value chain)	Primarily through overall "case management" of utilization	Managed care via case manager; partially supplants arms-length market contracting; enhanced pre- and postdischarge services (visit, planning for hospital, ambulatory care, and long-term care); link to insurer enhances continuity between delivery and financing of care
7. McKesson's "value-adding partnership" (VAP) (with manufacturing, distribution, retailing, third party insurance, and consumers for prescription drugs) (separate ownership of value chain components, contract-based integration)	Dramatic reductions in cost of order processing; reduced costs of restocking orders through conscious redesign of shelves	Enhanced monitoring through computer database of clinical-biological effects of alternative drug combinations

Overcoming market imperfections	Management and internal factors	Environmental conditions
Response to physician market power	Internal "culture" linking organizational and physician interests	Cost sensitivity of purchasers; necessary supply of physicians
Potential for more competitive physician pricing through contract and capitation incentives	Contracting largely supplants internal hierarchy	
Simulates competitive market's price network	Minimal	Similar to Form 4
Minimal factor	Internal culture linking hospital and physician interests	Minimal factor
Minimal factor	Example: an internal corporate joint venture	Excess hospital bed capacity; increasing supply of PCPs
"Backward" integration by insured into delivery; exerts buyer bargaining power on providers to reduce costs of services	Can deliver the product through variety of tightly or loosely "coupled" market or ownership mechanisms	Cost sensitivity of purchasers; excess supply of physicians; limited reimbursement for long-term care; (health) insurance underwriting cycle
Minimal factor	Create management culture that monitors competitive dynamics throughout value chain and fixes weaknesses as they occur; use of computer systems and information technology for order entry, packing, shipping, shelf design (e.g., for quality assurance) (drug combination)	Increasing competition from large drug store chains; eroding market share of independent drug stores served by McKesson

---

What can the organization do to ensure that diversification does not threaten its basic character, identity, and values?

---

health, long-term care, health promotion) with its core activity (e.g., acute inpatient care), rather than simply diversify into new product lines.

2. What explicit criteria should be employed in evaluating major potential diversification and vertical integration opportunities? Are different criteria pertinent to diversification, as contrasted with vertical integration?

For example, might diversification initiatives be expected to earn greater profits than services added to enhance vertical integration? Which criteria should be used to decide when to divest, as well as when to add services?

Criteria could be developed in such areas as

- compatibility with mission and image;
- fit with system priorities;
- availability of expertise, management time, and other crucial resources;
- reporting relationships;
- financial return;
- evidence of demand/need; and
- prospective specification of integrative mechanisms.

Capital requirements and capital financing

The available literature tells us little about the following capital formation issues posed by vertical restructuring:

- The size, scope of services, or geographic distribution of facilities required for a delivery system to achieve an adequate degree of dominance or identity in its local or regional market (especially if it is located in a major metropolitan area) may necessitate a considerable amount of growth. Is the health services organization willing to make the major investments that may be required to build a dominant local and regional delivery system?
- Assuming that it would be desirable from the delivery system's perspective to add a particular business or service, where should the funds come from? Can mechanisms be developed to transform a portion of the economic benefits flowing to one component of the system to finance or subsidize another? In short, should

one look at interunit financial incentives? Alternatively, how will the capital markets respond to demands for equity and debt capital to support the development of such comprehensive systems?

- Will the creation of better control and coordination of referral flows and channels of distribution (e.g., postacute care in the case of the hospital) lower the total business risk of the vertically integrated system relative to that of single-product or single-level organizations (e.g., home health, long-term care, primary care physicians, multispecialty groups)? If total business risk in the system is lowered, to what extent will the consequent reduction in the cost of capital (required return on assets) be passed through in price benefits to payers rather than ploughed back into new investments in facilities and services?

Organizational processes, incentives, and responsibility/accountability

To integrate previously separate stages in the health care value chain, the system must develop a supportive organizational "culture" reinforced by communication processes (e.g., between clinical service line and functional managers), incentives, and a framework for responsibility and accountability. The key aim of such a culture is to promote the effectiveness, efficiency, and long-run return on capital of the delivery system as a whole, rather than only individual units making up that system.

How should the system address conflicts between systemwide (global) optimization and suboptimization by the individual units? For example, the cost-efficient size, scope of services, or location for a nursing home may not be what would best meet the needs of the system. Another example is the hospital that, to minimize DRG losses, seeks to discharge patients needing more intensive care than the system's nursing home wants to provide, given the level of reimbursement available to the nursing home. An extreme example is managed care plans where the factors required for success go far beyond the interests of the individual hospitals that first sponsored the plans. In fact, the basic goals of managed care and hospitals may conflict in very fundamental ways. This difference reflects the need to clarify the locus of responsibility for delivery system as well as individual unit results. Another related issue is the visibility of the performance of individual units that are part of a larger delivery system (e.g., the skilled nursing facility unit of an acute hospital).

What should be the reporting relationship of the administrators of the different types of facilities and programs that make up a vertically integrated delivery system in a given region? Should they report to the administrator of the hospital that serves as the organizational hub of the regional delivery system? To a regional administrator? To program specialists in the corporate office? To the corporate executive vice president for operations? Should the integrated system consider some form of matrix organization structure?

How should the system and/or components of the system respond to the fact that full or optimal integration may call for fundamental changes in operating systems and organization structures at the corporate or institutional level, or at both levels, that are difficult to implement (e.g., program budgeting, program versus functional organization structures, integration of clinical and financial data systems, and greater participation of physicians and other clinical professionals in management decision making)?

When a vertically integrated health care system is formed that bridges several previously freestanding levels of care (e.g., primary and specialty physician care, home health care, long-term care, and acute hospital inpatient care), what sorts of internal transfer pricing mechanisms are most appropriate between those different levels of care: short-run marginal cost of production, long-run fully allocated (with overhead) average cost, cost plus, or market prices for comparable services? Nonprice transfer arrangements (e.g., guaranteed swing bed capacity in the hospital for long-term care patients requiring subacute care) must also be designed among organizational units in the integrated system.

How can the organization encourage physician acceptance and support of mechanisms that contribute to clinical coordination and functional integration of patient care programs and services? Physicians tend to resist, for example, the establishment of medical director or other clinical administrative positions that act to integrate and provide leadership for programs that cut across specialties. Physicians often see specialists in integrative fields like geriatrics and rehabilitation as a

competitive threat. Physicians may also resist such concepts as case management and interdisciplinary patient assessment teams. Finally, because hospital medical staffs are organized along traditional medical specialty lines, they are not well structured to deal with many of the issues and needs of vertical integration (e.g., interdisciplinary program planning).

How can an adequate degree of administrative coordination and integration be achieved in a delivery system where some components are under neither common management nor common ownership? In effect, this question challenges the organization seeking to develop and maintain a vertically linked system to shape contracting and pricing incentives and "good will" relationships between separately owned entities that can substitute effectively for the authority and control structures embedded in a system whose components are all under common ownership.

Sequencing of expertise and resources

Because many of the organizations considering vertical integration are acute hospital systems, expertise may be lacking at both the corporate and institutional levels with regard to nonacute care programs and services. Yet expertise—in evaluating and negotiating acquisitions, joint ventures, or other arrangements, and in managing new services—is often the single most important ingredient in success. The system must ask itself: do we need to make a special effort to develop or assure the availability of expertise in areas other than acute care? How, and in what areas? One needs to recognize the great amount of management time required to acquire or start up a new service, especially one outside the scope of management's normal responsibilities.

Can the organization define priority areas such as ambulatory care, long-term care, or managed care to be acquired or established first in building vertically integrated delivery systems?

There may be significant "free-rider" problems in initiating vertically integrated delivery systems. In the long run, and over a sufficiently large population base, there are likely to be patient care benefits and total cost savings from a better coordinated comprehensive delivery system. The cost savings may be realized not only in direct production costs, but also in transaction costs (e.g., administrative costs, travel time, waiting time, and other "side costs" of patient care). Unless the organization leading the drive to integrate delivery can capture direct market share and financial gains to justify

---

Because hospital medical staffs are organized along traditional medical specialty lines, they are not well structured to deal with many of the issues and needs of vertical integration.

the costs of devising coordinated health care arrangements, efforts to implement vertical integration may be impeded because of concentrated costs and diffuse benefits. This reasoning suggests two corollary questions:

1. In areas where the organization has neither a dominant hospital nor sufficient resources to develop a dominant vertically integrated system, and so must collaborate with other organizations to this end, what strategies for allocating costs and benefits among "strategic partners" might work best?

2. What bargains can be struck between the dominant institution and the nondominant institutions involved in a nascent, vertically integrated system for sharing risks, costs, gains, and fixed-capital investment outlays?

Clinical and managerial perspectives on case mix measurement and quality assurance

The vertically integrated delivery system encourages a fundamental shift in clinical and managerial focus from (1) caring for and billing transactions for whichever patients present themselves to the organization's door at a given point in time, to (2) accepting broader responsibility for the continuity and coordination of patient care for a defined population. This population-based perspective applies to clinical and financial management, and raises the following questions:

- How does the organization measure and manage case mix and the quality of patient care processes and outcomes for persons over time, in contrast to the more familiar measures of case mix and quality, which are defined for discrete episodes of care?
- What is the relationship between the costs borne by the integrated system (which, in the case of an HMO, should be recouped in premiums charged) and the process and outcome quality of patient care?

CONCLUSION: THE INTEGRATIVE BALANCE

We do not have the knowledge to answer these managerial questions definitively at this point, but we can articulate many of the crucial challenges for vertically integrated arrangements. The key to success is to strike the "integrative balance," that is, to adopt the intra- or interorganizational forms that optimize the mix of strategic flexibility with production and transaction cost-efficiency, given the market conditions facing the organizational decision makers.

Management analysts of vertical integration have been discussing the strategic flexibility/cost control tradeoff for years, so to state the need for integrative balance has not been the thrust of this article. Rather, we have presented a fresh synthesis of the theory and have articulated the managerial implications of developing and sustaining vertically integrated health care systems.

REFERENCES

1. Porter, M.E. *Competitive Strategy.* New York, N.Y.: Free Press, 1980.
2. Harrigan, K.R. "Formulating Vertical Integration Strategies." *Academy of Management Review* 9 (1984): 638–52.
3. Mick, S.S., and Conrad, D.A. "The Decision to Integrate Vertically in Health Care Organizations." *Hospital and Health Services Administration* 33 (1988): 345–60.
4. Ouchi, W.G. "A Conceptual Framework for the Design of Organizational Control Mechanisms." *Management Science* 25 (1979): 833–48.
5. Pointer, D.D., Begun, J.W., and Luke, R.D. "Managing Inter-organizational Dependencies in the New Health Care Marketplace." *Hospital and Health Services Administration* 33 (1988): 167–77.
6. Conrad, D.A., et al. "Vertical Structures and Control in Health Care Markets: A Conceptual Framework and Empirical Review." *Medical Care Review* 45 (1988): 49–100.
7. Ross, A. "Organizational Challenges and Linkages Associated With Vertically Linked Health Organizations." In *Vertically Linked Health Organizations: The 1978 National Forum on Hospital and Health Affairs,* edited by B.J. Jaeger. Durham, N.C.: Department of Health Administration, Duke University, 1978.
8. Shortell, S.M., and Zajac, E.J. "Internal Corporate Joint Ventures: Development Process and Performance Outcomes." *Strategic Management Journal* 9 (1988): 527–42.
9. Hamel, G., Doz, Y.L., and Prahalad, C.K. "Collaborate With Your Competitors—and Win." *Harvard Business Review* 89 (1989): 133–39.
10. Johnston, R., and Lawrence, P.R. "Beyond Vertical Integration: The Rise of the Value-Adding Partnership." *Harvard Business Review* 88 (1988): 94–101.

Inter-organizational linkages in the health sector

Beaufort B. Longest, Jr.

A key element in the success of organizations in the health sector is the maintenance of effective interorganizational linkages with interdependent organizations. A conceptual framework is posited of three general classes of mechanisms through which these linkages are managed.

Health Care Manage Rev, 1990, 15(1), 17–28
© 1990 Aspen Publishers, Inc.

Organizations in the health sector typically maintain a variety of relationships with other organizations. Often, these interorganizational relationships involve a high degree of interdependence in that at least one of the organizations does not completely control all of the conditions necessary for the achievement of its purposes. For a particular focal organization, other organizations that can affect, or that are affected by, the achievement of its purposes are interdependent with it.[1] An organization in the health sector (e.g., a hospital or a health maintenance organization [HMO]) might maintain relationships with interdependent others as diverse as groups of consumers, agencies of government, or suppliers of the inputs it needs (see box, "Interdependencies between Organizations in the Health Sector"). Furthermore, a focal organization can be simultaneously involved in systems, joint ventures, partnerships, or any of a host of affiliations, consortia, and confederations, all of which entail interdependent relationships.

The multiplicity of potential interorganizational linkages suggests the need for a typology of the basic types available to managers in the health sector. For example, some linkages are simple market exchanges needed to acquire necessary resources or ensure markets for outputs. Some are more complex interorganizational linkages, voluntarily established, that range from loosely structured couplings to tight bureaucracies. Still other linkages are involuntary arrangements (from the focal organization's perspective) that guide relationships with regulators, fiscal intermediaries, or utilization management companies. Increasingly, a key element of success for organizations in the health sector is the ability of their managers to develop and maintain effective interorganizational linkages as a means of managing their organizations' interdependencies. This article posits a conceptual framework of three general classes of mechanisms through which health care organizations manage their interdependencies with other organizations: market transactions, voluntary interorganizational relationship transactions, and involuntary interorganizational relationship transactions. These categories of linkage mechanisms, each with a place in the management of interdependence between and

Beaufort B. Longest, Jr., *Ph.D., is Professor of both Health Services Administration and Business Administration and Director of both the Health Administration Program and the Health Policy Institute at the University of Pittsburgh.*

Interdependencies between Organizations in the Health Sector

In the health sector, focal organizations have potential interdependencies with organizations such as:

Accrediting agencies
Affiliated organizations
Alternative health systems
Competitors
Confederated organizations
Consortia members
Consumer representative (public and private)
Employee representatives (unions)
Fiscal intermediaries
Financial organizations (bond rating)
Foundations
Government (all levels)
Health maintenance organizations (HMOs)
Independent practice associations (IPAs)

Insurance companies
Joint venture partners
Media
Medical staff-hospital joint ventures (MeSHs)
Multiinstitutional systems
Other partners
Owners
Political groups
Preferred provider organizations (PPOs)
Suppliers (including capital, consumables, equipment, and human resources
Third party associations (TPAs)
Trade associations
Utilization management companies

---

among organizations in the health sector, are briefly summarized in the Appendix and more fully elaborated in subsequent sections of this article.

MARKET TRANSACTIONS

Market transactions are the most prevalent form of linkage with interdependent others for most organizations, and usually the simplest. By dealing with each other through market transactions, organizations buy needed resources and sell outputs. These transactions also occur between a focal organization and individuals such as its nonunionized employees and some patients. The transactions between a focal organization and its customers (and their advocates and representatives), suppliers, and employees, including physicians, can be relatively straightforward market exchanges (see box, "Interdependencies between Organizations in the Health Sector").

The application of exchange principles (most notably that organizations are calculative when it comes to their rewards and costs in exchanges) often results in the development of contracts that, even if only implicit, govern most market transactions by defining the conditions of exchanges between two or more parties. "This economic view of exchange relations, often criticized as overly calculative when applied to interpersonal relations, is highly applicable to the analysis of interorganizational relations, where the corporate entities have well-established mechanisms for monitoring rewards and costs."[2(p.357)] Contracts are used widely as supporting devices for managing linkages in a great variety of

interorganizational relationships. They are usually negotiated agreements between parties for the exchange of future benefits. Simple contracts can rest on the belief that each party will perform as agreed. More rigorous contracts can rely on specific terms that can be evaluated by third parties and that can serve as the basis for penalties to be assessed if performance is unsatisfactory.

Exchange relationships based on contracts may entail nothing more than an acceptable agreement with a supplier for some needed item or service or an agreement between a hospital and an HMO to provide certain services to a defined population. Contracts permit health care organizations to establish stable and predictable (albeit interdependent) relationships with the federal government for reimbursement for Medicare patients, state governments for reimbursement for Medicaid patients, and with commercial insurers for their subscribers. Contracts also permit the employment and utilization of a work force and the orderly acquisition of other needed resources.

Negotiating skills are the most important skills in managing organizational interdependencies through market transactions. *Negotiation*, also called bargaining, is "the process whereby two or more parties attempt to settle what each shall give and take, or perform and receive, in a transaction between them."[3(p.2)] In these interactions, the parties attempt to agree on a mutually acceptable outcome in a situation where their outcome preferences are usually negatively related. Indeed, if the preferences for outcomes are positively related, an agreement or contract can be reached almost automatically, although this relationship among interdependent organizations is rare. More typically among interdependent organizations, there are at least two sources of conflict that must be resolved through negotiations: (1) a division of resources, the "tangibles" of the negotiation, such as which organization will receive what quantity of money, goods, or services in exchange for what considerations, and (2) the resolution of problems of psychological dynamics and the satisfaction of personal preferences of the leaders of the organizations involved in the negotiations. These latter elements are the "intangibles" of the negotiation and can include such variables as appearing to win or lose, compete effectively, or cooperate fairly. Negotiations between interdependent organizations (e.g., a contract negotiation between a Blue Cross plan and a hospital) sometimes hinge more on the intangible issues than on the tangible resource issues.

Negotiations between interdependent organizations usually follow one of two strategic approaches: (1) cooperative, win-win strategies, or (2) competitive, win-lose, strategies. The nature of the negotiating strategy is a function of the interaction of several variables (see box, "Optimal Conditions for Cooperative and Competitive Negotiating Strategies").[4]

Whether interdependent organizations are engaged in cooperative or competitive negotiations, the process tends to proceed in five distinct phases. First, there is a *preparation phase* during which both sides assess the nature of their conflict of interest, establish their own goals and priorities, try to guess those of their opponent, and determine the negotiating strategy they plan to use. Second, there is an *entry phase* in which the sides make initial contact with each other, establish an agenda, rules, and procedures for the negotiation, and present their initial goals and priorities. The third phase can be called the *elaboration and education phase* and is characterized by both sides learning more about their opponent's stated goals and priorities and elaborating upon their own initially stated goals and priorities in light of what they learn. The fourth phase, called the *bargaining phase,* is the heart of the negotiating process and entails attempts by both sides to challenge their opponent's goals and logic, defend their own, search for ways to make compromises and tradeoffs, and invent alternative solutions. The final phase of the negotiating process is the *closure phase,* during which both sides seek to arrive at a basic agreement, consolidate the issues into a package, record the agreement in mutually satisfactory language, and begin planning for the implementation of the agreement.[4]

Table 1 contains an outline of tactics that can be used in both cooperative and competitive negotiating strategies in each of the phases of the process. Negotiations are often neither purely cooperative nor competitive, requiring a mixture of the tactics for successful results.

Optimal Conditions for Cooperative and Competitive Negotiating Strategies

Cooperative negotiating strategies	Competitive negotiating strategies
The tangible goals of both sides are to attain a specific settlement that is fair and reasonable.	The tangible goals of both sides are to attain a specific settlement or to get as much as they possibly can.
Sufficient resources are available in the environment for both sides to attain their tangible goals, more resources can be attained, or the problem can be redefined so that both sides can win.	Insufficient resources are available for both sides to attain their goals, or their desires to get as much as possible make it impossible for one or both parties to actually attain their goals.
Each side believes that it is possible for both sides to attain their goals through the negotiation process.	Both sides perceive that it is impossible for both of them to attain their goals.
The intangible goals of both sides are to establish a cooperative relationship and work together toward a settlement that maximizes their joint outcomes.	The intangible goals of both sides are to beat the other, keep the other from attaining its goals, humiliate the other, or refuse to make concessions in negotiating position.

TABLE 1

TACTICS IN COMPETITIVE AND COOPERATIVE NEGOTIATIONS

Phase of negotiation	Competitive tactics	Cooperative tactics
Preparation	Set specific goals, bottom lines, and opening bids; develop firm positions and competitive tactics to attain those goals at the expense of the other.	Develop general goals and broad objectives; cultivate good options; cultivate good relations of trust and openness with opponent to promote effective problem solving.
Entry-problem identification	State the problem in terms of the organization's preferred solution; publicly disguise or misrepresent organization needs and goals; don't let the other side know what's really important.	State the problem in terms of the underlying needs of both sides; represent organization needs accurately to the other side; listen carefully to understand their needs.
Elaboration or education	Disclose only that information necessary to support the organization's position, and have the other side understand it; hide possible vulnerabilities and weaknesses.	Disclose all information that may be pertinent to a problem, regardless of whose position it supports; expose vulnerabilities in order to protect them in the joint solution.
Bargaining	Include false issues, dummy options, or options of low priority in order to trade them away for what your side wants; make an early public commitment and stick to it.	Minimize the inclusion of false or dummy issues and stick to the major problems and concerns; avoid early and public commitments to preferred alternatives, in order to give all options full consideration.
Closure	Maximize own utilities while not caring about the other's; overvalue concessions to other; undervalue achieved gains; use "nibbling" strategy of taking issues off the table as favorable settlements are achieved.	Maximize solutions that have joint utility; be honest and candid in disclosing preferences; use "nothing is ever final until all issues are settled" strategy.

Source: Adapted with permission from Greenberger, D., et al. "Perception, Motivation, and Negotiation." In *Health Care Management: A Text in Organization Theory and Behavior*, edited by S.M. Shortell and A.D. Kaluzny. 2d ed. New York: Wiley, 1988, p. 134.

VOLUNTARY INTERORGANIZATIONAL RELATIONSHIP TRANSACTIONS

Voluntary interorganizational relationship transactions have become commonplace in the health sector as managers seek to secure and stabilize their organizations' places in turbulent and often hostile environments. Horizontal and vertical systems, joint ventures, partnerships, and various affiliations, consortia, and confederations are pervasive. They illustrate the range of voluntary interorganizational relationship transactions that managers of health care organizations are using to better manage their organizations' interdependencies.

These voluntary interorganizational relationship transactions can be classified into four types. Thompson has termed two of these linking mechanisms *co-opting* and *coalescing*.[5] Pointer, Begun, and Luke,[6] building on the earlier conceptualization of Eccles,[7] have added a third type, the *quasifirm. Ownership* is a fourth type of interorganizational transaction through which interdependencies are managed. Here, interdependencies that cannot be effectively managed through market transactions or one of the other forms of interorganizational transaction are brought inside the boundaries of the focal organization through ownership. This type of organizational transaction has been aptly labeled *consumption*.[8,2] Each of these categories of linkage represents relationships through which interorganizational interdependencies can be managed, each category has advantages and disadvantages, and each becomes relatively more complicated as one moves down the list.

Co-opting

This form of linkage involves the absorption of leadership elements from other organizations into the focal organization. Next to straightforward market transactions, co-opting mechanisms are often the most flexible and easiest linking processes to implement, two advantages that have made their use pervasive. In the health sector, this mechanism often takes one of two forms: (1) management contracts or (2) the placing of representatives of interdependent organizations on the focal organization's governing body. Management contracts, identified by Starkweather[8] as an example of co-opting, permit one organization to supply day-to-day management to another organization by agreement. In these arrangements management includes at least the chief executive officer, who reports to the governing body of the managed organization as well as to the managing organization. This is in contrast to the practice prevalent in many health care organizations of using outside contractors to manage individual departments and programs such as housekeeping, food service, or respiratory therapy.

Another common co-opting mechanism for achieving interorganizational coordination is the appointment of representatives from external organizations to positions in the focal organization, usually to a seat on the governing body. For example, a hospital system, interested in access to capital, may find considerable advantage in placing an investment banker on its governing body to gain that person's expertise in financial markets. Similarly, an HMO may find it advantageous to place members of its medical group on its board.

Coalescing

The health sector is replete with this type of linkage in such forms as joint ventures, partnerships, consortia, and federations. Its central feature is the partial pooling of resources by two or more organizations to pursue defined goals.[9] Glassman refers to this type of interorganizational relationship as *loose coupling*.[10] Loosely coupled interorganizational relationships link interdependent and mutually responsive organizations in ways that preserve their legal identities and autonomies and most of their functional autonomies.[11]

Next to straightforward market transactions, co-opting mechanisms are often the most flexible and easiest linking processes to implement, two advantages that have made their use pervasive.

These relationships are held together by stronger ties than those involved in market transactions, but the ties are less binding and less extensive than in ownership arrangements. Loosely coupled, or coalesced, organizational relationships can differ along a number of dimensions such as importance, permanence, and directionality:

First, loosely coupled relationships differ in terms of their relative importance to the success and viability of the participating organizations.[12] Health care facilities are embedded in a large number of interorganizational relationships; importance discriminates between those that are truly strategic and those that are not.

Second, loosely coupled relationships can be distinguished as to their degree of *permanence*. Some interorganizational relationships are of short duration, others are long term. Enduring relationships are necessary for organizations to achieve shared strategic purposes.[13]

Third, loosely coupled relationships vary in terms of their *directionality*. Organizations can be linked vertically, horizontally, or symbiotically.[14–16] Horizontal combinations entail interrelationships among similar organizations operating in the same industry which serve geographic markets with roughly equivalent products. Vertical combinations occur between organizations that operate along a chain of production where the output of one organization becomes the input of another. Such relationships are developed to secure inputs or dispose of outputs. In symbiotic combinations, organizations complement each other in the provision of services to customers and/or achieve joint competitive advantage in other areas (shared marketing or management or both). They occur between organizations operating in different segments of the same industry or in totally different industries. In either case, no significant amount of input/output is exchanged, and competition among such organizations is limited or nonexistent.[6(p.170)]

Joint ventures, increasingly prevalent in the health sector, "can be predicted by considerations of resource interdependence, competitive uncertainty, and conditions that make various forms of interdependence more or less problematic."[17(p.161)] Joint ventures between hospitals and their medical staffs or groups of the members of their medical staffs are especially commonplace. As has been noted:

> Hospitals and physicians are exploring new kinds of relationships through a variety of joint ventures. These range from highly formal activities such as hospital-sponsored group practices, health maintenance organizations sponsored by hospitals and their medical staffs, and preferred provider organizations (PPOs), to somewhat less formal arrangements involving leasing of space and equipment or providing ancillary services, computerized billing, financial analyses, and medical records services.[18(p.327)]

Major health care enterprises such as the Voluntary Hospitals of America and the American Health Care System, themselves loosely coupled networks of organizations, can enter into joint ventures with health insurance carriers for the development of a range of new alternative delivery system products. Trade associations are a particularly prevalent form of loosely coupled, (coalesced) structure in the health sector. For example, the American Hospital Association, comprising more than 5,000 member organizations, mounts a sophisticated political and lobbying activity on behalf of its member hospitals. Similarly, there are regional and state hospital associations that base affiliation on a geographical or state community of interests. As states have become increasingly involved in regulatory and control activities, state hospital associations have undertaken aggressive lobbying efforts on behalf of their members.

Quasifirm

The quasifirm is an interorganizational transaction lying between market relationships and ownership arrangements. A quasifirm has been defined as "a loosely coupled, enduring set of interorganizational relationships that are designed to achieve purposes of substantial importance to the viability of participating members."[19(p.13)] Such arrangements possess many of the characteristics of a true firm (shared goals, mutual dependency, task subdivision and specialization, bureaucratic structures, and formal coordinating and control mechanisms), but, critical to their distinction, ownership linkages are absent.

An example of a quasifirm arrangement is an arrangement in which an acute care general hospital, a large multispecialty group practice, a skilled nursing facility, and an insurance carrier collaborate in designing, producing, and marketing a managed care prod-

uct. In such an arrangement, the four organizations can continue to operate independently of one another in accomplishing other, perhaps even mutually exclusive, objectives. However, the collaborative activity may have significant strategic importance to the participating organizations, up to and including their survival.[6] The interdependencies among the participating organizations in this example are managed neither through purely market transactions nor through the bureaucratic mechanisms characteristic of ownership arrangements. Instead, the quasifirm configuration provides a means to accomplish strategic purposes that do not lend themselves to market transactions, and it also permits avoidance of the restrictions and diminution of autonomy and identity that would be associated with acquiring or merging with other interdependent organizations.

Ownership

The final category of voluntary interorganizational transaction for managing interdependencies is ownership. Thus far, most ownership arrangements in the health sector have been voluntary. However, hostile acquisitions and takeovers are possible in this sector of the economy, and more of them may be seen in the future. For now, this form of interorganizational transaction is more appropriately placed in the voluntary category. For example, a particular focal organization might voluntarily participate with other organizations in ownership of a new organizational entity created for some special purpose. (This mechanism may be only a small step beyond the quasifirm described above.) Or it could voluntarily merge with, acquire, or be acquired by another organization with which it is interdependent.

It is not unusual for organizations to create a new entity, sometimes called an umbrella organization, to span, but *not* to replace, the organizations forming it. Starkweather described two important subtypes of the umbrella corporation in regard to hospitals:

> One grants only limited authorities to the new corporation, but in these realms the umbrella corporation's decisions are final. These arrangements often deal with planning or allocation of services among otherwise distinct hospitals. There is usually no central management or central fiscal control. The other subtype grants the umbrella corporation more general and complete authority, usually exercised through unified management, policy, and fiscal control. This type is akin to the parent–subsidiary form found commonly in the business world. This arrangement re-

quires the participating hospitals to turn over all assets to the new corporation, and it in turn assumes their liabilities. Newly developed assets are typically owned by the umbrella corporation.[8](pp.37–38)

An extreme and often very complicated kind of voluntary interorganizational transaction designed to manage interdependence is absorption of or absorption by interdependent others through merger or consolidation. A *consolidation* is a formal combination of two or more organizations into a single new legal entity that has an identity separate from any of the preexisting institutions. A *merger* is a formal combination of two or more institutions into a single new legal entity that retains the identity of one of the preexisting organizations. Both consolidations and mergers, as interorganizational linkage mechanisms, involve an essential restructuring of organizational interdependence. The restructuring can be in several form. It can be a vertical integration where, for example, a nursing home merges with a hospital, the hospital gaining the ability to discharge patients to a less intensive level of care and the nursing home gaining a source of referrals. It can be a horizontal expansion, such as when two hospitals merge, resulting in a different capacity configuration or market. It can also be a diversification, where, for instance, a hospital absorbs a retail pharmacy chain, gaining a new source of revenue.

The most complex of these restructuring schemes is vertical integration. As a general business strategy, vertical integration is "the combination, under a single ownership, of two or more stages of production or distribution (or both) that are usually separate."[20](p.93) In the health sector, vertical integration usually involves "linking together different levels of care and assembling the human resources needed to render that care."[21](p.136) Vertical integration has distinct advantages and disadvantages. Advantages include

- reduced buying and selling costs,
- supply and raw materials assurance,
- improved coordination,
- enhanced technological capabilities, and
- higher entry barriers for competitors.

Disadvantages include

- high capital requirements,
- potential for unbalanced throughput,
- reduced flexibility and increased risk, and
- loss of specialization.[20]

The most important consideration, often sufficient to override the possible disadvantages of vertical integra-

tion, may well be the enhanced competitive position gained through the improved coordination afforded to interdependent organizations linked in this way. But this form of linkage is not suited to all health care organizations. For example, using a single hospital as the focal organization, there are two important aspects of vertical integration,

integration forward into the patient acquisition chain to achieve greater control of health plans and primary care physicians, or integration backward toward control of the continuum of care (long-term care, home health care, and so on). [In Coddington and Moore's view,] opportunities for successful forward integration are limited to a few players who begin with substantial market power. Opportunities for successful backward integration, however, are available to many health care systems in both large and small markets.[22](p.128)

Each ownership form of interorganizational transaction carries with it significant burdens for the participants. Varying degrees of autonomy are sacrificed, and the interdependencies among participating organizations, though bound by ownership, must still be managed if the relationships are to serve their purposes. Achieving effective linkages among the various units of such arrangements is a demanding management task. Adaptation of Porter's approach to developing effective linkages among business units of a diversified corporation suggests several ways of managing the necessary linkages among participants in such organizational configurations:

- *structural features* that cut across unit lines, such as partial centralization and interunit task forces or committees that facilitate communication;
- *management systems* with a cross-unit dimension in areas such as planning, control, incentives, capital budgeting, and management information systems;
- *human resource practices* that facilitate unit cooperation, such as cross-unit job rotation, management forums, and training; and
- *conflict resolution processes* that resolve conflicts and settle disputes among units.[15]

Effective linkages are particularly important and difficult within systems that have different boards for some or all units. The most efficacious mechanism in this situation may well be interlocking the boards to provide a stable structure through which coordinated activity and communication flow can be established and facilitated.

INVOLUNTARY INTERORGANIZATIONAL TRANSACTIONS

Some interdependencies among organizations in the health sector cannot be managed through market transactions or voluntary interorganizational transactions. Most notably, these involve regulatory agencies; however, such interdependencies may also include interactions with fiscal intermediaries and utilization management companies. The strategies outlined in this section are specific to interactions with regulatory bodies, but they may also be applicable in other involuntary interorganizational transactions, in modified form.

Despite all the deregulation rhetoric and even some action in the past decade, organizations in the health sector remain highly regulated. Regulation of provider organizations includes fiscal and utilization controls, controls on facilities and services, human resources, and quality.[23] Similarly, regulation of insurance carriers and their products by the states is extensive.

Regulated organizations bear an obviously interdependent relationship to the organizations that regulate them; but these interdependencies cannot legally be managed through market transactions, which, by definition, involve economic exchanges. Furthermore, the nature of the interdependent relationship between a particular regulated organization and its regulator is hardly suitable for the voluntary types of interorganizational transactions described in the previous section. These involuntary relationships require unique mechanisms for managing interdependence, although the existence of regulation does stimulate certain forms of voluntary interorganizational relationship transactions among regulated organizations. For example, one of the primary reasons for some of the coalescing activi-

---

Despite all the deregulation rhetoric and even some action in the past decade, organizations in the health sector remain highly regulated.

---

ties among organizations that have regulatory agencies in common is to gain a strong hand in dealing with the regulators and their regulations through shared expertise. In any industry, regulation encourages consolidation among the regulated for the purpose of developing counterregulatory expertise and power. However, here we are interested in the mechanisms for managing the interdependence between individual regulated organi-

zations and those organizations that regulate them. Ingenious strategies have been devised; many of them have at times been effective as means of managing this particular form of interdependence. Some of the more common ones have been described by Altman, Greene, and Sapolsky.[24] The synopses of these strategies presented below are adapted from this source.

The litigation strategy

The opportunity to litigate is an important mechanism available to a regulated organization for managing its relationships with regulators. Most regulatory decisions can be appealed in the courts, and the courts are very sensitive to procedural errors and infringements on due process rights. Regulators who overlook requirements for proper notice, public hearings, or the opportunity for a full consideration of issues invite litigation by the regulated. Also, regulators may lack the necessary resources for proper legal representation, or in some cases may have to rely on state legal staffs that are inexpert in health affairs. Another factor that facilitates the litigation strategy is the condition that some of the standards adopted by regulators in some domains are not rigorously substantiated by analysis or fact and thus are vulnerable to judicial scrutiny.

The political intervention strategy

While distasteful to many as a means of managing interrelationships with regulators, cultivation of supportive relationships with executive and legislative branches of government and with state and federal regulatory agencies can be effective protection for regulated organizations against overly enthusiastic or even dutiful regulators. It is no accident that hospitals have routinely placed prominent public officials and politically well-connected private citizens on their governing boards, that physicians are among the most generous political campaign contributors, or that well-connected consultants flourish in and around Washington, D.C., and the states' capitals.

The loaf-and-a-half strategy

This strategy, drawn from the pages of textbooks on negotiating strategy, involves a regulated organization initially seeking more than it expects to get get from the regulator. For example, by enlarging a project for which an organization is seeking a certificate of need approval from a state, the regulated organization gives the regulator the opportunity to play hardball by forcing the scaling back of a project without actually jeopardizing

Some relationships have strategic purposes and some do not; the ability to discern between them is crucial.

its essential elements. A common variation on this strategy is to offer regulators something they want (e.g., a commitment to provide care for indigent patients) in order to obtain approval for the elements of the project that the regulated organization is actually seeking.

The constituency strategy

Regulated organizations that gain the support of a politically powerful constituency are obviously less vulnerable to adverse regulatory decisions than those that do not. The constituency may have a religious, ethnic, geographical, or other basis. Regulated organizations may even be each other's constituents, agreeing to trade regulatory approval opportunities.

Beyond these widely used strategies lie some that are unethical or illegal or that can be used in such ways. While it is not a frequent occurrence, some regulated organizations have misused such strategies.

The data overload strategy

One advantage those in a regulated health care organization may have over their regulators is the ability to assemble and manipulate large volumes of complicated data. Thus, when challenged by a regulatory agency, the regulated organization may choose to flood the agency with technical data that may actually justify its position on a matter subject to regulation or may simply obscure the real issues at hand in an avalanche of paper and printouts.

The open job offer strategy

A well-worn but still potentially effective strategy is to attempt to buy off the regulators with the promise of attractive jobs. U.S. Patent Office examiners often become patent attorneys. A year or two with the Federal Communications Commission provides excellent training for lawyers seeking positions with law firms specializing in communications law. Organizations in the health sector also know this strategy. Regulators, particularly those in state agencies, often go to work for state hospital associations or major hospitals. Usually

these are very legitimate and appropriate transfers of knowledge and experience. However, sometimes they can represent repayment of a "debt" incurred in transactions between the regulator and the regulated.

The deception strategy

Clearly illegal and unethical, deception is possible in relationships between regulated and regulator organizations. The cost and scope of projects can be easily understated. Pertinent data can be fabricated or falsified. Projects can be altered after approval has been granted. The complexity of projects, their long lead times, the turnover of regulatory staff, and the difficulty government agencies have in coordinating their programs can prevent close scrutiny of regulated organizations and encourage cheating.

MANAGING INTERORGANIZATIONAL LINKAGES

Cross-cutting the market, voluntary, and involuntary interorganizational relationship transactions described in this article is the matter of the managerial skills necessary to establish efficacious and efficient linkages with interdependent organizations. These skills include: (1) skill in the discernment of the relative necessity for linkages with interdependent others, and (2) skill in choosing from a menu of possible linking mechanisms those most appropriate for each situation.

As a starting point, managers must realize that interdependencies among organizations are not equally important, nor are the interorganizational relationships developed to manage them. Some relationships have strategic purposes and some do not; the ability to discern between them is crucial. Interorganizational relationships that are relatively more important, in terms of their impact on the financial condition and competitive position of participating organizations, and relatively more *permanent*, if intended to be permanent, can be considered more strategic that those of less importance or those not expected to be permanent.[19] Managers must be more concerned with those relationships that involve a strategic purpose than with those that do not.

In judging importance, managers may find it useful to remember that there are several types of interdependence among organizations: pooled, sequential, or reciprocal.[5] *Pooled interdependence* occurs when organizations are related but do not bear a close connection; they simply contribute separately in some way to a larger whole. For example, a group of geographically dispersed nursing homes owned by a single corporation may be viewed as linked largely in the sense that each contributes to the overall performance of the corporation, but they have very little functional interdependence.

Sequential interdependence occurs when organizations bear a close and sequential connection. For example, the relationship between a health care provider organization and Blue Cross or some other fiscal intermediary is sequential in that the provider organization's cash flow depends upon the intermediary to process reimbursement for care provided to certain patients.

Reciprocal interdependence occurs when organizations bear a close relationship and the interdependence goes in both directions. For example, a vertically integrated health care system with acute care and long-term-care units exhibits reciprocal interdependence. The long-term-care beds are occupied by patients referred from the acute care beds; the acute care organization depends upon the long-term-care organization as a place to discharge certain patients. The acute care unit suffers if the long-term-care unit cannot accept a patient. Conversely, the long-term-care unit suffers if patients are not discharged to it from the acute care unit.

Effective management of interdependence generally is more important as it moves from pooled to sequential to reciprocal forms,[25] and the need for managerial attention to effective linkages also increases. Linkages at sequential or reciprocal levels are relatively more complex, because they involve issues such as the nature of the exchange relationships between participating organizations, which organizations will have the most power, the terms of the resource transactions between them, and how innovations will be developed and diffused between the organizations.[26]

Managers must realize that the choice of optimal linking mechanisms used to manage organizational interdependencies arises from the circumstances of a particular situation. Making a selection from the menu of possible ways to manage interdependencies with other organizations is among the most important and difficult decisions managers face. The decision to continue a straight market transaction when a voluntary interorganizational relationship transaction could cement far greater benefits for his or her organization can be a costly mistake for a manager. Conversely, a decision to manage an interdependency through a complex ownership strategy that sacrifices important and valuable legal and functional autonomies, when a simple market transaction would suffice, may be an even more costly mistake. Hence, great care must be exercised in choosing an option and implementing it for linkage with interdependent organizations in the health sector.

In making these choices, it must be remembered that interorganizational linkages are not achieved without costs. These costs must bear directly on the decisions about which options to choose. The obvious costs are time, personnel, and money needed to support the various linkage mechanisms. There is also the potential loss of some degree of autonomy. The less obvious but very important costs include what Porter has termed the "cost of compromise" and the "cost of inflexibility."[15]

The cost of compromise arises because effective linking across organizational boundaries may require that an activity be performed in a consistent way that may not be optimal for individual participants in the interorganizational relationship. From the manager's perspective, the cost of compromise can be reduced if an activity is designed for sharing. For example, two merger participants may find that using a new management information system designed to accommodate the needs of the new organization is better than using either or both of the systems previously used by the merging organizations. The cost of inflexibility is not an ongoing cost of interorganizational linkage efforts, but one that arises with the need for flexibility, usually in the form of difficulty in responding to a competitor's move or to a new market opportunity. In dealing with interorganizational interdependencies, organizations became increasingly complex and, consequently, inflexible. Managers faced with these costs must weigh them against the benefits to be gained from interorganizational linkages.

The future direction of organizations in the health sector is toward even more complex and pervasive interorganizational linkages. Therefore, it may well be that the skills of discerning the necessity for linkage with interdependent others and choosing the most appropriate from an expanding menu of linkage mechanisms are among the most valuable skills that health care managers can possess or cultivate.

REFERENCES

1. Freeman, R.E. *Strategic Management: A Stakeholder Approach.* New York: Ballinger, 1984.
2. Starkweather, D.B., and Cook, K.S. "Organization–Environment Relations." In *Health Care*

Management: A Text in Organization Theory and Behavior, edited by S.M. Shortell and A.D. Kaluzny. 2d ed. New York: Wiley, 1988.

3. Rubin, J., and Brown, B. *The Social Psychology of Bargaining and Negotiation.* New York: Academic Press, 1975.

4. Greenberger, D., et al. "Perception, Motivation, and Negotiation." In *Health Care Management: A Text in Organization Theory and Behavior,* edited by S.M. Shortell and A.D. Kaluzny. 2d ed. New York: Wiley, 1988.

5. Thompson, J.D. *Organizations in Action.* New York: McGraw-Hill, 1967.

6. Pointer, D.D., Begun, J.W., and Luke, R.D. "Managing Interorganizational Dependencies in the New Health Care Marketplace." *Hospital & Health Services Administration* 33 (1988): 167–77.

7. Eccles, R.G. "The Quasi-Firm in the Construction Industry." *Journal of Economic Behavior and Organization* 2 (1981): 335–57.

8. Starkweather, D.B. *Hospital Mergers in the Making.* Ann Arbor, Mich.: Health Administration Press, 1981.

9. Longest, B.B., Jr., and Klingensmith, J.M. "Coordination and Communication." In *Health Care Management: A Text in Organization Theory and Behavior,* edited by S.M. Shortell and A.D. Kaluzny. 2d ed. New York: Wiley, 1988.

10. Glassman, R.B. "Persistence and Loose Coupling in Living Systems." *Behavioral Science* 18, no. 2 (1973): 83–98.

11. Weick, K. "Educational Organizations as Loosely Coupled Systems." *Administrative Science Quarterly* 21, no. 1 (1976): 1–19.

12. Luke, R.D., and Kurowski, B. "Strategic Management." In *Health Care Management: A Text in Organization Theory and Behavior,* edited by S.M. Shortell and A.D. Kaluzny. New York: Wiley, 1983.

13. Shirely, R.C. "Limiting the Scope of Strategy: A Decision Based Approach." *Academy of Management Review* 7 (1982): 262–68.

14. Astley, W.G., and Fombrum, C. "Collective Strategy: The Social Ecology of Organizational Environments." *Academy of Management Review* 8 (1983): 576–87.

15. Porter, M.C. *Competitive Advantage: Creating and Sustaining Superior Performance.* New York: Free Press, 1985.

16. Pennings, J.M. "Strategically Interdependent Organizations." In *Handbook of Organizational Design,* edited by P.C. Nystrom and W.H. Starbuck, vol. 1, 433–55. New York: Oxford University Press, 1981.

17. Pfeffer, J., and Salanick, G.R. *The External Control of Organizations: A Resource Dependence Perspective.* New York: Harper & Row, 1978.

18. Shortell, S.M. "Public Policy and Managerial Implications." In *Hospital-Physician Joint Ventures,* edited by S.M. Shortell, T.M. Wickizer, and J.R.C. Wheeler. Ann Arbor, Mich: Health Administration Press, 1984.

19. Luke, R.D., Begun, J.W., and Pointer, D.D. "Quasi Firms: Strategic Interorganizational Forms in the Health Care Industry." *The Academy of Management Review* 14, no. 1 (1989): 9–19.

20. Buzzell, R.D. "Is Vertical Integration Profitable?" *Harvard Business Review* 61, no. 1 (1983): 92–102.

21. Goldsmith, J.C. *Can Hospitals Survive? The New Competitive Health Care Market.* Homewood, Ill.: Dow Jones-Irwin, 1981.

22. Coddington, D.C., and Moore, K.D. *Market-Driven Strategies in Health Care.* San Francisco: Jossey-Bass, 1987.

23. Kinzer, D.M. "Our Realistic Options in Health Regulation." *Frontiers of Health Services Management* 5, no. 1 (1988): 3–43.

24. Adapted with permission from Altman, D., Greene, R., and Sapolsky, H.M. *Health Planning and Regulation: The Decision-Making Process.* Ann Arbor, Mich.: Association of University Programs in Health Administration Press, 1981.

25. Bolman, L.G., and Deal, T.E. *Modern Approaches to Understanding and Managing Organizations.* San Francisco: Jossey-Bass, 1984.

26. Aldrich, H.E., and Whetton, D.A. "Organization-sets, Action-sets, and Networking: Making the Most of Simplicity." In *Handbook of Organizational Design,* edited by P.C. Nystrom and W.H. Starbuck, vol. 1, 385–408. New York: Oxford University Press, 1981.

APPENDIX

CATEGORIES OF LINKAGE MECHANISMS IN THE HEALTH SECTOR

MARKET TRANSACTIONS

Many, but not all, interdependent relationships stem from the necessity for a focal organization to enter economic exchanges with other organizations to obtain resources needed to conduct its affairs or a market for its outputs. These exchanges are market transactions. They, like market exchanges among all organizations in market economies, are governed by certain basic exchange principles. These principles hold that organizations engaging in exchange transactions seek exchanges that are mutually beneficial or rewarding. Furthermore, they hold that the organizations are calculative; that is, they make assessments of both relative rewards and costs. Relationships that produce greater utility by going beyond market transactions, as well as those that cannot be achieved through market transactions, are candidates for management through voluntary or involuntary interorganizational relationship transactions.

VOLUNTARY INTERORGANIZATIONAL RELATIONSHIP TRANSACTIONS

As relationships with other interdependent organizations become more important and sustained, there may be advantages to extending the relationship beyond a straightforward market transaction. In these situations, interdependent organizations can voluntarily seek to manage their interdependence through a variety of interorganizational relationship transactions. The voluntary dimension of these transactions is their most important distinguishing feature. It implies that the participating organizations have other choices as to how they manage their interdependence. They can simply continue to handle it through market transactions, they can choose to shift the interdependence to other organizations that are better able to meet their requirements or more amenable to meeting them, or they can seek to become independent of other organizations along a particular dimension.

INVOLUNTARY INTERORGANIZATIONAL RELATIONSHIP TRANSACTIONS

This class of mechanisms is a unique function of the necessity to interact with certain organizations involuntarily. Some relationships with interdependent others are precluded from market transactions, and the choice of interorganizational relationship transaction is limited or fixed by the interdependent other. These include relationships with government regulatory agencies, utilization management companies, or intermediaries, such as Blue Cross, in their roles as fiscal intermediaries for Medicare reimbursement.

Vertical integration strategies: More promising than diversification

Wende L. Fox

Investment in businesses outside of traditional hospital services can help providers withstand the ill effects of today's business climate. However, the typical diversification approach must be discarded. This article describes a different approach that has been used successfully in other industries— vertical integration.

The dire predictions are finally coming true. Average net operating margins for health care providers are now nearly zero after eroding gradually over the past four years: The traditional health care business is just breaking even today (see Figure 1).

The industry anticipated this profit decline in the early 1980s. A popular response was to invest in new, unrelated businesses that seemed to have brighter financial prospects than inpatient care, a tactic called "diversification strategy." Parent-holding corporations were created and boards of trustees recruited to spearhead this effort. Some of the industry's most talented financial, planning, and ancillary executives became dedicated to parent activities, encouraged that their careers were expanding beyond "just running a hospital." The holding companies invested in a wide range of health-related businesses—home health care, retail pharmacies, HMOs, helicopters for transporting trauma cases, nursing homes, urgent care centers, fitness centers, and others. The primary selection criterion seemed to be the fact that other providers were investing in a particular business segment. Unfortunately, the new businesses have been tough to manage, competition has been fierce, and break-even horizons have been longer than expected.

The result? Businesses that were not involved in inpatient care and that were developed under the diversification banner have not substantially contributed to health care corporate portfolios. Many new businesses never became substantial or profitable. In fact, the strategy has frequently backfired, particularly among smaller institutions, and the traditional business has been forced to subsidize the diversification venture. Needless to say, enthusiasm for provider diversification strategies dwindled by the mid-1980s.

The recent strategic thrust has been to strengthen the traditional business—a "back to basics" approach. An outgrowth of this traditional-business focus is the regional system, created by linking the assets of several geographically dispersed institutions. The three objectives of this strategy are (1) to use the combined strength of the linked institutions to create regional clinical "centers of excellence"; (2) to redesign operations to reduce costs; and (3) to offer broad geographic coverage

---

Wende L. Fox, *B.A., M.B.A., is a principal with the management consulting firm Booz, Allen & Hamilton. She specializes in the health care industry and has developed a concentration in strategic planning assignments for health care providers.*

FIGURE 1

TRENDS IN SOURCE OF NET MARGIN FOR ALL HOSPITALS

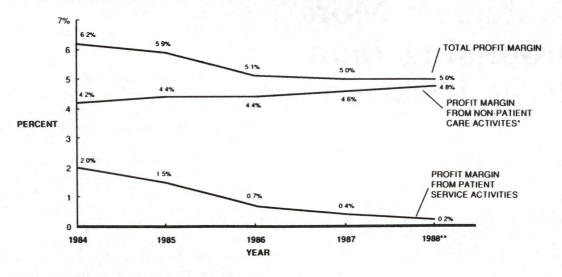

* Includes income from investments, contributions and diversified businesses
** Based on results for the first three quarters
Source *Economic Trends,* the Hospital Research and Educational Trust of the American Hospital Association, AHA Panel Survey

as a means of securing employer or insurance contractors. It is still true, however, that the systems are competing in a mature industry, a fact that is causing increasingly lackluster operating margins. As a result, renewed interest is starting to show in investments outside of traditional hospital services. Retirement centers suddenly look interesting.

There are two critical distinctions between vertical integration and the industry's diversification strategies of the early 1980s. First, diversification implies an explicit move away from a declining core business. In contrast, the whole objective of vertical integration is to support the core business. In fact, vertical integration does not create value in and of itself. Its value consists of the gains that it permits management to realize in the base business. Second, successful vertical integration need not involve complete ownership of a new business. Partnerships, joint ventures, and even contractual arrangements can often yield the same result.

This article describes the vertical integration concept, explores its benefits for the health care industry and suggests an approach to successful strategy development.

THE CONCEPT OF VERTICAL INTEGRATION

This sounds all too familiar, as if the same problematic cycle is in the midst of being repeated. Before the industry risks reliving the same disappointing outcome, Booz, Allen & Hamilton suggests that senior management challenge the whole notion of diversification. Diversification focuses on the attractiveness of the new business, not on its strategic fit with or impact on the core hospital business. The whole idea is to move away from and reduce dependency on the care business. In fact, new venture performance is measured independently of core business performance. There are two basic problems with this approach: It has not worked in any other industry that has been studied and, worse, it actually creates perverse incentives.

Experiences in other industries

In 1986, Booz, Allen & Hamilton cosponsored a review of 218 randomly selected public acquisitions made by Fortune 500 companies to determine the value of investments in new businesses. Changes in shareholder value were compared with the strategic fit between the acquiring company (the bidder) and the purchased company (the target).

Four categories were created to classify degree of strategic fit:

1. Unrelated—there was no fit between the bidder and the target.
2. Opportunity-intensive—the target gave the bidder access to new markets and new customers for existing products.
3. Resource-intensive—the target gave the bidder new resources and products that could be applied to existing markets and customers.
4. Identical—the target and the bidder had very similar access to customers or markets and resources.

The results show that, on average, acquisitions of businesses with no strategic fit decreased shareholder value (see Figure 2). Among those with strategic fit, the acquisitions that give existing products access to new markets and customers—that is, they provided new distribution channels—created the most shareholder value. The same holds true in health care. Consider how many health care organizations lost money in health-related businesses that did not materially benefit from hospital distribution channels or products: fitness centers, insurance, and retail pharmacies, to name just a few.

FIGURE 2

EFFECT OF TYPE OF FIT ON VALUE CREATED (218 MERGERS, 1962 TO 1983)

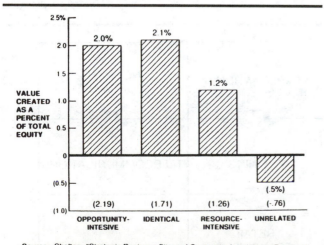

Source: Shelton, "Strategic Business Fits and Corporate Acquisition: Empirical Evidence," 1986

Perverse incentives

In diversification, parent companies select new ventures if they think the businesses can be managed profitably on a stand-alone basis. This is a perverse incentive because the real goal is to contribute to the success of the enterprise as a whole, using new ventures to support the core business of acute inpatient care. Consider some examples.

One system's physician practice-management venture is just reaching the point where it's breaking even: Support for further investment is mixed. However, viewing physician practice-management as a stand-alone business is shortsighted. The admissions generated by physicians recruited into the practice

---

Booz, Allen & Hamilton suggests taking a new approach when selecting, structuring, and measuring the performance of new business ventures.

---

management program contribute more than $4 million in incremental revenue to the acute care business. Practice volume gains for affiliated practice contribute an additional $2 million. Even assuming marginal costs of 5%, the program is generating approximately $3 million in incremental income. Thus, to cut the program because it is not independently profitable would hurt the acute care business.

Another common venture is an insurance product such as a health maintenance organization (HMO). An HMO purchases hospital services at a discount in order to be competitive; however, the first customers are often employers whose employees already use the hospital. In addition, the profit margin for the insurance product—if it even exists—is often lower than the discount rate the HMO gives to the hospital.

Many parent corporations provide financial, legal, consulting, or other management services to other hospitals—sometimes even competitors—for cost plus a modest markup. On paper, the management services business appears to be profitable. However, services are time-consuming for the organization's most talented senior executives, who should instead be focused on the tough issues of the core business.

Booz, Allen & Hamilton suggests taking a new approach when selecting, structuring, and measuring the performance of new business ventures. This approach, which has been used successfully in other industries, is called vertical integration.

Vertical integration is an approach that other maturing industries have used to secure and retain customers for the traditional business (see Figure 3). There are two types of vertical integration: "upstream" and "downstream." Upstream vertical integration entails securing control over raw materials or supplies that differentiate the core business product. Such control helps to ensure availability, establish a cost advantage, regulate quality, and gain exclusive access to those differentiating supplies. For example,

- IBM's contract with Microsoft locks in access to a superior operating system, and IBM's controlling interest in Intel ensures access to semiconductors.
- Automobile manufacturers have begun to invest in companies with expertise in the integrated electronics that can improve automobile performance.

Downstream vertical integration entails securing control over distribution channels that provide advantageous access to customers. The new distribution option not only helps to differentiate the commodity but also keeps the enterprise aware of customers' changing needs and purchase criteria. For example:

- Agricultural cooperatives have invested in the packaging and distribution of products made primarily from a single crop (e.g., the cranberry cooperative's development of Ocean Spray and the orange growers' licensing of Sunkist).
- Oil-exporting countries own retail chains of gas stations in oil-importing countries in an effort to lock up demand for crude oil.
- Muffler manufacturers have created specialty retail outlets to distribute their products. The outlets feature service and convenience (e.g., Midas, Speedy, Carx).

The health care industry exhibits some of the characteristics that provided opportunities for successful vertical integration in other maturing industries. First, certain resources and supplies that are critical to delivering services are scarce (e.g., RNs, organs for transplant, blood), and many are very expensive (e.g., implants, patented pharmaceuticals). This situation creates an opportunity for upstream vertical integration that either creates a barrier to competition or secures margins. Second, the decision on which hospital should be used, which used to be the sole responsibility of physicians, is now being shared by patients, employers, and insurers. This creates an opportunity for downstream vertical integration of new distribution channels that serve the need of these new "customers."

In health care, an academic medical center's participation in the commercialization of its basic research capabilities (such as Johns Hopkins' Dome Corporation) is an example of upstream vertical integration.

FIGURE 3

INDUSTRY EXAMPLES

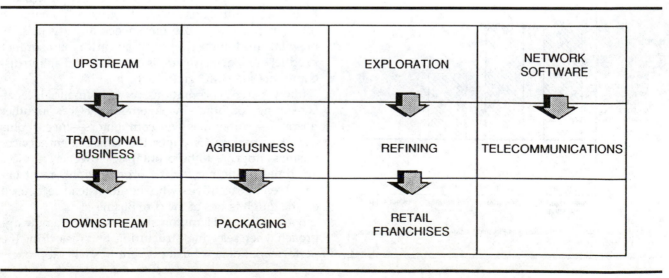

FIGURE 4

THE RELATIONSHIP OF VERTICAL INTEGRATION AND HORIZONTAL INTEGRATION

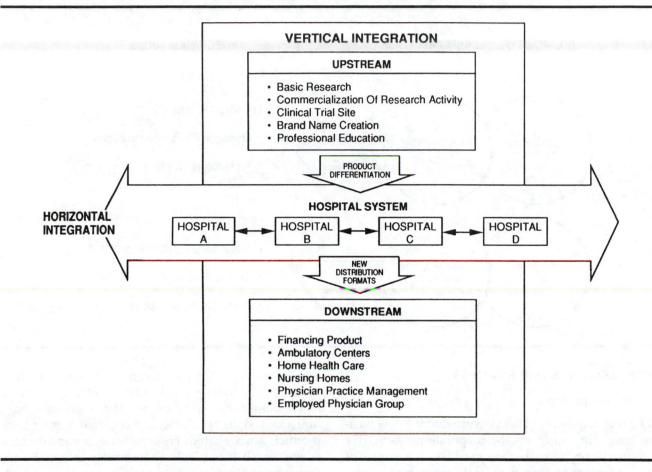

Another example is a hospital's participation in clinical trials for a new drug or medical product. These initiatives allow health care organizations to be the first or one of the first providers of a new clinical technology.

Examples of downstream vertical integration along distribution channels in health care include off-site ambulatory center development, primary care physician sponsorship, physician practice management, and financing product development.

Vertical integration, whether upstream or downstream, can also bolster the current strategy of creating regional systems, which is a form of "horizontal integration." Such systems link the inpatient assets of several hospitals to gain geographic advantage. A framework for thinking about how vertical and horizontal integration relate to each other is illustrated in Figure 4.

The specific vertical integration pursuits selected will depend on the support needs of the acute care business (see Figure 5). For example, an academic medical center's goal of becoming a regional cancer center might lead to the creation of off-site diagnostic centers, through joint ventures with oncologists or local community hospitals as well as through arrangements with pharmaceutical firms for clinical trials of new chemotherapy agents. On the other hand, a community hospital might focus its efforts on developing a distribution network of managed physician practices and proximate ambulatory care outlets.

The key, of course, is to select new business pursuits that can contribute to core business performance. These activities must then be managed and evaluated in a way that permits them to realize their potential contribution. There are seven requirements for developing a vertical integration strategy that meets these objectives.

FIGURE 5

INFLUENCE OF SUPPORT NEEDS ON SELECTION OF VERTICAL INTEGRATION PURSUITS

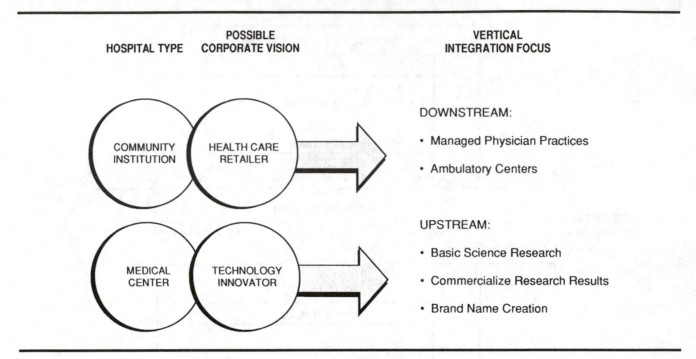

REQUIREMENTS FOR SUCCESS

Support the mission

The first requirement is to ensure that the new business materially supports the corporate mission. This alignment is necessary both to justify the investment of top management talent, time, and corporate resources and to sustain support through difficult times, such as an unprofitable startup or difficult negotiations.

To fulfill this requirement, a hospital needs to develop a clear and specific mission statement that is based on its individual strengths. In years past, hospitals' mission statements were virtually identical. The vertical integration strategy should reinforce these strengths. By following this approach, senior executives will be able to resist temptations that plague the health care industry: to play "keep up with the Joneses," or to select a new business that talented middle or senior management members are personally interested in running.

Link to and leverage strengths

Second, it is important to pursue only opportunities that link to and leverage the existing strengths of the core business. Otherwise, the new venture has little hope of establishing a competitive advantage in its market. Linkage exists when such things as technology, functional skills, customer access, management, or products can be shared across both the core and the new businesses. It is particularly important in health care that current distribution channels be powerful enough to direct current customers to the new services. Even when acquisition is involved, this correlation is important. Ideally, the acquired–developed enterprise will be more successful because of what the hospital brings to it.

Market financial evaluation

The third requirement is to conduct a rigorous market and financial evaluation of any proposed vertical integration pursuit to make certain that it is likely to support the base business materially. Common errors can be avoided by applying the following criteria:

- The basis for demand assumptions should include qualitative as well as quantitative analysis. That is, the concept should be market-tested with potential customers or partners.

- Bold steps must be taken. The tendency in the risk-averse hospital environment is to test the waters by making small investments. Often the result is that the new venture is undercapitalized and does not stand a chance of contributing materially to the enterprise.
- Financial operating projections must be realistic. This seems almost too obvious to state. However, champions of the strategy often underestimate investment needs and expenses, to the detriment of the project.

Sharing the risk

The fourth requirement is to find a way to share the risk of vertical integration with outside experts. The vertical integration objective of controlling resources, supplies, or distribution channels can often be realized through partnership or contractual relationships. Unfortunately, the health care industry has been biased toward internal development and complete ownership of new businesses, strategies that tie up capital and expose the sponsor to all of the risks of the new undertaking.

Other industries have used distribution partnerships to unite the complementary skills and resources of two or more parties in a way that provides the most attractive product or service to the customer without overexposing the sponsors. McDonald's, for example, gives its franchisees a national brand name, real estate development, and operations start-up expertise. Its franchisees, in turn, provide familiarity with local markets and day-to-day management of perishable product assembly. Another example is Giorgio Perfume. Giorgio provides brand name and product manufacturing. Upscale retailers provide local reputation, sales force, and inventory management. Upscale magazines provide access to target customers. In all cases, the manufacturer's or sponsor's partner provides local access.

The management structure should be tailored to the needs of the new business.

Implementation of distribution arrangements is certainly more complex for health care providers than for other industries. First and foremost, a customer's primary initial contacts are with private physicians, who have traditionally been independent agents. As such, physicians have few obligations or incentives to refer exclusively to one provider. Furthermore, there are legal problems with many of the schemes that have been conceived to create such incentives. The growth of managed-care insurance products creates a second, equally independent initial contact for customers. In addition, many employers are beginning to direct employees' health care purchases. Thus providers should consider multiple partners when trying to establish controlled distribution channels.

Management structure

Fifth, the management structure should be tailored to the needs of the new business. It should be based on the operating culture and types of talent required for the new business, and it should reflect the degree of coordination necessary for core business activities. Management expertise required for core and new businesses are often different; they can even be opposite. Thus management may need to be recruited from outside the core industry. However, the degree of interdependency between the new business and the core business often makes it unhealthy for these new managers to be separated from the core business. In this case, a shell parent corporation may exist for legal purposes, but management and governance are consolidated.

Customer needs

The sixth requirement is to ensure that vertical integration strategies keep up with customer needs. A strategy is useful only to the extent that it meaningfully differentiates the core "commodity" in the eyes of the customer. As medical treatments, technology, and the preferred methods of purchase change over time, so must the vertical integration vehicles employed.

Measurement

The seventh and final requirement for successful vertical integration is to measure new businesses based on their value to the enterprise as a whole, rather than on their profitability as stand-alone entities. Of course, this value must outweigh both the direct and indirect costs, including the diversion of existing senior management time and attention from the tough issues of the core business. So that management can periodically evaluate whether the venture will be maintained or divested, return on investment targets should be specific, and performance criteria should be enforced.

If the expectations are not met, management can adjust the partnership or contractual arrangements or divest the venture. Because casualties are to be expected even among ventures that are developed as part of a sound strategy, hospitals must be willing to divest. Nonfinancial justifications for maintaining a failed venture, such as enhanced community image, must be rejected.

A RATIONAL APPROACH TO VERTICAL INTEGRATION

When developing a vertical integration strategy, attention must be given to each of the seven success requirements just described—that is, alignment with the corporate mission, linkage and leverage of existing strengths, rigorous evaluation of market and financial potential, securing outside expertise as needed, establishing an appropriate management structure, keeping up with customers, and implementing meaningful criteria of success. A four-step approach is recommended.

Portfolio analysis

A vertical integration strategy begins with a thorough evaluation of any noncore businesses that are currently in the enterprise's portfolio. This is a useful first step to ensure that the often difficult decision to divest unsuccessful ventures is made at the same time when new business pursuits are being considered. On the other hand, some currently unprofitable businesses may turn out to be strategically appropriate entities that need operational restructuring. Information gained during this process about "lessons learned" can help to plot a more successful course.

Prospect identification

The second step is to identify businesses to be considered for a major integration undertaking. This list would be the result of a careful review of the core enterprise's strategic direction, combined with an understanding of the regional market's current and evolving supply and distribution channels.

Success potential

The third step is a careful evaluation of the potential for successfully entering each business in light of market and competitive considerations. Critical to this step is a realistic assessment of what is required in order to succeed. The organization must determine whether it really could succeed in this new venture, either alone or with a partner.

Business plan

The last step is the development of a vertical integration business plan that combines nonacute businesses retained from the current portfolio, divestiture plans, and new ventures. It should describe a clear procedure for developing and managing these nonacute businesses, including determination of relationships with outside parties; the types of new talent required; the roles, responsibilities, and authority of senior executives; corporate structures; and integrated management and governance processes. In addition, the plan should serve as an implementation road map that establishes work steps, assigns responsibilities, and sets time targets. Lastly, the plan should set targets for growth and profitability and include criteria by which to evaluate periodically whether the business will be maintained or divested.

This top-to-bottom approach will ensure that vertical integration strategies support broad corporate objectives. Meticulous venture selection and attractiveness analysis guarantee that ventures will have at least a reasonable likelihood of success.

• • •

In the future, the attitude toward participation in health care businesses outside the core enterprise will be one of focus and control. Providers will make fewer but larger commitments in new areas. They will aim to control and not just participate. Providers will manage and measure each business with the goal of maximizing the whole enterprise's performance. Almost as a necessary consequence, current small or unprofitable efforts outside the core business will be divested. Even successful ventures that are not compatible with corporate missions will be sold.

Providers who take the risk of vertical integration will withstand many of the ills of a commodity business. Vertical integration can help providers to have more control over their futures and brighter financial prospects.

Corporate diversification: Expectations and outcomes

Jan P. Clement

A review of the research concerning the diversification experience of firms in other industries shows that expectations of higher profit rates and lower risk are not entirely realistic. However, there are many ways in which the probability of financially successful diversification may be increased.

Health Care Manage Rev, 1988, 13(2), 7–13
© 1988 Aspen Publishers, Inc.

Business strategy is perceived by many health care managers as crucial to the survival of their organizations. Strategy, which is a proactive plan, should change with significant environmental changes. Health care organizations have recently responded to major transformations in reimbursement and competition by integrating horizontally, reducing costs, integrating vertically, entering joint ventures, or diversifying the service or product mix of the institution. Lately, the horizontal integration strategy, which dominated health care during the 1970s, appears to be waning in popularity. One of the more popular replacement strategies is diversification.

By adopting a strategy of diversification, health care organizations hope to realize one or more of several purported benefits. Diversification may be beneficial if it allows a firm to escape a declining industry or over-dependence on a single market, move into more profitable businesses, avoid business cycles by increasing the number of revenue sources, realize economies of scope, or lower debt financing costs. When these benefits are achieved, lower costs or higher revenues, which increase profits, or less variability of costs and revenues, which lowers total risk, may also be expected. Although diversification may not be undertaken solely for financial reasons, actually achieving these two financial expectations may ensure the organization's continued ability to provide services.

As yet, it is difficult to tell whether these expectations are realized in actual financial outcomes of health care organizations. Since diversification is a relatively recent phenomenon in health care, there has been little research to evaluate its profit and risk consequences. Instead, the health care literature consists primarily of anecdotes and selective references to other industries. This incomplete picture cannot provide adequate guidance for an industry exceedingly interested in diversifying.

As a result, it is instructive for managers deliberating diversification moves to consider the financial outcomes of diversification reported for large for-profit industrial and consumer products firms. The effects have been evaluated more systematically and extensively among these firms. In addition, the profit outcomes should be especially evident among these firms

Jan P. Clement, *Ph.D., is an Assistant Professor in the Department of Health Services Management and Policy at the University of Michigan, Ann Arbor, where she teaches accounting and finance.*

because they must at least approximate profit maximization. Finally, their experience is particularly interesting because diversification is more prevalent now and has been used longer by managers of for-profit firms. Although health care firms are currently much less diversified than most of the for-profit firms studied and diversification itself is not well defined, the experience of for-profit firms engaged in various levels and types of diversification can help health care managers decide whether to diversify, as well as aiding them in formulating realistic expectations and resource allocation strategies.

In this article, the evidence on the profit and risk effects of diversification for for-profit firms and business units as reported in the empirical literature is used to derive five lessons for health care managers. The review of literature from three academic areas—strategy, industrial organization economics, and finance— is comprehensive and focuses on empirical testing rather than theories or unsupported promises. In contrast to the previous selective reviews contained in the health care literature, the breadth of the current review permits the various findings to be linked; in addition, results that by themselves may be somewhat misleading can be examined in the context of other research findings.

The literature summary is organized by the five lessons drawn from the empirical research. Two lessons concern the profit and risk effects of diversification; three concern variables that managers can evaluate or influence to increase the chances of financially successful diversification.

PROFIT AND RISK OUTCOMES

Two lessons regarding the profit and risk outcomes of diversification can be derived from the literature. First, diversification does not guarantee higher profitability. Second, diversification does not reduce total risk.

Profitability

Research findings concerning the profit effect of diversification are mixed. In studies in which diversification is the only independent variable, the profit rate outcome depends on how diversification is measured. In general, researchers do not report a positive relationship between measures that quantify the extent of diversification and the firm's accounting profitability. This is true whether three quantitative measures of diversification are evaluated[1] or whether one measure

is evaluated.[2] The result is consistent over two widely separated study periods (1947-1957 and 1975-1977).

The same is true when diversification is defined in terms of a conglomerate firm, a highly diversified firm usually operating in several industries. For example, Weston and Mansinghka[3] compared accounting profit rates of conglomerate and nonconglomerate firms in 1968 and found no significant differences in four profit rates. In similar studies, Melicher and Rush[4] found no profit rate differences from 1966-1971 and Reid[5] found no differences in 1969. When Holzmann, Copeland, and Hayya[6] averaged accounting performance data for 20 years (1951-1970), they found conglomerates had significantly lower profit rates than nonconglomerates.

Similar results are obtained when finance researchers examine the returns to shareholders from conglomerate firms. Shareholder measures are especially interesting because they reflect the firm's long-term prospects by incorporating all publicly available information about a firm. Accounting return rates, on the other hand, are shorter-term measures of profitability that constitute one signal of the firm's prospects.

Three studies are representative of the research concerning shareholder returns. Mason and Goudzwaard[7] report that from 1962 through 1967, the accumulated stockholder wealth performance of 22 conglomerate firms was inferior to the performance of 22 simulated portfolios mirroring the asset structures of the firms. The result is consistent for three portfolio strategies— self-management, outside management (mutual funds), and buy and hold—even after allowing for transactions costs and taxes. Comparisons by Melicher and Rush[8] of conglomerates and nonconglomerates on continuously compounded monthly stock returns and excess returns (above those required to compensate the shareholder for systematic risk) for 1966 through 1971 produce no statistically significant differences. Finally, Beattie[9] found no excess returns in his case study of conglomerates whose degree of diversification was large and whose industry entry was rapid.

In contrast, when diversification is the only variable investigated for its effect on the firm's profit rate and when diversification is measured with Rumelt's[10,11] classifications, some types of diversification are associated with higher firm accounting profit rates than others. Unlike other measures of diversification, Rumelt's nine-category classification scheme examines both the firm's commitment to diversification and the way new activities relate to existing ones. Both Rumelt[12,13] and Montgomery,[14] in similar studies of over 100 large firms, report superior performance by constrained diversified firms, that is, those firms building on a single perceived strength. The study periods span over 25 years (1951-1969 and 1955-1974, and 1975-1977, respectively).

The superiority of the related type of diversification (i.e., diversification that directly uses the firm's existing assets and skills) is not supported, however, when the related-unrelated dichotomous diversification classification is investigated. Palepu[15] discovered no cross-sectional accounting profit rate differences between related and unrelated diversified firms from 1973 through 1979. From a cross-sectional investigation of risk-adjusted shareholder returns, Michel and Shaked[16] conclude that shareholders of unrelated diversified firms earned significantly higher risk-adjusted returns from January 1, 1976, through December 31, 1980, than those of related diversified firms. In sum, investors in their sample of large unrelated diversified firms were more than adequately compensated for their risk bearing.

Diversification does not guarantee higher profits for large for-profit firms.

The primary lesson from this evidence is that diversification does not guarantee higher profits for large for-profit firms. It is difficult, however, to draw many other conclusions because of the diverse findings and measures of diversification and return, and because of the small sample sizes of some of the studies (e.g., Beattie, and Michel and Shaked). Nevertheless, based on the results from research using the Rumelt diversification measure, which is best at differentiating types of diversification, it is likely that carefully selected projects, such as those that build on one central strength of the firm, may be more profitable than other types. Higher profitability results from generating fewer new expenses or more revenues than other diversifying investment projects.

Risk

The risk outcomes of diversification for large for-profit firms are clearer than the profitability outcomes. Contrary to the expectation of lower risk, higher total (the variance or standard deviation of return rates) and

systematic (the covariance of the return rate with the return rate on a market index) shareholder risks are generally associated with corporate diversification. Four studies are most representative of research in this area. All evaluate a single independent variable, diversification. Because risk determined from accounting profit rates has rarely been evaluated for its association with corporate diversification, that relationship is not discussed here.

Two of the shareholder risk studies are cross-sectional and two examine risk as firms become more diversified over time. Both cross-sectional studies report that higher systematic risk is associated with conglomerates than with nonconglomerates, but the authors disagree on total risk differences. Weston, Smith, and Shrieves[17] report that the mean systematic risk (beta) of conglomerates was twice as high as that of a random sample of mutual funds from 1960-1969. From 1966 through 1971, and during two subperiods, betas were significantly higher for Melicher and Rush's[18] conglomerates than for nonconglomerates. Similarly, Weston, Smith, and Shrieves report significantly higher total risk for conglomerates than for mutual funds. Melicher and Rush, however, note no significant differences in total risk between their conglomerate and nonconglomerate samples.

Similar results were obtained longitudinally by Beattie[19] and Joehnk and Neilsen.[20] They report increased systematic risk as firms become more diversified over time.

In sum, the majority of the evidence shows that both systematic and total risk are higher for diversified firms than for nondiversified firms. Thus, the lesson is that diversification does not decrease risk; countercyclical businesses that could lower the overall risk of the firm are hard to find.

SUCCESSFUL DIVERSIFICATION

The research summarized above, which provides differing evidence on whether there is a relationship between diversification and the firm's accounting profit rates or shareholder return rates, as well as evidence of a zero or positive association between diversification and risk, is noteworthy because it emphasizes that diversification is not the panacea that its popularity among some health care managers and consultants seems to imply. Although diversification itself is not sufficient to improve financial outcomes, there are other variables identified in some research that may be important to the success of diversification projects. By influencing or explicitly evaluating these variables, managers can increase the likelihood of realizing financial benefits from diversifying investments. Findings concerning these variables provide three more lessons for health care managers. Because the majority of the research concerns accounting profit rate effects, discussion focuses there.

Some types of diversification may be better

Evidence derived from applying Rumelt's refined diversification typology indicates that managers can transfer some skills from business to business or can share assets among businesses as long as the businesses build on a single identifiable strength. Since the other quantitative and categorical diversification measures are not so finely partitioned, they are unable to capture this important characteristic of some diversification activities. Therefore, it is reasonable at this point to conclude that some types of related diversification, namely constrained, result in better firm performance as measured by accounting profit rates.

Financial benefits from diversification may take time

Managers must be patient. Diversifying investments usually take time to yield financial benefits. The role of the length of time that a firm has been diversified is not obvious. Nonetheless, four studies supply some evidence on this variable's importance. Rumelt's[21] findings that constrained diversified firms outperform other firms on accounting profit rates are based on diversification classifications of his sample firms after examining their activities over the prior decade. The firm's activities were not recently adopted. Second, Palepu[22] reports superior profit rate growth (although not cross-sectional profit rates) for related versus unrelated diversified firms. Third, Weston, and Mansinghka[23] record significantly lower accounting profit rates for conglomerate firms in 1958. However, by 1968, the conglomerates had caught up with other firms. Fourth, Reid[24] replicated the Weston and Mansinghka study for 1960-1969. He found significantly lower performance by conglomerate firms in 1960, and conglomerate improvement on three of four profit rate measures by 1969. Taken together, these research findings provide some evidence that time improves the performance of both related and unrelated diversifying investments, and does so more for related investments.

Biggadike's[25] research on 68 diversifying new businesses launched by Fortune 200 firms in the late 1960s and early 1970s underscores the importance of time for accounting profit rate performance. During the first four years of operation, almost all the new businesses experienced negative return on investment and cash flow-investment ratios. There was some improvement from the first two to the second two years. Biggadike attributes that to sales growth, not declining outlays. Despite the improvement over the first four years of operation, on average, surviving new businesses do not become profitable until their eighth year. Based on their performance for the first 8 years, it is only 10 or 12 years after inception that their projected profit rates will reach those of the firm's mature businesses.

These findings are useful for tempering unrealistic expectations. But even though Biggadike argues persuasively for the importance of revenue growth for the success of new investments, the potential role of historical investment cost and depreciation accounting in accentuating the findings should not be forgotten. Insufficient data are provided to determine the extent to which these factors may influence outcomes.

In sum, in contrast to cross-sectional examinations of firm profit rates, the research in which time is evaluated shows that these projects are not soon profitable; rather, it takes time for revenues to grow. Managers expecting quick profits will only be disappointed. It is also important to note that these findings do not examine whether the profits earned are sufficient to justify incurring the risk of the project or the wait. Nor should they be interpreted to mean that diversifying investments should not be periodically evaluated and possibly divested.

Market conditions are critical to financial success

Before and after adopting diversifying investment projects, managers must explicitly evaluate the effect of market variables on the investment. In addition to the type and length of diversification, market conditions have been shown to significantly affect accounting profit rates. Three market characteristics, high market growth, high market share, and low competition, are repeatedly shown to be associated with higher accounting profit rates for for-profit firms.[26]

For two of these variables, market competition and market growth, however, the story is different for new businesses, according to Biggadike.[27] In his sample, new businesses entering markets characterized by low competition were less profitable during their early

> *The environmental or market conditions that a firm or new business faces affect its accounting profit rate.*

years than those entering more competitive markets. Although established firms seem to be protected by the barriers to entry that may be found in less competitive markets, such barriers hurt the performance of new businesses. In addition, among Biggadike's new businesses, those entering moderate-growth markets fared better than those entering low- and high-growth markets, perhaps because of lower marketing outlays.

The difficulty of entering less competitive markets as well as the importance of market share are supported by Montgomery's[28] comparison of high and low diversifiers in her sample of 128 large firms. The markets of low diversifiers are less competitive than those of high diversifiers. In addition, low diversifiers have higher market shares, which is consistent with operating in less competitive markets, and, perhaps, having less motivation to diversify.

The environmental or market conditions that a firm or new business faces affect its accounting profit rate. Barriers to entry that may be present, such as in noncompetitive markets, protect an existing firm's revenues but make revenues for a new business harder to generate or make costs higher. In a rapidly growing market, revenues may be higher, but costs may also be higher. Finally, both old and new businesses with high market shares perform best, probably because volume is sufficient to cover or exceed fixed costs.

FINANCIAL ANALYSES

Although the empirical literature concerning the effect of diversification on profitability and risk is not extensive, and much of the research is limited because it only examines surviving firms or projects, the results are consistent enough for five lessons to be derived. Certainly the lessons derived from the research findings are not particularly new or glamorous but they should be incorporated into initial and follow-up financial analyses of diversification projects. However, along with some other popular strategic concepts, they are frequently forgotten or ignored in financial analyses.

Initial and periodic discounted cash flow (net present value, or NPV) analyses of the diversification investment are among the best means to increase the chances for financially successful diversification. In this analysis, incremental cash inflows less outflows received over the life of the project are discounted to reflect their current period equivalent or present value. The model for the analysis is as follows:

$$NPV = \sum_{t=0}^{n} \frac{C_t}{(1+k)^t}$$

where C_t = the expected net incremental cash flow from the project in year t; k = the required rate of return; and n = the life of the project, generally in years.

Although most finance texts concentrate on the analysis before a project is adopted, the same type of analysis can be useful at various points after a project has begun. Periodic analyses can include new information and unanticipated environmental changes. Results from follow-up analyses may suggest divestment or continuation.

Market conditions variables, which are sometimes not fully considered in these analyses, are useful in projecting both incremental cash inflows and outflows. For example, cash inflows are likely to be low for new entrants to highly competitive and noncompetitive markets, when the firm expects a low market share, and in a slowly growing market.

The type of diversification also affects cash inflows and outflows. When diversification builds on a firm's strengths, cash inflows may be larger and start sooner than when other types of diversification are practiced. Cash outflows are correspondingly lower because assets and skills may be transferable to new businesses, and few additional outflows may be needed. When only one strength is to be transferred, as with constrained diversification, it may be easier to identify that strength and accomplish the transfer. In sum, when evaluating diversification investments, like other investments, the effects of important variables on cash flows are incorporated in the NPV model. For the analyses to be valid, however, managers must manage the investments as planned after the initial investment is made.

Time, the last variable important to the success of diversification, is a critical component of the NPV analysis. The arrival of net cash flows is plotted and their time value is explicitly considered. Near-term flows are valued more highly in this analysis, but negative net cash flows during the early years of a project may be outweighed by later discounted positive cash flows. To create value, only projects with a positive NPV are accepted. For these projects, the wait for positive flows is worthwhile. Positive NPV projects will be reflected in shareholder returns and accounting profit rates.

Note also that the risk of the investment project is important in determining k, the required rate of return. In general, k increases as systematic (market) risk increases. To attain the same positive NPV as low-risk projects, higher net cash inflows are required for riskier projects. The details of the determination of k are beyond the scope of this article but are found in standard finance textbooks.

In long-run competitive equilibrium, all projects have a zero NPV. Therefore, a nonzero NPV merits further attention and evaluation. "Smart managers do not accept positive (or negative) NPVs unless they can explain them."[29] Checking for market opportunities where market conditions indicate deviations from long-run equilibrium and looking at the firm's abilities to exploit these opportunities may explain nonzero NPVs. It is also possible that making errors, making overly optimistic projections, or ignoring a project's risk are responsible for positive NPVs. Further investigation of nonzero NPVs is always warranted.

• • •

Diversification is in early stages of development and implementation by health care organizations. As a result, systematic evaluations of its financial effects have, with rare exception, not been undertaken. However, from the summary of the comprehensive review of research on the profitability and risk effects of diversification for large for-profit firms, several lessons for the health care industry can be learned. Diversification does not guarantee higher profitability; diversification does not reduce financial risk; some types of diversification may be better than others; financial benefits from diversification may take time; and market conditions are critical to financial success. In addition, discounted cash flow analysis that explicitly evaluates market variables and the firm's abilities increases the potential for success in diversification. Thus it may be seen that "successful performance is the outcome of market opportunity combined with the capacity to take advantage of that opportunity."[30]

REFERENCES

1. Gort, M. *Diversification and Integration in American Industry.* Princeton, N.J.: Princeton University Press, 1962.
2. Montgomery, C.A. "Diversification, Market Structure and Firm Performance: An Extension of Rumelt's Model." Ph.D. diss., Purdue University, 1979.
3. Weston, J.F., and Mansinghka, S.K. "Tests of the Efficiency Performance of Conglomerate Firms." *Journal of Finance* 26 (1971): 919-36.
4. Melicher, R.W., and Rush, D.F. "The Performance of Conglomerate Firms: Recent Risk and Return Experience." *Journal of Finance* 28 (1973): 381-88.
5. Reid, S.R. "A Reply to the Weston/Mansinghka Criticisms Dealing with Conglomerate Mergers." *Journal of Finance* 26 (1971): 937-46.
6. Holzmann, O.J., Copeland, R.M., and Hayya, J. "Income Measures of Conglomerate Performance." *Quarterly Review of Economics and Business* 15 (1975): 67-78.
7. Mason, R.H., and Goudzwaard, M.B. "Performance of Conglomerate Firms: A Portfolio Approach." *Journal of Finance* 31 (1976): 39-48.
8. Melicher and Rush, "The Performance of Conglomerate Firms."
9. Beattie, D.L. "Conglomerate Diversification and Performance: A Survey and Time Series Analysis." *Applied Economics* 12 (1980): 251-73.
10. Rumelt, R.P. *Strategy, Structure and Economic Performance.* Boston: Harvard University Graduate School of Business Administration, 1974.
11. Rumelt, R.P. "Diversification Strategy and Profitability." *Strategic Management Journal* 3 (1982): 359-69.
12. Ibid.
13. Rumelt, *Strategy, Structure and Economic Performance.*
14. Montgomery, "Diversification, Market Structure and Firm Performance."
15. Palepu, K. "Diversification Strategy, Profit Performance and the Entropy Measure." *Strategic Management Journal* 6 (1985): 239-55.
16. Michel, A., and Shaked, I. "Does Business Diversification Affect Performance?" *Financial Management* 13 (Winter 1984): 18-25.
17. Weston, J.F., Smith, K.V., and Shrieves, R.E. "Conglomerate Performance Using the Capital Asset Pricing Model." *Review of Economics and Statistics* 54 (1972): 357-63.
18. Melicher and Rush, "The Performance of Conglomerate Firms."

19. Beattie, "Conglomerate Diversification."
20. Joehnk, M.D. and Neilsen, J.F. "The Effects of Conglomerate Merger Activity on Systematic Risk." *Journal of Financial and Quantitative Analysis* 9 (1974): 215-25.
21. Rumelt, *Strategy, Structure and Economic Performance*.
22. Palepu, "Diversification Strategy, Profit Performance and the Entropy Measure."
23. Weston and Mansinghka, "Tests of the Efficiency Performance of Conglomerate Firms."
24. Reid, "A Reply to the Weston/Mansinghka Criticisms."
25. Biggadike, E.R. *Corporate Diversification: Entry, Strategy, and Performance*. Cambridge, Mass.: Harvard University Press, 1976.
26. Montgomery, "Diversification, Market Structure and Firm Performance."
27. Biggadike, *Corporate Diversification*.
28. Montgomery, "Diversification, Market Structure and Firm Performance."
29. Myers, S.C. "Finance Theory and Financial Strategy." In *Readings on Strategic Management*, edited by A.C. Hax. Cambridge, Mass.: Ballinger, 1984, p. 181.
30. Christensen, H.K., and Montgomery, C.A. "Corporate Economic Performance: Diversification Strategy Versus Market Structure." *Strategic Management Journal* 2 (1981): 339.

The case for hospital diversification into long-term care

Carole W. Giardina,
Myron D. Fottler,
Richard M. Shewchuk,
and
Daniel B. Hill

Since the market for long-term care (LTC) services is expected to grow rapidly in the years ahead, the case for hospital diversification into LTC is a strong one. This article discusses the major LTC diversification options, the cost of entry, potential profitability, potential problems, and recommendations for implementing them.

Health Care Manage Rev, 1990, 15(1), 71–82
© 1990 Aspen Publishers, Inc.

Hospitals today operate in an environment that has undergone great change in recent years due to cost-containment measures such as Medicare's Prospective Payment System (PPS), the increased power of bargaining units such as preferred provider organizations (PPOs) and the growth of alternatives to acute hospital care. These changes have forced hospitals to search for new markets for expansion. One market that has been discussed frequently for hospital entry is the long-term care (LTC) market. This article will explore the benefits that can accrue to a hospital from LTC diversification, the potential pitfalls of such diversification, and the means of most effectively implementing such diversification.

This article is based on an exhaustive search of the current literature as well as on over 20 interviews conducted in the Birmingham, Alabama area in 1987 and 1988. In addition, the first author has had many years of experience as a nursing home administrator. Since there has been little empirical research in this area, most of the articles reviewed were conceptual in nature or were addressed to a practitioner audience. Interviews were conducted with hospital planners, hospital administrators, nursing home administrators, corporate officials of large nursing home chains, an official of the Alabama Nursing Home Association, an administrator in the Alabama Medicaid Office, an official in the swing-bed demonstration projects at the Health Care Financing Administration (HCFA), the director of a Birmingham comprehensive outpatient rehabilitative facility, and the director of the Center for Aging at the University of Alabama at Birmingham. The interviews

Carole W. Giardina, *M.H.A., is a Ph.D. candidate in Administration-Health Services at the University of Alabama at Birmingham and an Assistant Professor at the School of Business, Samford University.*

Myron D. Fottler, *Ph.D., is a Professor and Director of the Ph.D. Program in Administration-Health Services at the University of Alabama at Birmingham.*

Richard M. Shewchuk, *Ph.D., is an Assistant Professor and Director of Gerontology in the School of Health Related Professions at the University of Alabama at Birmingham.*

Daniel B. Hill, *Ph.D., is an Associate Professor of Health Care Administration in the School of Health Related Professions at the University of Alabama at Birmingham.*

The authors thank Teresa Burgess, Julie Shoemaker, and Larry Walls at the University of Alabama at Birmingham for their assistance in the preparation of this article.

focused on reasons for diversification, cost of entry and potential profitability of each diversification option, and recommendations concerning the management of the diversification.

It should be noted that the authors use the term *diversification* to describe the entry of a hospital into nonacute care areas. This is, of course, *related diversification*. Some readers may believe that the term *vertical integration* is more appropriate to describe the efforts of the hospital to control other aspects of the health care continuum. However, the authors view this article as an effort to describe the benefits that can accrue to a hospital from entry into the LTC marketplace; therefore, the concept of related diversification is more appropriate.

BACKGROUND

In 1953, the American Hospital Association (AHA) endorsed the cost-based principle of reimbursement for hospital care.[1,2] It is interesting to note that at that time, cost-based reimbursement was already the most common basis for the payment plans of Blue Cross, the nation's preeminent carrier of health care insurance. In 1965, Congress enacted the Medicare program to improve accessibility of health care to the elderly. One of the tenets of the Medicare program was that providers be paid on a reasonable cost basis.

However, evidence accumulated indicating that cost-based reimbursement systems, as implemented under Medicare, provided little incentive for the provider to

---

It is evident that LTC involves a multifaceted array of services that includes skilled nursing care, domiciliary care, retirement housing, home health care, and wellness programs.

---

control its costs. Under the retrospective payment scheme, Medicare inpatient hospital expenditures averaged an increase of 20% per year between 1966 and 1972.[3] Although the hospital industry experienced rapid growth during the period, funding problems for the Medicare entitlement program grew to crisis proportions.[4]

By the mid-1970s, a major concern of public policy makers was how to contain these costs. Certificate-of-need (CON) laws were passed to control the construction of new hospital beds, and various review agencies,

such as the Professional Standards Review Organization, were empowered to deny reimbursement claims for unnecessary care. However, the most dramatic means of controlling hospital costs evolved from the 1982 passage of the Tax Equity and Fiscal Responsibility Act (TEFRA), which mandated that the reimbursement system be changed from a cost-based system to a PPS.[3]

Under the PPS, Medicare payments to hospitals are made at a predetermined, specified rate for each admission diagnosis. PPS reimburses the hospital at the rate established for each patient diagnosis regardless of patient length of stay. It has served as a strong incentive for hospitals to discharge patients as early as possible. Studies have shown that patients have been discharged "sicker and quicker" from hospitals since the PPS was instituted.[5]

Furthermore, cost control measures implemented under PPS have resulted in a dramatic decrease in hospital occupancy rates. Between 1983 and 1985, there was a 10% decline in hospital census levels.[6] Nationwide, occupancy rates declined from 76.6% in 1975 to 64.1% in 1985.[6] A study by Johns Hopkins University and the Joint Commission on Accreditation of Healthcare Organizations (Joint Commission) reported that 100 hospitals per year are expected to close until supply–demand equilibrium is reached.[7]

The altered reimbursement rules have also made it attractive for Medicare recipients to seek health care outside the traditional hospital setting. Other competitors have entered the health care market and have forced hospitals to compete for patients not only with each other but also with alternative delivery systems such as free-standing emergency centers, diagnostic centers, and outpatient one-day-surgery centers.

The growth in health maintenance organizations (HMOs) and PPOs is another reason for the pervasive decline in hospital occupancy rates. The number of HMO subscribers increased from 9.1 million in 1980 to 14 million in 1984 and was projected to increase to 30 million by 1990.[8] A survey by InterStudy in 1986 found that there were 25.8 million HMO enrollees.[9] Since HMOs emphasize preventative medicine and careful screening prior to hospital admission, hospital admissions for HMO subscribers are 40% lower than for subscribers to a typical fee-for-service group (although some of the lower admission rates can be attributed to favorable selection of subscribers).[10] PPOs have adversely affected hospital revenues by using their purchasing powers to persuade hospitals to grant them favorable terms.

FIGURE 1

A CONTINUUM OF LONG-TERM CARE OPTIONS FOR HOSPITAL DIVERSIFICATION

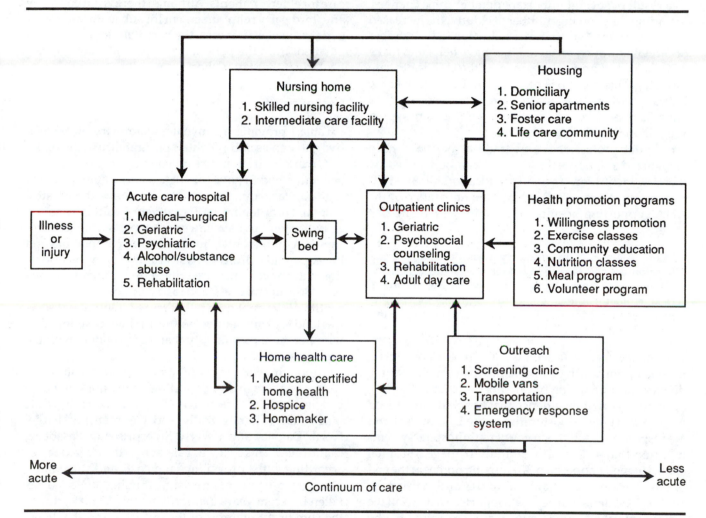

The decline in hospital census as well as the emphasis on continued cost control mechanisms can be expected to create a need for hospitals to seek new markets in order to maintain their viability. LTC presents a growing and potentially profitable market that can help satisfy this need.

THE LTC MARKET

LTC services have been defined as

providing diagnostic, preventive, therapeutic, rehabilitative, supportive and maintenance services for individuals who have chronic physical and/or mental impairments in a variety of institutional and noninstitutional health care settings, including the home, with the goal as promoting

the optimum level of physical, social, and psychological functioning.[11(p.2)]

From this definition, it is evident that LTC involves a multifaceted array of services that includes skilled nursing care, domiciliary care, retirement housing, home health care, and wellness programs (see Figure 1). A hospital patient can be viewed as progressing through a continuum of care as he or she makes a recovery from an illness or injury. The hospital or hospital system that chooses to enter the LTC market can select from among the various components of this continuum. These components should be viewed as a reciprocal system through which patients feed from one component to another as their physical or mental conditions change. This allows the hospital to capture the revenue from any point in the continuum.

The demand for LTC services is expected to increase as a result of several important demographic changes, including the growing number of elderly, the increased incidence of morbidity, and a reduction in the number of caregivers. Such social realities have helped to make LTC the fastest growing segment of the U.S. health care industry. This growth is best seen in the nursing home industry, where the expenditures for these services have increased from $24 billion in 1981 to a projected $56 billion in 1990.[12]

Hospital professional and trade associations have recognized the opportunities that can be realized by member institutions from diversification into the LTC continuum. A proposed policy statement drafted by the AHA supporting hospital interest in the LTC market states:

> Multiple strategies are necessary in view of limited access to resources and availability of services. Innovative delivery and financing mechanisms must be initiated and examined in relation to their ability to ensure that the comprehensive care needs of all older adults are met in an effective and efficient manner.[13(p.1)]

This policy also states that LTC "offers hospitals a unique opportunity to lead in the restructuring of the delivery and financing of care for the elderly."[13(p.2)]

There is growing evidence that hospitals are indeed seeing emerging opportunities in the LTC market and are responding. A 1987 survey of multihospital systems reported that 42% of 213 centrally managed hospital chains owned or operated 329 nursing homes at the end of 1985.[14] A study by Shewchuk and Giardina using the 1986 AHA Annual Survey Data reported that 18% of the hospitals in the United States that were accredited by the Joint Commission as acute care hospitals had nursing home units, and 22% provided geriatric services.[15]

Hospital diversification into LTC is often initiated when the hospital purchases an existing nursing home or other LTC service. The various state CON laws, as well as Medicaid restrictions against issuing any new provider agreements, prohibit the unrestricted addition of nursing home beds and the establishment of comprehensive outpatient rehabilitative facilities (CORFs) and home health care agencies in many states. These barriers can be circumvented to some degree by small rural hospitals with the use of acute care beds as swing beds; the extension of this concept to urban hospitals is under study. Other hospitals have developed the concepts of subacute care and transitional beds as a means of retaining the geriatric patient for longer periods. Respite care and geriatric psychiatric units are additional means of providing skilled nursing care for elderly patients. Although there is not generally any third party reimbursement for subacute, respite, or geriatric psychiatric care, the hospital can often obtain payment from the patient or the patient's family, particularly if the stay is short term.

Cost of entry

Table 1 provides a convenient summary of the relative entry costs and potential profitability in the major LTC markets. It should be noted that inpatient services generally tend to have the highest cost of entry, due to high capital requirements, but also have the greatest potential profitability. Alternatively, health promotion activities tend to have lower entry costs (due to lower capital requirements), but have more competitors and lower potential profits. Physical and geographical location and convenience are critical determinants of success. Housing markets tend to have high entry costs, but profitability is not generally assured. Outpatient services tend to exhibit either medium or high costs together with potential profitability that varies widely with the specific services.

Although there is wide variation in construction costs, the average cost of adding a new nursing home bed is $29,000. This is based on estimates by Dale Mackenzie (Charles Bailly and Company of Fargo, North Dakota) and Beverly Enterprises of Pasadena, California.[16] This cost will vary across the United States according to the prevailing land costs and wage rates. The purchase price of an existing nursing home bed has fallen in recent years to approximately $23,000, due to the slim profit margins of the industry and the divesture of less profitable facilities by Beverly Enterprises, the industry leader.[17] The cost of constructing retirement housing will vary according to the degree of amenities offered.

It should be noted that, if a hospital has chronic low-occupancy levels, it might be possible to convert existing hospital beds to nursing home beds, domiciliary beds, or retirement apartments. Excess capacity in the hospital's physical and occupational therapy departments could be used for outpatient rehabilitation; the cost of conversion is minor in comparison to the cost of new construction. A hospital that wishes to choose the conversion option, however, should check the respective state's CON laws, since it might prove difficult to change any converted beds back to acute care beds.

TABLE 1

HOSPITAL COST OF ENTRY AND POTENTIAL PROFITABILITY IN MAJOR LONG-TERM CARE MARKETS

Cost of entry	Inpatient services	Housing	Outpatient services	Health promotion
High	Skilled nursing*	Retirement housing	Homemaker Durable medical equipment	
	Intermediate nursing* Rehabilitation* Geriatric unit Alzheimer unit* AIDS unit Psychiatric unit* Alcohol/substance abuse	Life-care community Domiciliary Senior apartments	Mobile van*	
Medium	Swing-beds clinics*	Foster care	Home health care rehabilitation* Geriatric Adult day care Meals-on-wheels Nutrition psychological counseling hospice	Screening Emergency response system
Low				Wellness program Mobile vans Transportation Exercise class Nutrition class Community education Meal program Volunteer program

* Estimated profitable or break even by at least 80% of the 753 hospital CEO respondents to an American Hospital Association Survey. See "Diversification: More Black Ink." *Hospitals* 62 (1988): 36–42.

Potential profitability

Obviously, there are numerous contingencies associated with the profitability of various LTC markets. The profit margin of long-term institutional care is a function of the patient mix, the cost of construction, the state Medicaid rate, and the quality or intensity of services provided.[18,19] There is wide variation in the Medicaid rates and their formulas for compensation across states. Hospital-based nursing homes have the potential to be more profitable than free-standing nursing homes, since hospital-based nursing homes are reimbursed at a higher rate by Medicare.[20] Likewise, swing beds are not profitable unless hospitals can keep marginal costs from increasing with volume.[21] The rehabilitative services of a CORF are usually fully reimbursed and offer

excellent potential for profitability. The rehabilitation industry, however, has seen a market growth in recent years and may be reaching saturation levels in some areas.

There are 14,400 certified nursing homes in the United States,[22] many of which are profitable because of tight cost-control measures. A study of a sample of American nursing homes by Johnson showed that many facilities earned a return of 5% to 7% on gross sales and up to 15% on investment.[19] The number of uncollectible accounts is generally low in nursing homes, due to the more thorough screening permitted the nursing home administrator because of the lower turnover rate of patients. Most nursing homes' bad debts are only 1% to 2% of revenues, compared with the 5% to 7% in hospitals. Cash flow is usually more of a problem, due to the often lengthy wait for reimbursement.[19] However, it should be pointed out that limited state Medicaid budgets and escalating wage rates have cut into nursing home profitability in recent years. The increase in the minimum wage proposed by the Bush administration could further strain state Medicaid budgets and consequently erode nursing home profits, since these facilities are staffed in large part by unskilled staff.

Retirement housing, congregate care retirement communities (CCRCs), and lifecare communities have experienced well-publicized financial problems in recent years. The high inflation rates of the late 1970s and early 1980s, poorly estimated actuarial figures, and a lack of understanding of the market caused many large projects to fail.[23] In a study by Ruchlin, it was found that CCRCs were showing an improved financial position, although in many instances income and equity deficits were reported.[24] This market is projected to grow as demand for retirement centers is bolstered by the growing acceptance and increasing number of elderly who can afford retirement housing. Generally, elderly

people with annual incomes of $20,000 or more can afford this option.[25] In 1985, 5.6 million elderly households had incomes of $20,000 or more; it is projected that by the year 2001, that figure will rise 34% to 7.5 million.[25] However, since a large capital investment is required for a hospital to expand into the retirement community industry, hospitals should evaluate this option very carefully before deciding to implement it. In particular, the hospitals should be certain that their market area has a sufficient number of elderly with relatively high incomes.

HOSPITAL BENEFITS FROM LONG-TERM CARE DIVERSIFICATION

Why should a hospital, with its large fixed capital expenses and staff of well-paid professionals, want to enter the LTC market, which has inherent risks and low reimbursement ceilings? There are several possible reasons. First, there is a need, as suggested earlier, for hospitals to diversify to offset revenue loss from declining acute care census. Second, the LTC market is a

FIGURE 2

A MODEL OF HOSPITAL BENEFITS FROM LONG-TERM CARE DIVERSIFICATION

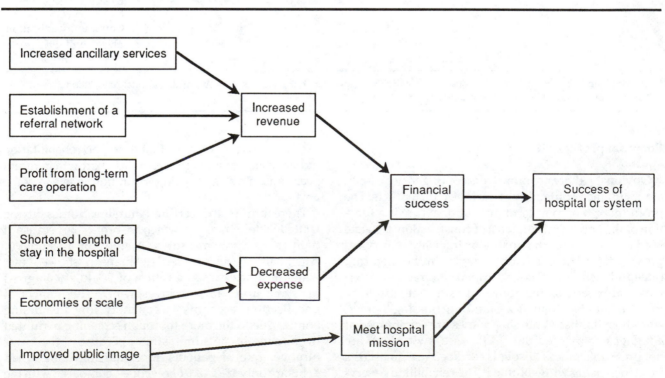

growing and potentially profitable enterprise. There are several benefits from hospital entry into LTC, and they should be thought of as interacting with each other. These are summarized in Figure 2.

Hospitals should examine profitability from LTC diversification in more ways than by simply isolating the profitability from the actual operation of the nursing home, retirement housing, home health care agency, or other long-term venture. Indeed the hospital may lose money on the actual operation of the LTC component and yet still find LTC diversification profitable. The indirect synergistic benefits that accrue to the hospital from using such diversification as a form of vertical integration may outweigh and offset the direct loss on the nursing home beds or other LTC services.

With the constraints of diagnosis related groups (DRGs), an obvious benefit of LTC diversification is decreased length of stay for the acute care Medicare patient. Under PPS, the hospital has an incentive to discharge the patient as quickly as possible. With the emphasis on cost-containment measures,[5] it has been noted that the hospital is reluctant to provide acute care to Medicare recipients who are *outliers* as defined under the DRG regulations. Outliers are DRG patients for whom the cost of providing a service significantly exceeds its reimbursement due to the intensity of service required, the length of stay, or both.[26] The hospital also tends to decrease lengths of stay by discharging patients as rapidly as possible, reducing the use of services during stays, and transferring Medicare recipients to nursing homes and public hospitals.

If the hospital were to have ready access to nursing home beds, it could discharge patients even more quickly. By building up its extended care services, the hospital would be in a position to move the patient out of the acute care setting faster and more efficiently.[27] In addition, this would lessen the problem of dealing with a heavy care patient whom local nursing homes might prefer not to admit because of the cost of care. If the patient's condition worsens after discharge, the patient could possibly be treated in the LTC facility, avoiding readmission.

Another benefit that the hospital can derive from diversification into LTC is increased revenue from charges for ancillary services such as physical therapy, lab work, and the provision of various supplies. Although Medicaid does not cover ancillary services, Medicare will reimburse charges under some circumstances. Also, some families can afford to pay for uncovered services. Most of these services are now provided on a limited basis by nursing homes through contracts

with various consulting groups or independent laboratories. If a hospital owned a nursing home, it would be able to capture this market and generate more services for its therapy departments and laboratories. Kovner and Richardson indicated that hospitals with swing beds have reported ancillary charges ranging from $30 to $50 per swing-bed day.[28] This revenue is in addition to any per diem charges for basic nursing services and board.

A third benefit realized by hospitals that choose to diversify into LTC is economies of scale. The organization can spread certain fixed costs over more patient days or services. The additions of swing bed or nursing home days in a small rural hospital with a low census could help support the more expensive care in the acute care sections.

The hospital can also benefit from the establishment of a referral network. Patients discharged to a nursing home or to another LTC service tend to be readmitted to the hospital, as illustrated in Figure 1. A study of 197 discharged nursing home patients showed that 33% of the patients died in the facility, 28% transferred to their home, 32% transferred to hospitals, and 7% transferred to other nursing homes.[29] If a hospital owned a nursing home, it would have a virtually "captive" market on these transfers back to the hospital.[30] This could result in significant numbers of hospital admissions. Although about one fourth of the patients readmitted to the hospital in the nursing home discharge study died,[29] they were revenue-producing patients, regardless of their length of stay.

Another benefit that the hospital can derive from diversification into LTC is increased revenue from charges for ancillary services such as physical therapy, lab work, and the provision of various supplies.

The provision of nursing home and other LTC services could also benefit the hospital by improving its public image. According to Brody,[27] the hospital will benefit from providing long-term care by becoming more responsive to the needs of its patients, by bonding people to the institution, and by enabling the hospital to deny the accusation that it is dumping patients without making provision for their care. Thus in providing this care, the hospital may be perceived as being more concerned about the welfare of its patients.

It should not be overlooked that hospitals may actually make a profit from their LTC operations. Hospital-based nursing homes are reimbursed at a higher rate for patients than are free-standing nursing homes.[20] If the state Medicaid rates are reasonable and if the nursing home is able to attract a relatively high percentage of private-pay patients, the nursing home may be quite profitable. Long-term care options such as rehabilitation services have proven to be extremely advantageous to the hospital's bottom line.

The traditional acute care hospital has much to gain by entering the LTC market. Not only is the actual operation of the LTC service potentially profitable, but also the benefits derived from other areas can help the hospital meet both its financial goals and stated missions.

IMPLEMENTATION GUIDELINES

It should be remembered that there are inherent differences between the management required by an acute care hospital and that required by a nursing home, retirement home, home health care agency, or rehabilitation facility.[31] The astute hospital executive who wishes to diversify his or her hospital into the nursing home area would be well advised to hire an experienced nursing home administrator. Although the administrator of the hospital can legally also serve as the administrator of the nursing home, it might be advantageous to employ a full-time LTC administrator. The cost containment component of the job, as well as the government and reimbursement red tape, make this a time-consuming job that might be best delegated to a middle-management employee trained or experienced in this type of work. Other LTC options such as rehabilitation and retirement housing would require less attention but might best be delegated to an experienced manager when volume reaches a sufficient level to justify such an expense.

Cost control is of paramount importance in LTC; resources must be utilized as efficiently as possible in areas where reimbursement rates are low. Nursing homes, domiciliaries, and retirement housing are largely staffed with unskilled workers who receive minimal benefits. When possible, the hospital should try to maintain separate wage scales for the LTC facility and for the hospital. Nursing home, domiciliary, and retirement home charges, whether Medicaid or private, are not usually sufficient to provide more than the mandated essentials required by the licensing agencies.

As previously stated, one of the primary ways in which hospitals can benefit from diversification into LTC is through earlier discharge of the acute care patient. However, if the hospital utilizes its nursing home for only difficult-to-place, heavy-care patients, it will in effect be running a low-intensity hospital. Other than the limited benefits available under Medicare, reimbursement rates are not sufficiently high to cover the cost of patients requiring a large number of services. The hospital-based nursing home should attempt to place patients with high acuity levels in community nursing homes or should encourage discharge to the patient's home and should only accept those patients for whom unavailability of LTC beds will delay hospital discharge. The hospital-based nursing home should also try to attract as many low-care patients as possible from the community in order to offset the costs associated with those patients requiring more intensive care services.

Separate accounts must be maintained for the long-term facility under the Medicare and Medicaid provisions. An experienced LTC reimbursement accountant should be periodically retained as a consultant to compute the necessary cost reports. An accountant trained specifically in LTC reimbursement can save a facility a great deal of money.

Another recommendation is to market LTC services. The necessity of doing so might be questioned, especially in particular nursing home services, because most nursing homes and many other LTC facilities maintain between 95% and 100% occupancy. However, it is important to remember the nature of the LTC market. In a system where Medicaid, the primary third party payer, often reimburses at less than cost, it is necessary to maintain as advantageous a patient mix as possible. The marketing should be aimed at the private-pay market. Indeed, it is well documented that the nursing home administrator will first fill all possible beds with private-pay patients (who can be charged whatever the market will bear) and then fill the remaining beds with Medicaid patients.[32] Private-pay patients are needed to offset the economic losses from the sometimes heavy-care Medicaid patients.

Marketing in an LTC facility is done primarily through two groups: hospital social workers and physicians. It is inefficient to market to the public at large through the various media, because no one wishes to know about LTC services, in particular nursing home services, until the need for them arises. This is due in part to the view of LTC facilities as places that maintain people until death. When the need does arise, the social workers and the patient's physician often help guide the patient and his or her family to an appropriate nursing home.

The hospital may choose a focused strategy for LTC diversification. Many LTC facilities specialize in caring for people who have Alzheimer's disease or in posthospital rehabilitation. A survey of the market should be made to ascertain in what particular areas services are deficient, how these needs are currently being addressed, and how the hospital might address LTC needs.

Procedures should be implemented to evaluate the LTC diversification. The hospital's cost-accounting data should be examined to determine the profitability of the long-term facility in terms of not only its individual profitability, but also its effect on overall hospital profitability. Statistics should be studied to determine if the average length of stay in the hospital has decreased as a result of the diversification. Discharge records should be analyzed to see if there are increased internal referrals due to the presence of LTC facilities.

It should be pointed out that not every hospital should consider LTC diversification. The primary candidates for entry into LTC are those with high Medicare census. The economic status of the elderly in the market area is another factor that should be considered.

An area that can affect an American hospital's profit from LTC diversification is government regulation. Changes in reimbursement policy can affect the operation of the long-term facilities either negatively or positively. Doing something about the cost of LTC is currently a hot topic; it is a major theme in both the Republican and the Democratic parties. However, the immense cost of implementing such programs and their consequent requirements for additional revenues may serve to keep any meaningful LTC program from being passed. It is also important to watch for changes in the CON laws. If a state decides to increase CON nursing home bed limits, the hospital might choose to build rather than purchase an existing LTC facility.

DIVERSIFICATION OPTIONS

This article has already dealt with many of the advantages and disadvantages of the various types of LTC options. Table 2 lists these advantages and disadvantages in a brief overview of the major choices for the hospital and the factors influencing each selection. These options are also discussed in the section below.

TABLE 2

FACTORS INFLUENCING LTC DIVERSIFICATION

LTC option	Market variables	Risk	Reimbursement climate	Advantages	Disadvantages
Nursing homes	% of elderly in population, affluence of elderly, competition	High (construction or purchase costs required)	Depends on state	Earlier hospital discharge, referral network, ancillary charges, economics of scale	Reimbursement is often low, requires a great deal of attention
Retirement housing, life care, CRCs	Affluence of elderly	High (need good market survey)	Not applicable	Ties residents to hospital	Very costly to build
Domiciliaries, assisted living, personal care	% of elderly in population, affluence of elderly	High because of construction costs	Not applicable	Referrals, ties residents to hospital, economies of scale	Target market is usually small
Home health care	Degree of market saturation	Medium (low capital intensity)	Good	Flexible staffing, referral network	Potential market saturation
Wellness programs, health promotion	Not applicable except to determine if other hospitals are doing this	Low	Not applicable	Good will, referral network	Poor financial return
Outpatient rehabilitation	% of elderly in population, proximity to industries	Medium (purchase of equipment, employment of staff)	Excellent	Referral network, flexible staffing (if existing therapists can be used)	Potential market saturation

Nursing homes

There are basically two types of nursing homes: skilled and intermediate care. A combination of both is needed: the skilled beds provide care for those patients with higher levels of acuity, and the intermediate care facility beds offset the high costs of operating the skilled beds. Private-pay or self-pay patients can go in either type of bed, but Medicare patients are limited to the skilled beds.

Nursing homes offer moderate profit opportunity depending on the generosity of the Medicaid program, the availability of private-pay patients, and the acuity levels of the patients. A hospital that considers this option would be well advised to do a market study to determine if there are a sufficient number of relatively affluent elderly in the market area for the nursing home to attract better-paying patients. The competition from free-standing nursing homes should be evaluated. While many families would give preference to placing their patients in hospital-based nursing homes (because of the proximity of emergency personnel), the hospital may still find that free-standing nursing homes can undercut them in price. Unlike hospital services, many families shop around for the best price for nursing home services.

Retirement housing

Retirement housing offers the opportunity for good profit if it is done correctly. Because of the large risk and the lack of reimbursement in this area, it is especially important that a good market survey be conducted. It is also important to know if there are sufficient elderly in the area who desire and can afford this service. The facility should be built with the demographic characteristics of the target population in mind. For instance, a luxury facility will be beyond the means of many elderly. Services should be priced appropriately: Too high a price will make it unaffordable to most elderly, but too low a price will make it unprofitable. The cost will have to be borne entirely by the resident and his or her family, although there are some provisions for low-cost housing for the lower-income elderly.

Nursing homes offer moderate profit opportunity depending on the generosity of the Medicaid program, the availability of private-pay patients, and the acuity levels of the patients.

Domiciliaries

Domiciliaries offer some advantages over nursing homes. One advantage is that no CON is required. Another advantage is that the staffing requirements are much lower than for certified nursing homes. At the same time, charges for domiciliary care are usually about two thirds of what a private patient pays in a nursing home. However, it should be remembered that there is no reimbursement for these services, and the cost will have to be borne by the family. Moreover, since many of the potential patients are able to be maintained in the home under a caregiver's supervision, only a small fraction of the target market will elect to enter a domiciliary.

Home health care

Home health care offers a good profit opportunity depending on the degree of competition in the marketplace. The advantages of home health care are that it is not capital intensive and that staffing can be somewhat flexible, depending on the patient case load. Also, Medicare reimbursement is quite good.

However, it is important to determine if the market is saturated before selecting this option. Too many competitors will simply split the market more ways. Although the hospital will have a ready source of referrals from its own discharges, additional patients are usually necessary to make this area profitable.

Health promotion

There is little revenue to be obtained from this source, although expenses are usually relatively low. This option should be viewed more as a public-image promotion than as a profit-making venture; it can create good, positive feedback for the hospital at a minimal cost.

Rehabilitation

Outpatient rehabilitation is a potentially excellent source of profit. CORFs are reimbursed at relatively high rates for Medicare patients. This has been mandated as a means of avoiding more costly inpatient services. Also, insurance companies that offer workers' compensation insurance usually pay well to rehabilitate injured employees. An additional benefit of choosing this type of care is that the capital outlay can be relatively small, providing that the hospital has existing space that can be converted to this use.

The section above presents a brief summary of the various options. The scope of this article precludes a more detailed discussion. However, it should be remembered that the main tenet of this article is that each of these options should be examined not only for what it can contribute directly to the hospital's bottom line, but also for what indirect benefits it presents to the hospital. Ultimately, these synergistic benefits are what is of value to the hospital.

A good example of how a hospital can benefit from LTC diversification can be found at a hospital in a large city in the Southeast. This hospital recently completed a new facility. The old hospital was converted into retirement housing and domiciliary care. In addition, the hospital purchased a nursing home across the street from the old hospital. Home health care, outpatient rehabilitation, and wellness programs were also added. An experienced nursing home administrator was employed to manage the nursing home, domiciliary, and retirement housing. While the hospital is not making large profits from its LTC services, it has been able to maintain a high occupancy rate and to have the highest percentage of Medicare patients of any hospital in that city.

•   •   •

As shown in this article, the market for LTC services is growing. Not only is the number of elderly increasing, but also this population uses a disproportionate share of American health care resources. For example, in 1985, 42% of all hospital inpatient days were used by the 11.7% of the population over the age of 65.[13] Long-term care insurance, long discussed and now becoming a reality, will help to give the elderly additional purchasing power.

However, the advantages from the growth in the need for these services must be tempered with the reality of relatively low levels of third party reimbursement. It is important that a hospital administration view the addition of LTC services not only in terms of their individual contribution to the hospital, but also in terms of the synergistic effect they will have with existing hospital services as a result of vertical integration. Diversification efforts into LTC that result in an immediate, direct, and significant increase in profits are relatively rare, because many services are not presently reimbursable.[33] It should also be remembered that the potential benefits from LTC diversification will have to be weighed against the opportunity costs of not investing in other areas. But if the success of diversification is also measured in terms of patient referrals, medical staff satisfaction and commitment, and community service, then success is more likely.

The astute health care executive may find that diversification into long-term care can enhance hospital market share. Given careful screening and selection, objective market and economic analysis, and well-managed implementation, such diversification can provide positive synergistic benefit for the hospital.

REFERENCES

1. Somers, H.M., and Somers, A.R. *Medicare and Hospitals.* Washington, D.C.: Brookings Institution, 1967.
2. Meyers, R. *Passing the Health Care Buck: Who Pays the Hidden Cost?* Washington, D.C.: American Enterprise Institute, 1979.
3. Lave, J.R. "Hospital Reimbursement Under Medicare." *Healthcare Financial Management* 38, no. 7 (1984): 62–74.
4. Ruther, M., and Dobson, A. "Equal Treatment and Unequal Benefits: A Reexamination of the Use of Medicare Services by Race, 1967–1976." *Health Care Financing Review* 2, no. 3 (1981): 55–83.
5. Broyles, R.S., and Reilly, B.J. "National Health Insurance: A New Imperative." *Journal of Medical Systems* 8, no. 4 (1984): 331–350.
6. American Hospital Association. *Annual Survey.* Chicago: AHA Data Center, 1985.
7. Thompson, D.M. "Nursing Homes Show Versatility in Hospital Services." *Journal of the American Health Care Association* 12 (1986): 10–14.
8. Reisler, M. "Business in Richmond Attacks Health Care Costs." *Harvard Business Review* 63, no. 1 (1985): 145–155.
9. InterStudy. *National HMO Census.* Excelsior, Minn.: InterStudy, 1986.
10. Manning, W.G. "A Controlled Trial of the Effect of Prepaid Group Practice on Use of Services." *New England Journal of Medicine* 310 (1984): 1505–10.
11. Health Resources Administration, Division of Long-term Care. *The Future of Long-term Care in the United States—The Report of the Task Force.* Washington, D.C.: GPO, 1977.
12. Rudensky, M. "Manor Care Mapping Strategy as Long-Term Care Heats Up." *Modern Healthcare* 16 (1986): 98–100.
13. American Hospital Association. *Proposed Policy and Statement on Care for the Elderly.* Chicago: Section for Aging and Long-Term Care Services, 1986.
14. Graham, J. "Not for Profits More Diversified Than for Profits." *Modern Healthcare* 17, no. 16 (1987): 40.
15. Shewchuk, R., and Giardina, C.W. "Hospital Diversification Into Long-Term Care" Manuscript, The University of Alabama at Birmingham, 1986.
16. Finkler, S.A. "The Swing-Bed Alternative: Cost Issues." In *Swing Beds: Assessing Flexible Health Care in Rural Communities.* Washington, D.C.: Brookings Institution, 1987.

17. Wagner, L. "Nursing Home Giants Pull Back, Smaller Chains Advance as Industry Profits Plunge." *Modern Healthcare* 18, no. 23 (1988): 40–50, 54–55.

18. Fottler, M.D., Smith, H.L., and James, W.L. "Profits and Patient Care Quality in Nursing Homes." *The Gerontologist* 21 (1981): 532–38.

19. Johnson, D.E. "Hospitals Build, Buy Nursing Homes to Increase Share of Local Market." *Modern Healthcare* 17, no. 1 (1987): 74–77.

20. DeAngelis, P.L. "Hospital Based SNFs: An Alternative to Empty Beds." *Healthcare Financial Management* 41, no. 8 (1987): 60–66.

21. Weiner, J.M. "Swing-Beds: Policy Issues Raised by Current Law and the Robert Wood Johnson Demonstration." In *Swing-Beds: Assessing Flexible Healthcare in Rural Communities.* Washington, D.C.: Brookings Institution, 1987.

22. National Center for Health Statistics. "Nursing Home Characteristics: Preliminary Data from the 1985 National Nursing Home Survey." *Advanced Data from Vital and Health Statistics.* No. 131. DHHS Pub. No. (PHS) 87-1250. Hyattsville, Md.: Public Health Service, 1987.

23. Sumichrast, M.J.E. "Lifecare: A Growing Market." *Healthcare Strategic Management* 3, no. 8 (1985): 13–15.

24. Ruchlin, H.S. "Are CCRCs Facing a Promising Future or Potential Problems?" *Healthcare Financial Management* 41, no. 10 (1987): 54–61.

25. Graham, J. "Demand Should Foster Rapid Growth in Retirement Center Industry." *Modern Healthcare* 17, no. 9 (1987): 52, 58.

26. Smith, H.L., and Fottler, M.D. *Prospective Payment.* Rockville, Md.: Aspen Systems, 1985.

27. Riffer, J. "Extended Care Units Viewed as Problem Solvers." *Hospitals* 60, no. 1 (1986): 75.

28. Kovner, A.R., and Richardson, H. "The Robert Wood Johnson Demonstration Program." In *Swing-Beds: Assessing Flexible Health Care in Rural Communities.* Washington, D.C.: Brookings Institution, 1987.

29. Lewis, M.A., Cretin, S., and Kane, R.L. "The Natural History of Nursing Home Patients." *The Gerontologist* 25 (1985): 382–88.

30. Kenkel, P.J. "More Hospitals Enter Long-Term Care Business." *Modern Healthcare* 17 , no. 24 (1987): 30–31.

31. Monroe, S.M. "Nursing Home Diversification Requires Caution by Hospitals." *Healthcare Financial Management* 42, no. 12 (1988): 25–33.

32. Scanlon, W.J., and Feder, J. "The Long-Term Care Marketplace: An Overview." *Healthcare Financial Management* 38, no. 1 (1984): 18–36.

33. Larkin, M. "Payment Questions Could Stall New LTC Ventures." *Hospitals* 62, no. 15 (1988): 69.

Strategic acquisitions by academic medical centers: The Jefferson experience as operational paradigm

Gordon F. Schwartz
and
Catherine T. Stone

As capital investments in the health care industry have changed in popularity, mergers and acquisitions of and by hospitals have created supersystems of health care that are based on the assumption that economies of scale offer greater protection from a variety of forces. The acquisition of West Park (Jefferson Park) Hospital by Thomas Jefferson University and the infusion of Jefferson management into Methodist Hospital have provided the institution with unique opportunities to broaden its population base for acute care admissions and to permit greater diversification within the entire health care market.

Health Care Manage Rev, 1991, 16(2), 39–47

The popular song, "Staying Alive," from the 1977 movie, *Saturday Night Fever*, may be aptly and appropriately considered the theme song of today's health care industry.[1] Health care has grown from a pre-Medicare cottage industry to one that currently commands more than ten percent of the country's gross national product. Needy, benevolent, independent institutions have become multilayered systems run by top business talent, and business school attitudes, measures of performance, and philosophies have invaded the previously isolated and insular not-for-profit health care industry, including the university hospitals.[2]

HISTORIC PERSPECTIVE

Until recently, the infusion of Medicare dollars provided a ready source of capital for both not-for-profit and proprietary hospitals as these institutions were reimbursed for their direct patient costs and received a premium for equity and depreciation. Exploiting this windfall, the for-profit hospital sector expanded from 5.0 percent of available inpatient beds in 1965 to 10.4 percent in 1985, and financial markets rewarded these proprietary public companies with price-earnings multiples that were 1.96 times the overall stock market average.[3]

Not until the mid 1970s did the advent of Certificate of Need (CON) legislation dampen the exponential growth of hospital beds and services. However, the not-for-profit hospitals, including the major university hospitals associated with medical schools, were late to capitalize on these opportunities, since not-for-profit implied nonprofit to most institutional boards of trustees, and sound fiscal responsibility implied no better than a break-even income statement.

Gordon F. Schwartz, *M.D., M.B.A., is Professor of Surgery at Jefferson Medical College, Thomas Jefferson University, Philadelphia, Pennsylvania.*

Catherine T. Stone, *C.P.A., M.B.A., was a graduate student in the Management Department, Wharton School, University of Pennsylvania, Philadelphia, Pennsylvania, at the time that this article was written.*

The authors would like to acknowledge the enthusiastic support and assistance of members of the senior administrative staff of Thomas Jefferson University Hospital in the preparation of this manuscript. Special thanks are proffered to Thomas J. Lewis, III, Executive Director and Chief Operating Officer; Trevor A. Fisk, Associate Executive Director, Marketing and Planning; Harry S. Owens, Associate Executive Director for Financial Affairs; Max Goodman, Assistant Executive Director and Administrator, Jefferson Park Hospital—Children's Rehabilitation Hospital; and Kevin R. Hannifan, Chief Executive Officer, Methodist Hospital.

In the early 1980s, however, several federal responses to growing health care expenses forced hospitals to re-examine their strategies for success and even survival. Medicare reimbursement was revamped, and no longer were hospitals reimbursed according to their costs. Diagnosis related groups (DRGs) and prospective payment systems (PPS) were introduced to force efficiencies in hospital management; almost simultaneously, although the numbers of inpatient hospital days increased, they did so at a decreasing rate, indicating a shift from growth to maturity within the industry. The delivery of health care began to change from an acute-care hospital focus to a variety of medical ventures, in which the hospital was only one part of the overall system. To ensure their continued flow of patients, hospitals began to concentrate on specific, diverse activities, with special programs initiated to capture identifiable segments of the entire health care market.[4]

INVESTMENT STRATEGIES

In the windfall growth years before DRGs and PPS, acquisitions of hospitals by both for-profit chains were rampant, and supersystems of health care that would dominate the field were predicted by 1990. The abrupt change in the system made buyers into sellers overnight, and by 1987, the major publicly held health care companies had programs of divestiture instead of departments of acquisitions. Suddenly, the attractiveness of the health industry was replaced by wary forecasts of service demands, pricing structures, changing reimbursement systems, and cost predictions far into the future, recognizing the dramatic shifts in these projections might be provoked by unforeseen technologic advances, changes in the economic climate, or by shifts in societal demands. Because capital investment shapes the competitive position of an organization within its own defined market segments, how well capital is allotted and managed unquestionably influences the cost and pricing structure of an institution and, in turn, its ability to compete successfully within its industry.[5]

The key to merger and acquisition strategy, especially in today's health care industry, is the ability to achieve together what cannot be done alone.

Investment strategy that most closely complements the extant core business becomes the least risky and most secure. Within the not-for-profit sector, especially the university hospital, this translates into acute, usually inpatient, care as the safest bet. Diversification into a portfolio of revenue producing projects, such as long-term or psychiatric care, or special programs, such as substance abuse, "wellness," and women's services, creates a variety of different risks, each higher than that of the core business. Entry barriers are few or none, along with an apparent lack of product (service) differentiation, so that the level of competition is increased further. Managerial competence within the core, inpatient, hospital segment does not imply the same success in new ventures where experience is limited. However, diversification becomes beneficial if it allows an institution to escape overdependence on a single or declining market (inpatient care), to move into more profitable areas (ambulatory surgery, cardiac rehabilitation), to realize economies of scope or scale, or to reduce debt-financing costs. Whether diversified within a single hospital or by mergers with medical groups, clinics, rehabilitation centers, even childcare centers, the synergy created makes the whole greater than the sum of its parts. The key to merger and acquisition strategy, especially in today's health care industry, is the ability to achieve together what cannot be done alone.

Implicit in strategic decisions within the business community are the basic concepts of complementing the corporate mission and creating shareholder value. These are no less valid strategic considerations within not-for-profit or university hospital systems, even if the shareholders go by other names and the value is other than financial. The basic decisions take two divergent paths: should the institution pursue investments that will generate lower immediate returns but will create major future opportunities, or should only less risky opportunities with greater immediate returns be embraced?

The valuations of targets for capital investment in the health care industry are conceptually no different from those that would be confronted by any major business as a new acquisition might be contemplated. However, there are unique concerns inherent within the health care industry, requiring additional or different emphasis than those existing in the general business community.[6]

The present value of incremental cash flows may permit the quantifiable measurement of institutional assets, but the intangible assets of a hospital must be factored into any determination of overall value. These are, by definition, more difficult to appraise, but perceptions of the hospital's reputation in the community and the quality of the medical staff are crucial components of acquisition decisions.

Institutions must also measure their acquisition opportunities against their own corporate hurdle rates to evaluate the opportunity costs of the funds being invested. The strategic value of the investment opportunity must be evaluated most carefully to measure the "fit" of any capital venture, especially because no truly established market exists for not-for-profit organizations.[7] Failure to determine relative values often interferes with the successful completion of such tax-exempt mergers. The strength of the medical staff, the regulatory environment, presence of nearby alternative delivery systems, and management capability are especially important in this particular market, sometimes outweighing the historical and strictly financial bases of asset valuation.[8]

Additionally, because financial resources are finite, choices must be made. Not every investment with a projected positive net present value is a suitable choice for a university hospital, even though this argument may be advanced for many large businesses with relatively easy access to debt. Within the limitations of current and projected capital, investments must be selected with the greatest likelihood of market success. Not every opportunity that creates value is affordable in this context, depending upon current discretionary cash flows and institutional borrowing capacity.[9]

The health care industry exhibits additional idiosyncrasies that complicate management decisions. Although patients may be the ultimate users of health care services, there are two separate but dramatically important layers insinuated between the consumer and the hospital—the physicians, who produce revenue by admitting their patients to the hospital, and third party insurers, who bear the majority of the costs of those services. As hospital acquisitions are anticipated and planned, medical staff leaders, who historically are not conversant with the financial intricacies of the current medical care industry, must be made part of the decision-making process so that those decisions will be supported.[10] Important issues to physicians are effects on the perceived quality of patient care, medical staff access, and existing and future physician contracts with the institution. The relevance of lengths of stay, resources used, and third party reimbursement policies and prohibitions must be made an ingredient of sound medical decisions.[11]

Now that the Federal Trade Commission has become active in the review of hospital mergers from the perspective of antitrust legislation, an additional concern faces anticipated acquisitions of medical facilities.[12,13] Different messages are being received as apparently similar transactions have triggered contradictory judicial decisions in different venues.[14] Mergers to reduce costs and improve service have been disallowed because they lessen competition, so that market definitions become crucial. Whether mergers force other competing hospitals to lower prices or whether they reduce patient choice are conflicting questions addressed by the antitrust vigilantes. Competition within the health industry is protected by antitrust legislation, and physicians and not-for-profit institutions are no longer immune from prosecution for perceived antitrust violations.[15,16]

THOMAS JEFFERSON UNIVERSITY

From its modest inception in 1824 as the Jefferson Medical College of Philadelphia, Jefferson has emerged as the largest private medical school in the United States and one of Philadelphia's largest employers. Thomas Jefferson University was created in 1969 and comprises the medical school, Jefferson Medical College, the College of Graduate Studies, the College of Allied Health Sciences, and Thomas Jefferson University Hospital (TJUH). The university hospital has approximately 700 beds, 400 of which were replaced within a new plant in 1978. University assets in 1988 were valued at almost $500 million, and hospital operations accounted for almost $255 million of the University's $400 million revenues in the same year.[17] The Health Services Division of the University includes, in addition to the university hospital, the Children's Rehabilitation Hospital (CRH), formerly located on its own grounds near the city's boundaries with the western Main Line, but now occupying one floor of Jefferson Park Hospital, and Jefferson Park Hospital (JPH), formerly West Park Hospital, as well as for-profit subsidiaries, such as a pharmacy, a realty company (medical office building), and home health care services.

Additional explicit financial constraints challenge the urban teaching hospitals such as TJUH. Because they provide medical care to many indigent patients, they are jeopardized by the unwillingness and inability of local governments to pay what might be considered their fair, timely share of the costs of this care. In addition, university hospitals provide capital intensive, tertiary care to the very sickest of patients. The requirements of this sophisticated care include the support of resident teaching programs, and, therefore, engender greater per bed costs than are experienced by nonteaching community hospitals.

In spite of these unique financial difficulties facing urban university hospitals, Jefferson's loyal volunteer and salaried attending physicians, many of whom are well known outside the Philadelphia area and who attract large numbers of adequately insured patients from wide geographical areas, and the University's group of extremely capable professional medical managers, have together helped Jefferson attain its enviable fiscal position. The ability of the faculty to attract patients from afar is not only sustainable, but also essential to the institution's success. In 1988, of the six university hospitals in Philadelphia (Hahnemann University Hospital, Thomas Jefferson University Hospital, the Hospital of the Medical College of Pennsylvania, the Hospital of the University of Pennsylvania, Temple University Hospital, and the Hospital of the Philadelphia College of Osteopathic Medicine), only Hahnemann and Jefferson demonstrated a net income from operations.[18] Jefferson's net income from operations was over $16 million, with almost 24,000 inpatient admissions and over 200,000 patient days. TJUH currently operates in excess of capacity, far exceeding the national and regional average daily hospital occupancy rate of 65 percent. Nevertheless, demographic variables, legislative and regulatory changes in payments for services, and even such mundane events as physician retirement threaten the institution's competitive advantage. Because "brand loyalty" is not a characteristic of the health care industry, and medical decisions are largely a one-time, one-event "purchase," the vagaries of health care demand affirmative, often bold, decisions.

JEFFERSON PARK (WEST PARK) HOSPITAL

The Challenge

The Jefferson-owned CRH, a 40-bed chronic care pediatric facility, was originally located on nine acres of commercially valuable property (fair market value approximately $3 million) at Philadelphia's western boundary. In 1987, the buildings were in need of significant refurbishing, with costs estimated at $4 to $6 million.

Concurrently, West Park Hospital (WPH), a 131-bed, not-for-profit, community hospital was floundering two blocks away. On this site for about 25 years, WPH had tried to compete with other more prestigious hospitals in the affluent western suburbs but had been unsuccessful in attracting a large enough volume of privately insured or self-pay patients to remain solvent. Most WPH physicians had another hospital appointment, so that as its financial difficulties mounted and needed maintenance was postponed, attending physicians became even less comfortable admitting their patients, and difficulties begat difficulties. Even though only 100 beds were staffed, occupancy fell as low as 40 percent of this number. Additionally, lax management policies made third party reimbursements difficult to collect, and WPH went further into debt. Adding even further to the hospital's problems, an unfavorably publicized late-term abortion resulting in the criminal prosecution of one of the members of the medical staff tarnished the hospital image, and both physicians and patients were reluctant to be associated with the institution.

The Solution

Gasping for survival, struggling to meet its biweekly payroll, the hospital's board of trustees searched for a white knight to rescue the institution from bankruptcy. Several West Park physicians also held Jefferson appointments, so that Jefferson was among the hospitals approached. Readily apparent were the

Gasping for survival, struggling to meet its biweekly payroll, the hospital's board of trustees searched for a white knight to rescue the institution from bankruptcy.

benefits that would accrue to WPH by an association with Jefferson; its prestige would be restored, a financially secure institution would guarantee payment of its debts and reorganize its management, and additional influential Jefferson physicians might be willing to admit their patients. Above all, the viability of the hospital would be assured.

Why should Jefferson risk its enviable position at the top of the Philadelphia hospital heap to bail out WPH? At first glance, it might appear to be a no-win situation. Nevertheless, several immediate and long-term strategic benefits fell into place as the situation was reviewed, and Jefferson entered into an affiliation agreement with the board of WPH in November of 1987. This agreement effectively replaced the management of WPH with Jefferson-trained and experienced personnel and elected Jefferson trustees to a majority position on the governing board. Included in the agreement was a name change, Jefferson Park Hospital, to identify its Thomas Jefferson University connection.[19]

Children's Rehabilitation Hospital

Probably the most significant immediate benefit was related to the proximity of CRH. By relocating CRH to Jefferson Park, refurbishing expenses would be limited to those needed to modernize enough space at JPH to accommodate the patients from CRH. Renovating one floor of JPH for these 40 patients saved between $3 and $5 million. (The renovations cost about $1 million to complete.) Although retaining its own license, the transfer of CRH to the Jefferson Park facility virtually guaranteed the occupancy of between 30 and 40 beds daily, almost the entire pre-acquisition occupancy of West Park. By sharing services such as housekeeping, maintenance, security, dietary, and medical records, economies of scale between JPH and CRH saved about $800,000 in the first year. Additionally, the site occupied previously by CRH is available for sale for commercial development; because of Jefferson's tax-exempt status, the only costs incurred to maintain that property until an appropriate sale price can be obtained are relatively modest expenses for liability insurance and security.

Overflow Patients

Because TJUH is operating virtually at capacity, overflow "Jefferson" patients may be admitted to JPH in lieu of the main university hospital but as an equivalent facility, without the prior stigma attached to West Park. Physicians on the TJUH staff have been urged to consider JPH, especially for their patients who live in that neighborhood or in the contiguous suburbs.

A smaller benefit to Jefferson was the expectation that patients initially admitted to JPH who needed tertiary care would be transferred to TJUH. Although patients are currently being transferred with greater frequency than before the acquisition, the loyalties and referral patterns of former West Park physicians who had dual appointments to other university hospitals in Philadelphia (e.g., Hahnemann or Medical College of Pennsylvania) have been slow to change. It will still take some time to influence these well-established patterns of referral to favor TJUH.

Economic Benefits

A major strategic benefit to Jefferson from the acquisition of JPH is related to forecasts of third party payor policy decisions. Because TJUH is the University's focal point for the introduction and exploitation of advances in technology and other clinical research activities, as well as being a tertiary care center, its costs are high. Insurance plans, especially managed care plans such as health maintenance organizations (HMOs), are reluctant and unwilling to pay this premium if equivalent care can be delivered in a lower-cost setting (i.e., in a community hospital). Price differentiation within the university hospital for similar services, but for different medically intensive illnesses, is all but impossible to implement, but JPH as a separate, satellite institution may respond to these economic constraints and deliver Jefferson care at a significantly lower cost. Direct price competition with suburban community hospitals becomes a reality.

Cosmetic surgery is one such example. Many patients undergoing these procedures are self-pay—not covered by any insurance plan. Because these healthy patients are undergoing elective surgery with predictably short lengths of stay, a bundled package of hospital services may be offered to them at a favorable rate, much less than the same procedure would cost if performed at TJUH. There are advantages to the surgeons, as well, using the same team of operating room and floor nurses, who become familiar with techniques and care plans, and these efficiencies ultimately transfer to the patient as better-managed and more comfortable, comforting care.

With respect to capacity, the acquisition of JPH has given Jefferson more inpatient beds, albeit at a satellite location. Because Philadelphia area hospital beds are not used to capacity, with average hospital census about 65 percent, it has been virtually impossible for TJUH to convince regulatory authorities to permit an increase in its own capacity, regardless of its current excess need. Not only does JPH provide additional needed room for expansion of inpatient capacity, but it also provides room for negotiation for additional beds at the central Philadelphia (Center City) location. Although it is not currently likely that a direct bed-for-bed exchange could made, it is possible that a compromise could be reached so that, for example, the closing of $2x$ beds at JPH could release x beds for new construction at the university hospital. Although not part of Jefferson's current strategic plan, however, this option is a consideration that might be raised in response to unforeseen changes in regional health care systems that occur in the next several years. So long as there is CON regulation in Pennsylvania, it will be difficult to convince regulatory authorities to permit an increase in capacity at TJUH, but it is considered likely that the CON law will be abandoned in the near future. Moreover, several Philadelphia area hospitals have recently filed for Chapter 11 bankruptcy protection, so that the regional decrease in the number of inpatient beds is almost a certainty.

Care of the Chronically Ill

A significant problem for every hospital, and especially for tertiary care facilities, more vexing now that third party reimbursement (Medicare) is related to the diagnosis, but not yet to the actual severity of the illness, is the care of the chronically ill. These patients may require university hospital care when acutely ill, but when their condition improves, they became problems for disposition. The patients occupy expensive tertiary care beds, but their needs become less acute and less intensive, and the cost of their care prohibitively exceeds their medical requirements. The hospital is forced to accept the economic burden of this care. Although the same framework exists, and patient care still may not be reimbursed past a given point, the ability to transfer patients from TJUH to WPH without sacrificing quality of care becomes a means of minimizing institutional losses from non-reimbursed care, because daily costs at WPH are significantly lower than those at TJUH.

Two types of patients are currently being transferred from TJUH to JPH—long-term patients requiring placement or requiring a lower level of care, and patients seen in the emergency department at TJUH for whom an extended wait for a bed is likely. The majority of this latter group have been medical patients not already under the care of a Jefferson physician, or patients of the pulmonary division. (The pulmonary division at TJUH manages the critical care units at JPH.) In 1989, 49 extended care patients were transferred from TJUH to JPH, and in the past 6 months, 104 patients were transferred from the emergency department of TJUH to JPH. Additionally, the Foot and Ankle Center has been opened at JPH as a satellite of an existing center at TJUH. Approximately 60 outpatients are currently seen weekly, and both inpatient and outpatient activity is growing steadily.

Emergency Department

Emergency care has been another emerging specialty within medicine, as residency programs in this discipline have developed, and large institutions have developed networks of referrals, funnelling major trauma cases and other ultra-acute, life-threatening problems to designated and approved trauma centers, such as TJUH. Strengthening the emergency department at JPH by the appointment of certified specialists in emergency medicine and fortifying its association with Jefferson's Trauma Center establishes a university presence where it had not been extant previously. The emergency department at JPH represents strategic access to this acute care referral network, Between 1983 and 1987, as the number of inpatient admissions at JPH fell precariously, visits to the emergency department increased by 79 percent, and further increases are projected.

Patient Population

The community adjacent to JPH is demographically diverse but includes a disproportionately large number of elderly patients, living in nearby high-rise apartment buildings and several senior citizen retirement homes in the neighborhood. These patients find it difficult and intimidating to come by bus or taxi to Center City TJUH for their health care, and if quality care were convenient, they would almost certainly choose their neighborhood hospital (JPH), recognizing that TJUH would be their back-up should the need for tertiary care arise. As the geriatric care delivered by JPH increases, educational and research programs that are initiated at TJUH and Jefferson Medical College in this subspecialty of internal medicine may be expanded to JPH or even located at JPH as a primary base.

Although short-term effects of the acquisition can be readily appreciated, the long-term effects of the WPH acquisition are perhaps more important to Jefferson's overall business strategy, and more easily understood by examining JPH's location within the Delaware Valley. Philadelphia is currently a shrinking city, plagued by numerous problems resulting in major population shifts to the suburbs, including individuals who, in other large urban areas such as Boston, Chicago, Houston, or Manhattan, would choose to live as well as work within the city limits. Concurrently, significant population growth is occurring at the outer edges of the suburbs, with relocation of businesses to large industrial parks that have competed successfully for

A generation of well-trained university hospital residents in all specialties has moved to the suburbs with the population . . . .

what would have always been considered city businesses, by virtue of lower local taxes, ease of parking, and fewer threats of urban violence. As the population disperses peripherally from the city, it is foreseeable that Center City hospitals, even university hospitals offering sophisticated care previously not generally available in the general community hospitals, will ultimately lose a larger proportion of patients to local hospitals, except for those problems that absolutely require tertiary care. A generation of well-trained university hospital residents in all specialties has moved to the suburbs with the population, so that university hospitals no longer have a monopoly on competent physicians and quality care.

It is in response to these changes that Jefferson Park may offer the University competitive advantages not otherwise available. JPH is located only blocks from an expressway exit, it is directly available to the western suburbs, and it has easily accessible parking, so that the intricacies of negotiating Center City traffic are avoidable. As the University's programs expand to the JPH location, university care can be merged with the community in a manner that is not available even at hospitals that are current teaching affiliates of the University. This creates the synergy that business strategists offer as the reasons for the success of corporate mergers. Even for those patients who require their care at TJUH (e.g., open-heart surgery, transplantation, radiation therapy), whatever preliminary preadmission testing is necessary may be performed at JPH, acquiescing to the patient's convenience but also assuring the rapid transfer of data within the same institution. Preoperative and postoperative outpatient care for patients undergoing surgery at TJUH may be accomplished at JPH by the establishment of office space for TJUH medical staff physicians; patients and their doctors may meet half-way, again making the trip convenient for the patient, but assuring continuity of care that may not be as efficiently performed by sending the patient too quickly back to his neighborhood referring physician.

Developing programs that are physician intensive but not technology driven—such as mental health care, preventive medicine, and primary care—may be better suited to the JPH environment than to the university hospital, for both patient comfort and economic concerns. As third party "pass-through" allowances for resident education fall, cost-conscious care becomes paramount, so new, untested educational programs that can be accomplished in a lower-cost setting become more easily justified. Burdening entrepreneurial ventures with actual prorated accounting allocations for overhead, professional staff, etc., virtually guarantees their failure. At least in a lower-cost setting, institutional managers will be less uncomfortable with these adjustments to generally accepted accounting principles as new programs are conceived and implemented.

It is still too early to judge the wisdom of the West Park/Jefferson Park acquisition. The acquisition was favorably influenced by the CRH situation; thus, from that point of view alone, the deal has been initially worthwhile. While Jefferson Park does not yet carry its own weight, the acquisition is little more than one year old. Break-even is forecast by the end of the third full year of management, fiscal year 1991. Fortunately, Jefferson's shoulders are broad enough, based upon its current financial strengths, and the strategic decisions are sound enough, to warrant a reasonable time to allow JPH to percolate. Jefferson's current management team has been consistently successful, and there is no reason to doubt its continued achievements in these areas in which it has already proved itself so competent.

METHODIST HOSPITAL

A 250-bed acute care hospital in South Philadelphia, Methodist Hospital had been affiliated with Jefferson Medical College since 1950 for the undergraduate education of students in medicine, surgery, orthopedics, and obstetrics and gynecology, and graduate education (residency affiliations) in these same specialties. Because program consolidation dictated by outside reviewers (Residency Review Committees) required the residencies in these specialties to anticipate withdrawing from Methodist Hospital, the rotation of medical students to the institution was similarly jeopardized. Concurrently, because of a major quarrel between the administration and the medical staff, leading to a decreased census as physicians admitted their patients elsewhere, Methodist's financial position became endangered. Management turnover did not improve the situation, and Jefferson's entire affiliation with Methodist Hospital was threatened.

As Methodist's separation from Jefferson became more likely, both institutions reassessed their positions and searched for a way to strengthen instead of terminate this traditional alliance. Jefferson examined its own position in Methodist's service area, South Philadelphia. A marketing study demonstrated that this catchment area represented a significant source of patients for TJUH, more TJUH inpatients (12 percent) coming from South Philadelphia than from any other single geographical area. Together, Methodist and TJUH had an almost 40 percent market share in South Philadelphia; when questioned, residents of the area listed Methodist as their preferred hospital, then Jefferson, despite the presence of several other community hospitals in this neighborhood. Because of the longstanding affiliation, a number of Jefferson physicians also admitted patients to Methodist, and vice versa. TJUH was also the preferred referral institution for clinical services not available at Methodist, such as open-heart surgery, radiation therapy, and cardiac catheterization, and about 175 inpatients annually had been transferred from Methodist to TJUH for tertiary care.

Armed with this information, Methodist's strategic importance to Thomas Jefferson University became more clear. As Methodist began to look elsewhere for a medical school affiliation, Jefferson began to see Methodist in a different light, better as partner than as competitor. A means was sought that would benefit both institutions, satisfying Jefferson Medical College's requirements for excellence in patient care and medical education, fortifying TJUH's patient base and potential for diversification, and relieving Methodist's management concerns. Because of Methodist's endowment restrictions, unlike West Park/Jefferson Park, a straightforward acquisition was not possible, but a "preferred affiliation" agreement was the structure and jargon that could be used to formalize this association.[20,21] (This unusual term was coined to denote a greater than standard affiliation but does not have any legal implications.) As structured, Methodist would retain its free-standing status, but the Health Services Division of Thomas Jefferson University, now including TJUH, CRH, and JPH, would become Methodist's management team. The chief executive officer (CEO) of Methodist Hospital would become a Jefferson employee; additionally, 4 of the 15 board members at Methodist would be appointed by Jefferson. Furthermore, from the educational viewpoint, chiefs of the clinical services at Methodist would be chosen with the approval of the respective department chairmen at Jefferson, strengthening both undergraduate and graduate education and more likely satisfying the requirements of the Residency Review Committees in the clinical specialties.

As the bond between Jefferson and Methodist strengthens, although their corporate identities have not merged, their goals have become more unified. For example, one of TJUH's significant referral sources has been southern New Jersey, from the Delaware River to the Atlantic Ocean; the segment of this area spreading eastward had also been a secondary source of patients for Methodist. Instead of the two institutions vying for these patients, those not needing Jefferson's more specialized care may be "shortstopped" at Methodist, yet still retained within the Jefferson physician/management/education network.

As with JPH, managed care programs that balk at the cost of tertiary care facilities if less costly community hospital beds are equally suitable may be accommodated at Methodist. Actually a second tier of care is present currently at Methodist, since it is less expensive than the university hospital but provides more sophisticated (and more costly) care than Jefferson Park. Methodist retains its individual status and mission as a community hospital, rather than as a Jefferson satellite. Even closer geographically to TJUH than JPH, but in a different direction, Methodist extends Jefferson's contiguous sphere of care south and east, as JPH extends it to the west. Adding Methodist, Jefferson becomes the largest system of acute care under common management in the Philadelphia/Delaware Valley region, and domination of the regional health care market becomes a greater reality. Anticipating the inevitable tighter squeeze for health care dollars by both vertical and horizontal integration of health services, Jefferson has achieved the luxury of time to assess priorities more carefully, rather than reacting only to the perils of each financial imbroglio as it presents. Jefferson's diversification into innovative programs is facilitated by these economies of scale, and medical markets may be more effectively segmented, maximizing utilization and efficiency within all of the individual entities that compose the entire Health Services Division of Thomas Jefferson University.

•   •   •

Capital investments in the health care industry have waxed and waned in popularity, initially expanding to capture virtually unlimited resources and then shrink-

Mergers and acquisitions of and by hospitals have created supersystems of health care on the assumption that economies of scale inevitably provide greater protection.

ing as these assets were more grudgingly allotted by federal and local governments and private industry. Mergers and acquisitions of and by hospitals have created supersystems of health care on the assumption that economies of scale inevitably provide greater protection, whether from direct market competitors, from regulatory agencies whose agendas seem to change according to political whim, from unforeseen scientific advances that render existing techniques obsolete, or from unforeseen social forces that propel demographic diversity. University hospitals have been relatively late entries into this arena of strategic management, sanctifying their nonprofit status by shibboleths of academic integrity until the survival of their scholarly undertakings has been threatened by financial failure.

The senior officers of Thomas Jefferson University have led the Philadelphia academic medical community in the quest to combine competent medical practice with proficient administrative skills. The acquisition of West Park/Jefferson Park Hospital and the "preferred affiliation" with Methodist Hospital have provided Jefferson with unique opportunities to broaden its population base for acute care inpatient admissions and open the window of opportunity for greater diversification within the health care market. How well Jefferson succeeds in these two ventures will influence its own future decisions as well as those of other academic medical centers as they plot their courses through the uncharted but indisputably hazardous waters of the 1990s.

REFERENCES

1. Gibb, B., Gibb, R., and Gibb, M. (The "BeeGees"). "Staying Alive", from *Saturday Night Fever*, Paramount Pictures, Hollywood, 1977.
2. Pauly, M.V. "Health Care Issues and American Economic Growth: Innovation in Financing Health Care." Paper presented at the 1988 Karl Eller Business/Academic Dialogue, Tucson, Ariz., December, 1988.
3. Mieling, T.W. "Market Overview." *Topics in Health Care Financing* 15, no. 4 (1989): 1–8.
4. Clement, J.P. "Corporate Diversification: Expectations and Outcomes." *Health Care Management Review* (1988): 7–12.
5. Wilks, C.L.F., and Choi, T. "Changing Criteria for Hospital Acquisitions." *Health Care Management Review* 13, no. (1988): 23–34.
6. Gordon, D.C., and Londal, D.F. "Guidelines to Capital Investment." *Topics in Health Care Financing* 15, no. 4 (1989): 9–17.
7. Pheil, D.P. "Looking to Acquire, Merge? Do Your Homework." *Hospitals* 61 (1987): 80.
8. Plimpton, C.G. "Keys to Formulating a Successful Business Combination." *Topics in Health Care Financing* 14, no. 4 (1988): 18–24.
9. Livingston, C.O. "Recent Developments Affecting Mergers and Acquisitions." *Topics in Health Care Financing* 14, no. 4 (1988): 53–59.
10. McFall, S.L., Shortell, S.M., and Manheim, L.M. "HCA's Acquisition Process: The Physician's Role and Perspective." *Health Care Management Review* 13, no. 2 (1988): 23–34.
11. Bergman, J.T., and McIntyre, B.J. "Structuring the Transaction." *Topics in Health Care Financing* 15, no. 4 (1989): 41–9.
12. Groner, C. "Hospital Mergers, Health Planning, and the Antitrust Law." *Journal of Legal Medicine* 7 (1986): 471–519.
13. Blackstone, E.A., and Fuhr, J.P., Jr. "Hospital Mergers and Antitrust: An Economic Analysis." *Journal Health Politics, Policy & Law* 14 (1989): 383–403.
14. Holthaus, D. "Rockford Merger: All in Favor, Say Nay." *Hospitals* 63 (1989): 58–9.
15. Bryant, L.E., Jr. "Should Not-for-Profit Organizations Be Exempt From Antitrust Laws?" *Healthcare Financial Management* 42 (1988): 70–85.
16. Shields, G.B. "Legal Aspects of Health Care Mergers and Acquisitions." *Topics in Health Care Financing* 15, no. 4 (1989): 62–73.
17. Thomas Jefferson University. "Thomas Jefferson University and the Community." In 1988 *Annual Report, Thomas Jefferson University*. Philadelphia, Penn.: Thomas Jefferson University, 1988.
18. Gaul, G.M. "A Grim Prognosis for Region's Hospitals." *Philadelphia (Sunday) Inquirer*, 5 March 1989: 1, 20.
19. Russell, A. *Benefits to TJU Health Services Division from Jefferson Park Linkage*. Philadelphia, Penn.: Thomas Jefferson University. Internal communication, 1 May 1989.
20. "Thomas Jefferson University and Methodist Hospital Agree to Preferred Affiliation." *New Directions* (Thomas Jefferson University) 9 May 1988: p. 1.
21. Thomas Jefferson University. *Methodist Hospital Planning Brief*. Philadelphia, Penn.: Thomas Jefferson University, 1988.

Hospital acquisition or management contract: A theory of strategic choice

Michael A. Morrisey
and
Jeffrey A. Alexander

Differences in the mission of the hospital and the multihospital system are key elements underlying the development of a management contract. Preliminary analysis suggests that the number of potential new acquisitions is severely limited, that contract management is not a stepping stone to acquisition, and that many recent management contracts appear to be attempts to overcome problems beyond the hospital's and the contractor's direct control.

Health Care Manage Rev, 1987, 12(4), 21–30
© 1987 Aspen Publishers, Inc.

The past decade has seen a fundamental change in the organization of the hospital industry. Multihospital systems grew by acquisition and management contract to become major forces in the delivery of hospital care. Throughout this period, however, there has been little systematic effort to explain the different conditions under which hospitals are being acquired by systems, entering into management contracts, or remaining freestanding. This article develops a unified theory of why these various options are chosen and offers a preliminary test of the model. It thereby offers managers and board members, as well as industry analysts, insight into the potential growth or divestiture of systems, addressing in particular the likely course of management contracts in relation to other affiliation options, such as acquisition.

ACQUISITIONS

The economics literature identifies three general motives for the acquisition of one firm by another. These are increased efficiency, the attainment of monopoly power, and tax considerations.[1] Increased efficiency is the broadest category. It can include better management in one firm and lower production costs as a result of economies of scale, economies of scope, or synergy. Monopoly power allows the merged firm to raise its prices above costs because of a lack of competing hospitals. Tax considerations relate to the ability of a profitable enterprise to acquire an unprofitable firm and use its accrued tax credits and depreciation to reduce the overall tax liability of the com-

Michael A. Morrisey, *Ph.D., is an Associate Professor in the School of Public Health at the University of Alabama at Birmingham. He has published in the areas of hospital–physician relationships, health maintenance organizations, and rate setting, and is examining the effects of Medicare prospective payment and employee initiatives to control health benefits costs.*

Jeffrey A. Alexander, *Ph.D., is an Associate Professor in the School of Health Related Professions at the University of Alabama at Birmingham. He has published in the area of multihospital systems, and his current efforts are directed toward issues of hospital restructuring.*

The research on which this article is based was funded by grant HS 05264 from the National Center for Health Services Research and Health Care Technology Assessment. The data contained herein were collected while the authors were with the Hospital Research and Educational Trust in Chicago, Illinois.

bined firm. For purposes of analysis an acquisition has occurred whenever a hospital has become owned, leased, or sponsored by a multihospital system. The system may be investor owned, organized as a religious or other nonprofit firm, or created by the state or local government.

The health services literature focuses on efficiency as the rationale for acquisitions by hospital systems. Writers on the subject have identified at least three general advantages system hospitals have compared to independent hospitals.[2-6] These include economic benefits such as economies of scale in providing medical services and access to capital; improved personnel and management benefits such as the ability to recruit, train, and retain high-quality medical and administrative staffs, expand referral networks, and provide access to administrative specialists to assist in coping with increasingly complex environments; and community benefits such as improved access and quality of care through enhanced resources, lower costs, and improved planning.

Ermann and Gabel have reviewed the literature on the effects of systems on hospital performance.[7] They conclude that systems make more efficient use of labor, have lower costs of capital, and have higher overall costs than independent hospitals. Differences in other outcomes are either nonexistent or contradictory. These findings, as has been argued elsewhere,[8] may result from the matched hospital design used in most studies. These studies have ignored why hospitals and systems have affiliated. Thus, if systems do not randomly choose hospitals, the approach to comparing performance is biased toward finding no differences.

CONTRACT MANAGEMENT

A management contract exists when the governing body of a hospital assigns the duties of managing the day-to-day operations of the institution to an organization other than the hospital. The board retains full control over hospital policy. A freestanding hospital, while also having its own fully autonomous governing board, has a management staff composed of hospital employees reporting exclusively to the hospital board.

Rationales for contract management have been less well developed in the literature, but a few authors have developed rationales for the existence of management contracts. Richards sees them as a mecha-

nism by which hospitals can acquire new management depth and experience.[9] The management firm is seen as able to take full advantage of economies of scale in recruiting management talent, developing and implementing cost accounting and accounts receivable techniques, and recommending and implementing strategic plans for the hospital. Brown and Money have noted that a contract provides the flexibility to bring in the necessary expertise to address the hospital's specific problems of marketing, physician relations, financing, or personnel management.[10]

On the other hand, Rundall and Lambert maintain that a major concern with contract management is that the management company will negotiate from a position of knowledge to buy financially distressed hospitals and change their missions from community service or services to the disadvantaged to those services that can cover the costs of the institution.[11]

While the literature is sparse, there is a growing body of knowledge on the strategies management contractors use in hospitals and on the performance of hospitals under contract. One could infer that the performance outcomes were largely the objectives the hospitals desired when they retained the management firm. They offer clues to the rationales for entry into contracts.

Wheeler and Zuckerman examined the process and effects of management contracts in 21 hospitals.[12] They found that in the first one to two years the firms concentrated on improving the financial position of the hospital through improved accounts receivable and pricing decisions, as well as changes in accounting and management information systems. In the second and third years attention focused on staff recruitment and retention. Subsequent years' activities focused on strategic planning and marketing of the hospitals' services. Kralewski et al. examined 20 pairs of matched hospitals run by nonprofit contract management firms.[13] The contract appears, over time, to restore the operating margin of managed hospitals to industry norms. In addition, the contract-managed hospitals exhibited a greater reliance on debt financing than did freestanding hospitals.

Alexander and Rundall examined 80 contract-managed hospitals and found contract-managed hospitals to operate somewhat more efficiently, to offer more inpatient services, and to refrain more often from cutting back on Medicare and Medicaid program participation than freestanding hospitals.[14] Levitz and

Brooke examined the relative performance of system-affiliated and freestanding hospitals in Iowa. While finding significant differences between freestanding and system hospitals with respect to profitability, pricing policy, labor productivity and staffing, they found virtually no differences between system-owned and contract-managed institutions.[15]

Hospital system executives present a mixed view of the desirability of entering into management contracts.

To further compound the ambiguity of outcome, hospital system executives themselves present a mixed view of the desirability of entering into management contracts. A series of interviews the authors conducted with system executives revealed a general disinclination to enter into management contracts on the part of most investor-owned systems. Most indicated that they did not encourage management contracts because they tended to be unprofitable ventures, largely because the system could not exercise enough control over the operations of the managed hospitals. The dissenting executive of an investor-owned system indicated that his system had a relatively large number of contracts in place, that they were profitable, and that some would likely result in acquisitions. However, he said that no contract was signed with the expectation that the hospital would eventually be acquired. Nonprofit-system executives were generally more interested in contract management than their investor-owned system counterparts. Some saw the contracts as adding to the system's bottom line. Others, particularly religious systems, saw management contracts as furthering their missions of maintaining or expanding a network of religious-based health care.

In short, the empirical literature is less than definitive as to the desirability of contract management relative to system ownership or freestanding status. Furthermore, there is no evidence on the extent or underlying conditions of hospitals' conversion from contract-managed to system-owned status.

THEORY

As with any theory, the theory of acquisition and contract management draws on the complexity of in-

dividual acquisitions or management contracts to identify the threads of commonality that run through a range of cases. The discussion begins with an analysis of a system's decision to acquire a hospital and is then expanded to include examination of the management contract. This analysis is based on an assumption of profit-maximizing hospitals and systems, which can be relaxed to include a broader look at the rationales for acquisition and contract management in nonprofit organizations.

Profit-maximizing firms

Acquisitions

The acquisition decision of the profit-maximizing system is essentially a comparison of the proposed sales price of the hospital with the expected net present value of its income stream. If the sales price is below the system's estimate of the hospital's net present value, the system acquires the hospital. Net present value, as calculated in equation 1, is simply the sum of expected revenue (R) in each time period (i) minus the expected costs in each period (C_i) over the expected life of the hospital (T). Because each time period is farther removed from the sales date (i = 0), the value of the revenue and costs in each period is discounted by the opportunity cost of funds $(1 + r)^i$, where r is the interest rate. (While calculations that allow for uncertainty, changing interest rates, and other complexities are available, they obscure the central issue.)

$$NPV = \sum_{i=1}^{T} (R_i - C_i)/(1 + r)^i \qquad (1)$$

A system will acquire a hospital only if it believes that the stream of net revenue exceeds the asking price of the hospital. The hospital will sell only if the system's bid exceeds its own calculations of net present value. Differences in bids and asking prices arise because of differences in R, C, or r. The system and the hospital may have differing views as to the growth of the market for hospital services, which would affect expected revenues and perhaps costs. The system may expect to have lower costs of operating the hospital and thus may expect to receive a larger net revenue flow than the current owner. Indeed, this is the presumed raison d'être of the system. Finally, the system may have a lower cost of capital than the hospital, perhaps because of lower risk of bankruptcy.

The system's calculation is actually more complex than the hospital's because the system must consider the indirect effects on its other member hospitals. It may acquire a teaching hospital, for example, predominantly because the perceived high quality and access to the full spectrum of services will increase the profits of all the system's hospitals.[16]

The net present value formula identifies the idealized information players on both sides of the acquisition will seek. However, that decision rule is driven by the estimates and expectations of the participants. Those estimates of revenues and costs are based on the future strength of the hospital's market and the relative abilities of the hospital's and the system's management. Figure 1 summarizes these market and management forces and their hypothesized effects on acquisition. Market factors are those elements beyond the control of the hospital. They include the composition of the population in the community and its growth, payment systems used by government and private insurers, regulation, and prices of labor and other inputs. Management factors are those elements of operation over which the board and its administrative and clinical agents have control. These include staffing, pricing, collectibles, services offered, marketing, and strategic planning.

FIGURE 1

THE ACQUISITION DECISION

Market Factors

	Favorable	Unfavorable
Strong	???	freestanding
Weak	acquired	???

(Management factors)

If a hospital is in an unfavorable market and is run by skilled, highly competent management, as in the upper right quadrant of Figure 1, it is unlikely to be acquired. Under these conditions, it is unlikely that the system can do anything to improve the hospital's performance. Alternatively, in the lower left quadrant, a poorly run hospital in a desirable market is likely to be acquired, because there are typically a wide variety of things the new owner can do to increase the hospital's profitability. In the remaining quadrants the acquisition decision depends on the relative divergence in expectations between the system and the hospital.

Management contracts

In this profit-maximizing model, contract management will appear only because of a divergence in expectations about the future desirability of the market; specifically, the hospital's view must be more optimistic than the system's. If expectations of the market are identical, the system will simply use its lower expected operating costs to offer a price acceptable to the hospital. On the other hand, if the hospital has sufficiently higher market expectations it will reject the buy-out option. It will, however, be able to acquire the management expertise through contract. The hospital will pay the price for the management contract and keep the remaining flow of net revenue for itself.

In this scenario there is little incentive for the system to enter the contract for the purpose of eventually acquiring the hospital. Unless the management firm is constrained from undertaking its best efforts it will have no basis on which to offer a price in excess of the hospital's estimate of net present value. Indeed, since management skill is the scarce resource, the system or management firm should be able to extract all the potential hospital profits through the contract—limited only by competition among management firms.

Nonprofit enterprises

Nonprofit secular and religious hospitals and systems differ from the foregoing profit-maximizing firms because of their missions. Their objectives may include care of the poor, provision of health care from a religious base, or provision of some services to the community that are not remunerative. Nonprofit organizations, however, have much in common with profit-maximizing firms. Specifically, without carefully managing resources and generating internal surpluses they are unable to devote resources to their missions.[17,18]

Acquisitions

A nonprofit system considering an acquisition must look at the same market and management factors as profit-oriented firms. Indeed, the interviews of system executives support this contention. Thus, the same decision model developed in Figure 1 is applicable, with the same implications for acquisition and contract management.

The weight that any given nonprofit system places on market variables, however, will generally be different from those used by profit-maximizing firms or other nonprofit systems. A Catholic system, for example, may give more weight to the number of Catholics in the community. Other systems may be particularly concerned about the services provided to the poor. These differences in mission have a number of implications for the model.

First, it implies that nonprofit systems will be more likely than for-profit systems to acquire hospitals in the lower right quadrant of Figure 1. That is, those systems will be willing in some instances to acquire hospitals in less economically favorable environments. They do so because their goals include significant objectives other than profit.

Second, and more fundamentally, the nature of the missions of acquiring and acquired firms now matter. An offer to buy a hospital at a price above the hospital's net present value may be commonly rejected because it will change the nature of the services provided by the institution. Therefore, systems and hospitals with similar missions are more likely to merge than are those with dissimilar objectives. For example, Catholic hospitals would merge with Catholic systems, private nonsecular hospitals would merge with private nonsecular systems, and so on.

Management contracts

In the context of incongruous missions, the management contract can be viewed as a mechanism for providing management expertise without abandoning the mission of the institution. Thus, regardless of the desirability of the local market, management contracts between organizations with different missions are expected. Examples include investor-owned systems managing religious, secular nonprofit, or government hospitals, or religious systems managing government, secular nonprofit, or other religious hospitals.

Some have argued that contract management may serve as a means to eventual acquisition. The theory offers some insight into the conditions under which such conversions may occur. First, it is obvious that only those hospitals that are candidates fo acquisition—those in the lower left quadrant of Figure 1—will be candidates for conversion. Second, the conversion will only be considered in situations of apparent mission conflict. If the missions had not been in conflict, the simple acquisition would have been less costly to orchestrate.

In this scenario the contract management period serves as a learning period for the hospital. It may discover that the management options available through contract are not sufficient to allow the hospital to capitalize on its market strength. That is, it may discover that the management deficiencies relate to board policy rather than operational decisions. Alternatively, the hospital board may discover that apparent differences in mission have little operational meaning in the provision of health care in this instance.

In principle the system can learn from the management contract as well. However, this learning is less valuable with respect to a future acquisition. First, the issue of mission conflict is irrelevant. The system knows its mission better than anyone and that mission would, of course, dominate after a subsequent acquisition. Second, the system can discover more about the hospital's market. It will discover either that the market is less desirable (implying no acquisition) or that it is even more desirable than originally thought (explaining why the hospital did not want to sell in the first place). Finally, the system can acquire more knowledge about the management problems of the institution. If the problems are worse than anticipated (implying greater opportunity for improve-

> *In the context of incongruous missions, the management contract can be viewed as a mechanism for providing management expertise without abandoning the mission of the institution.*

ment) the management firm can extract the profit by renegotiating the management contract, and an acquisition is unnecessary. Alternatively, the problems may be less severe than anticipated, in which case the management contract is quite remunerative and there is little incentive to acquire the institution.

Of course, these scenarios can be made more complex by including opportunistic behavior. While such forces can have major effects in individual transactions, over time mechanisms are developed to mitigate their effects.[19,20]

Testable implications

This model of acquisitions and management contracts has led to a number of hypotheses that are testable, at least in principle.

- Systems will acquire poorly managed hospitals located in favorable markets.
- Utility-maximizing (i.e., non-profit-maximizing) systems will acquire hospitals in less economically favorable markets than will profit-maximizing systems, on average.
- Acquisitions will be more likely to occur between systems and hospitals with similar missions.
- Contract management will exist only in hospitals with weak management. Market conditions are irrelevant.
- Contract management will lead to acquisition only in favorable markets.
- Contract management will more likely be between systems and hospitals with dissimilar missions.

PRELIMINARY TESTS

Several of these hypotheses can be subjected to preliminary tests on the basis of existing data. The data presented here are drawn primarily from the 1983 Multihospital System Validation Survey conducted by the American Hospital Association (AHA). This telephone survey of hospital system headquarters verified data collected from individual hospitals concerning the owned, leased, sponsored, or contract-managed status of the hospitals and the date they joined the system or changed status. It also identified additional system members. This discussion is limited to nonfederal, short-term, general acute care hospitals.

Table 1 presents data on the number of hospitals built or acquired by systems as of 1983. It was hy-

TABLE 1

HOSPITALS ACQUIRED BY MULTIHOSPITAL SYSTEMS

	Hospital ownership prior to acquisition			
	Investor owned	Religious	Secular nonprofit	Public
System ownership				
Investor owned	493	4	3	0
Religious	1	475	13	0
Secular nonprofit	10	103	234	8
Public	7	9	26	49

pothesized that hospital acquisition by systems would be more common when the system and the hospital had similar missions. Since information on the missions of organizations is not available, the ownership of the system and of the hospital prior to acquisitions were used as proxies. Thus, the investigators looked at whether the hospital or system was investor owned, religious, secular nonprofit, or run by a state or local government. While these ownership categories suggest some commonality of mission, there was substantial measurement error. For example, Catholic and Adventist hospitals do not have identical missions. Even hospitals that are legally investor owned may be owned and operated for objectives other than profit maximization. This may be the case for small for-profit hospitals owned by one or two physicians or local citizens. Nonetheless, the results provide striking support for the hypotheses. Ninety-six percent of investor-owned hospitals were acquired by investor-owned systems; 80 percent of religious hospitals were acquired by religious systems. Secular and public hospitals had similar experiences. The issue of similarity of mission appears to have been an essential element in hospital decisions to enter multihospital systems.

In contrast, it was argued that contract management was a mechanism to overcome conflicts over the goals of the hospital and the system. It was thought that contract management would be more prevalent when the hospital and the system had dissimilar missions. Table 2 supports this hypothesis to some extent. Generally the hospital is much more likely to be managed by a system with different goals. This is

TABLE 2

HOSPITALS CONTRACT MANAGED BY
MULTIHOSPITAL SYSTEMS

	Hospital ownership			
	Investor owned	Religious	Secular nonprofit	Public
System ownership				
Investor owned	31	7	132	130
Religious	1	36	20	30
Secular nonprofit	2	5	76	69
Public	0	0	0	0

particularly true with respect to hospitals managed by investor-owned systems where the conflict in goals is arguably most distinct. The diagonal elements of Table 2 offer partial support of the argument. The secular nonprofit and public hospital results are consistent with the theory, but the investor-owned and religious hospitals' contracts are not.

The mission conflict model has no role in the investor-owned hospital segment of the market. The investors' mission is achieved by selling at a price that exceeds the expected net present value. The explanation for the presence of these contracts is probably the profit-maximizing model, that is, the hospital recognizes management deficiencies but believes the expected net present value of the hospital exceeds the offered purchase price.

The results for religious hospitals refute the theory. However, it may be explained by measurement error. Jewish and Adventist systems do not necessarily have the same health care missions. Similarly, Catholic hospitals and systems run by different orders or dioceses may not have identical objectives. Therefore, it should be expected that some interreligious differences are reflected in the results.

The issue of conversion from contract management to ownership by a system is more difficult to test. It was hypothesized that this would occur only in favorable markets—and by extension—only in instances of mission conflicts. Table 3 presents data on the number of conversions from contract management to ownership from 1976–1982. The most interesting finding in Table 3 is its general lack of numbers. The data indicate that only 24 hospitals were converted

from contract management to system ownership during this period. This suggests that contracts are of long duration or that acquisition is not a primary motivation of management contracts.

Finally, as a test of the market and management hypotheses the investigators examined hospitals that were acquired by systems or were entering management contracts from 1982–1983. Market and management factors are truly multidimensional, but for this preliminary investigation single measures of each construct were examined.

A favorable market is defined as one in which there was no mandatory state rate-setting program and the five-year increase in county per capita income was in the top one-third of the sample counties. This was taken as indicative of community growth.

Management measures are always difficult to quantify because performance depends on the hospital's environment. Furthermore, because of the nonprofit nature of most hospitals and the accounting principle of valuing assets at book value, typical measures of, say, profitability or asset activity are suspect. Nevertheless, management was measured using the five-year change in the hospital's modified return on equity. (Due to limitations in the reported data modified return on equity was defined as net patient revenue divided by the unrestricted fund balance on the AHA Annual Survey.) Strongly managed hospitals were said to be in the top one-third of the distribution.

Table 4 summarizes the number of hospitals acquired by systems from 1982–1983. The cells of Table 4 and Table 5 are constructed on the arbitrary basis of

TABLE 3

MANAGEMENT CONTRACT CONVERTED TO
SYSTEM OWNERSHIP, 1976–1982

	Hospital ownership			
	Investor owned	Religious	Secular nonprofit	Public
System ownership				
Investor owned	8	0	3	3
Religious	0	3	3	1
Secular nonprofit	1	2	0	0
Public	0	0	0	0

TABLE 4

ACTUAL AND RANDOM DISTRIBUTION OF HOSPITAL ACQUISITIONS, 1982–1983

	Market factors	
	Favorable	Unfavorable
Management factors		
Strong	actual = 5 chance = 10 actual : chance = .5 II	actual = 9 chance = 20 actual : chance = .45 I
Weak	actual = 39 chance = 20 actual : chance = 1.95 III	actual = 37 chance = 40 actual : chance = .93 IV

favorable markets constituting one-third of all hospitals. Thus, the chance distribution of acquisitions and management contracts, respectively, is simply the number of acquisitions or contracts times the probability of being in each cell. Quadrant I of Table 4 is therefore $90 \times .67 \times .33 = 20$. It was hypothesized that profit-maximizing systems would seek to acquire hospitals in quadrant III, that is, those with weak management and favorable markets. This occurs almost twice as frequently as change would suggest. A corollary was that hospitals in unfavorable markets with strong management would least likely be acquired. As quadrant I indicates, this occurs only half as frequently as chance would allow, again giving preliminary confirmation of the model.

All systems, but particularly non-profit-maximizing firms, were hypothesized to seek acquisitions in quadrants II and IV. This was based on the expected revenues and costs associated with individual hospitals and, for non-profit-maximizing firms, on noneconomic factors. It appears from Table 4 that such actions tend to be biased toward weak management (quadrant IV) and away from favorable markets (quadrant II). The results in Table 4 are significant at the 99 percent confidence level using the Chi square test.

Table 5 presents the same comparisons for the 110 hospitals that entered into a management contract

during 1982 or 1983 and for which the requisite data were available. It was hypothesized that hospitals with weak management, regardless of market conditions, would seek to establish management contracts. This is found to be the case in quadrant IV but not in quadrant III. Quadrant I was anticipated to have few contracts as management was coping well with the market. Instead one finds one and one-half times as many contracts in place as one would expect by chance. Again, the pattern of results is different from that suggested by chance at the 99 percent statistical confidence level. In short, the preliminary evidence supporting the theory of contract management is mixed. One may observe, however, that the data suggest that hospital boards on many occasions seem to have entered into management contracts hoping that unfavorable market conditions could be overcome by new management. Similarly, it appears that hospital boards in favorable markets (quadrant III) have given up available earnings by not actively replacing weak management.

Comparisons between Table 4 and Table 5 are instructive. They point out the fundamental finding of this study. That is, acquisitions and management contracts occur under very different conditions. Acquisitions occur predominantly in poorly managed hospitals in favorable markets. Management con-

TABLE 5

ACTUAL AND RANDOM DISTRIBUTION OF HOSPITAL MANAGEMENT CONTRACTS, 1982–1983

	Market factors	
	Favorable	Unfavorable
Management factors		
Strong	actual = 6.0 chance = 12.2 actual : chance = .49 II	actual = 38.0 chance = 24.4 actual : chance = 1.56 I
Weak	actual = 16.0 chance = 24.4 actual : chance = .66 III	actual = 50.0 chance = 48.9 actual : chance = 1.02 IV

tracts exist primarily in unfavorable markets, and, ironically, are often instituted in situations where the previous management appears to have been reasonably strong. The comparisons also suggest that, if this theory is correct, the range of management contracts likely to result in system acquisitions is small.

DISCUSSION

The theory of hospital acquisition and contract management is based on the interaction of market factors in the hospital's environment and management factors indicating how well the hospital copes with its environment. Differences in the missions of the hospital and the system are key elements underlying the development of the management contract. Results of preliminary tests of the theory are generally consistent with the hypotheses developed. The theory, if borne out by more careful tests, offers a number of implications for the future of the hospital industry.

First, it suggests that a relatively limited number of hospitals will be attractive candidates for outright acquisition by multihospital systems. These hospitals are located in economically favorable markets and have weak management. It also suggests that in a divestiture, the hospitals in the relatively weakest markets will be sold or closed.

A relatively limited number of hospitals will be attractive candidates for outright acquisition by multihospital systems.

Second, the theory suggests that management contracts are stable organizational forms designed to provide operational efficiency without sacrificing the unique mission of the hospital. They do not appear to be stepping stones to system acquisition. However, while the theory suggests that management contracts will be used by hospitals with weak management, the simple data suggest that hospitals in weak markets, regardless of management strength, have entered into contracts. Whether this finding reflects the difficulty hospital boards have in separating market from management factors or whether it refutes the theory cannot be fully judged with the available data. If hospital boards become better judges of market and man-

agement factors, the use of contract management is likely to decline. In any case, the data suggest that a management contract may be a leading indicator of the eventual closure of the institution, not because of inept management by the contractual agents but because of deteriorating market conditions.

Third, the theory suggests that extreme care must be taken in analyzing performance differences between system-owned, contract-managed, and free-standing hospitals. If the theory is correct, matched sample comparisons should be based on the market, management, and mission of the institutions. The results of comparison studies, which have tended to find few differences, may simply reflect a comparison group deficiency.

Finally, the data, crude as they are, suggest that the theory should be subjected to further tests. More years of data and multivariate analyses of multiple measures of market and management factors will allow a solid basis for understanding system development and finding any true differences in performance. A particularly useful extension could involve the measurement difficulties hospital boards have in differentiating between poor markets and poor management.

REFERENCES

1. Copeland, T.E., and Weston, F. *Financial Theory and Corporate Policy.* 2d ed. Reading, Mass.: Addison-Wesley, 1983.
2. Lewin and Associates. *A Study of Investor-Owned Hospitals.* Chicago: Health Services Foundation, 1976.
3. Zuckerman, H. *Multi-Institutional Hospital Systems.* Chicago: Hospital Research and Educational Trust, 1979.
4. Mason, S. "Greater Access and Lower Costs with Multihospital Systems." *Hospital Financial Management* 35 (May 1980): 58–64.
5. Cooney, J., and Alexander, T. *Multihospital Systems: An Evaluation.* Chicago: Hospital Research and Educational Trust and Northwestern University, 1975.
6. DeVries, R. "Strength in Numbers." *Hospitals* 92 (March 1978): 81–89.
7. Ermann, D., and Gabel, J. "Multihospital Systems: Issues and Empirical Findings." *Health Affairs* 3, no. 3 (1984): 50–64.
8. Alexander, J.A., Lewis, B.L., and Morrisey, M.A. "Acquisition Strategies of Multihospital Systems." *Health Affairs* 4, no. 3 (1985): 49–66.
9. Richards, G. "The Growth of Contract Management." *Hospitals* 56, no. 19 (1982): 94–102.

10. Brown, M., and Money, W.H. "The Promise of Multi-hospital Management." *Hospital Progress* 56, no. 8 (1975): 36–42.

11. Rundall, T.G., and Lambert, W.K. "The Private Management of Public Hospitals." *Health Services Research* 19 (1984): 519–44.

12. Wheeler, J.R., and Zuckerman, H.S. "Hospital Management Contracts: Institutional and Community Perspectives." *Health Services Research* 19 (1984): 499–518.

13. Kralewski, J.E., et al. "The Effects of Contract Management on Hospital Performance." *Health Services Research* 19 (1984): 479–98.

14. Alexander, J.A., and Rundall, T.G. "Contract Management of Public Hospitals: An Assessment of Operating Performance." *Medical Care* 23, no. 3 (1985): 209–19.

15. Levitz, G.S., and Brooke, P.P., Jr. "Independent versus System-Affiliated Hospitals: A Comparative Analysis of Financial Performance, Cost and Productivity." *Health Services Research* 20 (1985): 315–40.

16. Alexander, J.A., Lewis, B.L., and Morrisey, M.A. "Acquisition Strategies of Multihospital Systems." *Health Affairs* 4, no. 3 (1985): 49–66.

17. Long, H.W. "Valuation As a Criterion in Not-For-Profit Decision-Making." *Health Care Management Review* 1, no. 3 (1976): 134–52.

18. Conrad, D.A. "Returns on Equity to Not-For-Profit Hospitals: Theory and Implementation." *Health Services Research* 19 (1984): 41–64.

19. Klein, B., Crawford, R.G., and Alchian, A.A. "Vertical Integration, Appropriable Rents, and the Competitive Contracting Process." *Journal of Law and Economics* 21 (1978): 297–326.

20. Williamson, O. *Markets and Hierarchies: Analysis and Antitrust Implications.* New York: Free Press, 1975.

Hospital alliances: Cooperative strategy in a competitive environment

Howard S. Zuckerman
and
Thomas A. D'Aunno

The resource dependence perspective is used to describe the formation of hospital alliances. Characteristics of alliances and their various strategies and structures are discussed. A life cycle model provides a framework for viewing the development and growth of alliances. Several dimensions for assessing alliance performance are proposed.

Health Care Manage Rev, 1990, 15(2), 21–30
Reproduced by permission of Delmar Publishers, Inc., from
Competitive Strategies in the Health Care Market, by Kronenfeld,
Amidon, and Toomey.

In adapting to changing environmental and industry conditions, hospitals have employed a range of interorganizational arrangements.[1,2] Among the forms of interorganizational activity is the hospital alliance or federation.

ALLIANCES DEFINED

Alliances are defined to consist of three or more organizations that pool resources to achieve stated objectives. Alliances are selective as to membership, using criteria to include or exclude additional members. This selectivity distinguishes alliances from trade associations, which typically encourage participation of virtually all organizations in a given field or industry. A distinctive feature of alliances is that their activities are coordinated and, to some extent, directed by a management group or organization.[3] Alliances may hold important advantages for their members. Unlike mergers and many joint ventures, for example, alliances involve no change in the corporate ownership of firms and, as a result, are easier both to enter and to leave. This may be one reason that, since the late 1970s, at least 15 hospital alliances have emerged, which include over 1,600 members.[4] Indeed, almost 30% of the nation's hospitals are members of alliances, and the number appears to be growing.

Hospital alliances (federations) should be examined for several reasons. Understanding hospital alliances is important to health care managers. Given the growth of alliances, knowledge of their behavior is becoming increasingly important, not only for hospital administrators but also for managers of a variety of organizations that interact with hospitals.

Furthermore, hospital alliances may increase the concentration of health care resources. Such concentra-

Howard S. Zuckerman, *Ph.D., is an Associate Professor in the Department of Health Services Management and Policy, School of Public Health, The University of Michigan. His primary areas of research, teaching, and publication have centered on the development, growth, strategies, structures, and performance of multiinstitutional organizations.*

Thomas A. D'Aunno, *Ph.D., is an Assistant Professor in the Department of Health Services Management and Policy, School of Public Health, The University of Michigan, and a Faculty Associate at the Institute for Social Research. His research, teaching, and publications have centered on the areas of organization–environment relations and interorganizational behavior and strategy.*

tion may raise questions for policymakers about the effects of alliances on the cost of, quality of, and access to health care.

Finally, hospital alliances are of interest to researchers and theorists concerned with organizational adaptation to environmental change such as that now occurring in health care, banking, transportation, and communications. Hospital alliances exemplify organizational strategies that involve cooperation among organizations rather than competition.[5]

CONCEPTUAL PERSPECTIVE: RESOURCE DEPENDENCE

Previous research on organizational federations has drawn largely from a conceptual perspective in organizational theory referred to as the resource exchange and dependence perspective.[1,3,6-10] This work has examined factors that facilitate the emergence of federations and factors that influence the autonomy of organizations in federations.

The resource (or external) dependence model assumes that, in the face of turbulent, complex, and constrained environmental conditions, organizations will not remain passive. Rather, they will develop strategies and structures designed to allow adaptation. Organizations will attempt to position themselves to reduce uncertainty, to reduce dependency, and to stabilize and manage the environment.[8,11,12] Organizations often cannot generate internally all of the necessary resources or functions; therefore, they enter into exchange relationships with other elements in the environment. The need to establish such interorganizational relationships is the essence of the resource dependence model. The model suggests that organizations adopt strategies to secure access to critical resources, to stabilize relations with the environment, and to enable survival. Furthermore, the model views organizations as capable of changing or influencing as well as simply responding to the environment.

However, organizations can reduce or manage dependence problems in several ways, including contractual arrangements, joint ventures,[13] mergers,[12] and interlocking boards of directors.[14,15] Why then might organizations form alliances or federations to deal with resource dependence instead of using some other strategy?

One answer is that, compared to other available strategies, alliances are relatively low cost in terms of managerial autonomy.[6] Secondly, alliances enable individual firms to band together, act as one, and thus increase their power in exchanges with suppliers of valued resources. By banding together, organizations can create an impression of size and strength; they appear to concentrate their resources and, in so doing, can more effectively bargain for their point of view with groups in the environment.

In comparison to looser coalitions of firms, alliances have the advantage of a management group that can act to develop and represent positions on issues confronting member organizations. In comparison to trade associations, federations may have fewer and less-diverse members, thereby making it somewhat easier to build consensus among them.

Another factor that may influence the emergence of alliances is the extent to which organizations share material interests. Consider, for instance, hospitals that are geographically dispersed and similar in terms of characteristics such as the kind of services they offer or the type of community in which they are located. Such hospitals are likely to face similar patterns of resource dependence and, as a result, have similar problems to solve. Likewise, organizations may share similar values, beliefs, or ideology that may serve as a basis on which an alliance or federation may emerge. Thus, there appear to be a number of factors that make alliances an attractive form of interorganizational collaboration aimed at reducing dependency while maintaining autonomy.

CHARACTERISTICS OF ALLIANCES

Alliances may be characterized along a number of dimensions, including stated purposes, basis of organization, structural forms, membership criteria, financing, and governance and management structure. The scope and nature of programs, services, and activities also serve to describe alliances.

Stated purposes

The stated purpose of alliances reflects the intent to secure for members the advantages of large size and scale while retaining individual ownership and control. Such stated purposes often seek to help members attract and retain needed human and financial resources; enhance access to capital; protect and strengthen market position; yield economies of scale through joint activities; develop new sources of revenue; contain costs; and provide management, consulting, and other services to members. Given the membership of these organizations, it is not surprising to find reference to assuring the continued viability of the voluntary, not-for-profit sector. Neither is it surprising to find concern with retaining the values and presence of particular religious denominations in the delivery of health care services. Some alliances espouse a political role, including lobbying and advocacy. A number of alliances seek to link delivery and financing of services, and thus include horizontal integration, vertical integration, diversification, and insurance products. This last statement of purpose may suggest a move from an association model to a more business-oriented role for the alliances.

Basis of organization

Alliances have been organized around several themes. Some are geographically defined: For example, Voluntary Hospitals of America (VHA) and American Healthcare System (AmHS) are national in scope, while SunHealth and the Yankee Alliance are regional. Other alliances are organized around common religious preferences, such as Consolidated Catholic Health Care (CCHC). Still others center on particular types of institutions—for example, the University Hospital Consortium (UHC). Premier Hospitals Alliance, which originated as the Consortium for Jewish Hospitals, now focuses on large, urban teaching hospitals. Thus, alliances have emerged around several organizing themes, each theme representing a common set of interests, beliefs, or dependencies.

Structural forms

Alliances have assumed a variety of structural forms. For example, some have been organized as rather loosely coupled consortia, with a high degree of autonomy and control retained by the individual members, seen in cases where members are unwilling or unable to make more substantial commitment. Others have been established as joint ventures among a group of hospitals or hospital systems. Still others are structured as nonprofit holding companies, serving as umbrella organizations within which various taxable and nontaxable subsidiaries may be created. A growing number of alliances are for-profit, taxable corporations or

cooperatives, again reflecting a shift in purpose and role and providing for flexibility in programmatic areas. Furthermore, the corporate or cooperative model allows for an equity position by the individual members, which is believed by some to be a useful mechanism to increase the degree of members' commitment to an alliance.

Membership criteria

Unlike traditional associations, membership in alliances is selective. Many alliances are composed of organizations that are already relatively large and strong. The more than 100 shareholders comprising VHA usually are at least 500-bed hospitals. AmHS is composed of over 30 shareholders, including some of the larger not-for-profit multihospital systems in the country. Large teaching hospitals, typically having more than 400 beds, dominate SunHealth, Premier Hospitals Alliance, and the UHC. As they evolved, the alliances developed explicit, often formal, criteria by which to assess potential new members. Such criteria often relate to various characteristics of potential members, such as mission, operating philosophy, size, revenues, management capability, financial status, market position, clinical reputation, and range of services offered.[16,17]

Several alliances have expanded their membership to include other organizations affiliated with the core shareholders. For example, SunHealth has been rapidly developing regional networks in the states served by its members,[18] while VHA has established regional partnerships for service delivery and business ventures.[19]

Financing

Costs of membership in alliances vary widely. Initial entry fees may range from a few thousand dollars to as much as $250,000. Annual costs also vary, but it is not uncommon to find expenditure levels of $25,000 to $60,000. In addition, there may be one-time assessments for new program initiatives and capitalization requirements to start new businesses.

Governance and management structure

The governing body of an alliance characteristically includes the chief executive officers (CEOs) of all member organizations. The board chairperson is elected from among the CEOs. The larger alliances also are likely to have executive committees or executive boards to guide the ongoing activities of the alliance,

---

As they evolved, the alliances developed explicit, often formal, criteria by which to assess potential new members.

with the full board meeting only periodically, perhaps two or three times per year. Governance of alliance subsidiary corporations tends to be more diverse, including other individuals from member organizations and, sometimes, external representatives. The size and scope of the management group will, of course, vary with the activities of the alliance.

Programs, services, and activities

Programs, services, and activities offered by or through the alliances cover a broad spectrum. They may be generally identified within six categories: economies of scale/cost containment; human and financial resources; influence; services to members; revenue generation; and market position. Each of these areas of activity is illustrated in the box, "Alliance Programs and Services."

Economies of scale/cost containment

Alliances seek to take advantage of their relatively large size to secure economies of scale for their members. To this end, virtually all the alliances have developed their own (or serve as a broker to provide access to) joint purchasing programs. Such programs are used to buy medical and surgical supplies, capital equipment, and pharmaceuticals. While some alliances use a diverse set of suppliers, others use preferred distributors or prime-supplier arrangements with particular vendors in efforts to secure volume discounts, better service, and limits on price increases. Some alliances also serve as brokers in providing support services to members, gaining pricing advantages for the members while reducing marketing costs to suppliers.[20] Economies of scale also are sought through insurance programs, which may include various types of liability coverage, malpractice coverage, workers' compensation, and risk management.

Human and financial resources

Acquisition/retention of needed resources is an area of activity in many alliances. Several alliances provide assistance to members in the recruitment of clinical and management personnel. Continuing education programs, especially for trustees and managers, are often available. Management development programs using external consultants or universities are also offered through some of the alliances. Some alliances have established councils or forums to provide for exchange of information among managers in various functional

---

Alliance Programs and Services

Economies of scale/cost containment:
   Purchasing
   Insurance programs

Resources, human and financial:
   Human:
      Recruitment
      Education and development
      Forums and councils
      Fringe benefits
   Financial:
      Access to capital
      Tax-exempt financing
      Bond insurance

Influence:
   Political lobbying
   Brand name promotion
   Image building

Services to members:
   Management:
      Marketing/planning
      Management engineering
      Consulting
      Feasibility studies
   Technical:
      Biomedical engineering
      Equipment maintenance
      Mobile computed tomography scanning

Revenue generation:
   Home health or DME
   Diversification
   Equity-ownership
   Cash management
   Investment opportunities

Market position:
   Vertical integration
   HMO or PPO
   Insurance products
   Regional networks

---

areas, such as finance, planning, and human resources, among others. These forums enable high-level functional specialists to work with their counterparts in other alliance member organizations.

Enhancing access to financial resources, particularly capital, is a programmatic area within several alliances. For example, alliances have developed bond insurance programs for their members as well as tax-exempt financing programs to provide members with access to capital at preferred rates. Several alliances are organizing venture capital investment opportunities as well.

Influence

A small number of alliances have made explicit attempts to increase their political power through efforts such as lobbying. For example, AmHS has established the American Healthcare Institute, located in Washington, D.C., the purpose of which is to develop and transmit AmHS philosophies and concerns through research, communications, and public affairs activity.[21] Several alliances have sought to enhance their images through marketing and advertising, and there is some evidence of alliance "brand-name" promotion.

Services to members

Management services are available to members in most alliances. Such services might include general consulting, management engineering, marketing, planning, financial feasibility studies, assistance in development of regional delivery networks, information systems, productivity management, and cost control programs. Several alliances are developing comparative databases to enable members to compare cost and performance with their peers.

Technical services are available in several alliances, particularly those whose members are geographically proximate. SunHealth, for example, offers biomedical engineering, plant and construction engineering, mobile computed tomography scanning, and maintenance and repair of high-technology medical imaging equipment.[22]

Revenue generation

Generation of new sources of revenue is yet another area of alliance activity. Several alliances have sought to broker joint ventures to develop home health care and durable-medical-equipment programs, with the profits from sales and leases to be shared by the members. Premier Hospitals Alliance and the UHC are seeking to capitalize on the characteristics of their members by enabling hospitals to serve as test sites for clinical trials and technological assessment.[23,24] Centralized cash management programs are another means to increase rates of return for members. Furthermore, several alliances have developed investment opportunities for member organizations.

Market position

An area currently receiving substantial attention is that of protecting and strengthening the market position of the alliances and their members. SunHealth and VHA, as noted above, are developing regional networks to link alliance members with other hospitals in a state or region. In the process, they enhance the market and the competitive positions of the participants. Several alliances have sought to provide vehicles for vertical integration and diversification in such areas as ambulatory surgery, chemical and alcohol dependency, mental health services, home health care, and ambulatory care. For example, CCHC, through a joint venture, seeks to assist members in developing congregate housing projects and services for the elderly. UHC and Premier, through the clinical research activities

---

An area currently receiving substantial attention is that of protecting and strengthening the market position of the alliances and their members.

---

noted above, aim to enhance the position of their members vis-à-vis other large teaching hospitals. Attempting to link delivery and financing on a national basis, VHA has entered into a joint venture with the Aetna Life Insurance Company to market health maintenance organizations (HMOs) and preferred provider organizations (PPOs) through VHA hospitals and is developing a network of PPOs with the International Brotherhood of Teamsters.[25] AmHS (having ended a joint venture with Provident Life and Accident Insurance Company) and SunHealth, rather than trying to build insurance programs for the alliance, are seeking to assist shareholders in the development of managed care products in their respective markets.[26,27]

DEVELOPMENT OF ALLIANCES

The literature on alliances and federations has centered primarily on why they emerge and what they do. Relatively less attention has focused on how alliances evolve and their behavior over time. The development of alliances may be cast in the context of a life cycle model. The model draws from the literature on life cycle models of individual firms[28–30] and development processes of multiunit organizations.[31,32] Such a model suggests that organizations move through predictable stages of growth, with one or more factors triggering such movement. Furthermore, each stage brings distinctive tasks to be addressed by the organization. The

TABLE 1

A LIFE CYCLE MODEL OF HOSPITAL ALLIANCES

Stage 1: Emergence of an alliance	Stage 2: Transition of an alliance	Stage 3: Maturity of alliance	Stage 4: Critical crossroads
Key factors in development at each stage			
Environment poses threat to and uncertainty about valued resources	Motivation to achieve purposes of the alliance	Willingness to put alliance interests first	Increased centralization and dependence on alliance motivates members to seek hierarchy or withdraw from alliance
Organizations share ideologies and similar dependencies	Increased dependence on alliance for valued resources	Members receive benefits from previous investments	
Examples of tasks at each stage			
Define purposes of the alliance	Hire or form a management group	Attain stated objectives	Manage decisions about future of the alliance
Develop membership criteria	Establish mechanisms for coordination and control	Sustain member commitment	

Reprinted with permission from the *Academy of Management Review* 12, no. 3 (1987): 538.

life cycle model of hospital alliances was recently proposed in some detail and is summarized in Table 1.[6]

Emergence

In the first or emergence stage, environmental threats and uncertainty lead organizations with similar ideologies and dependencies to seek or to form coalitions. In this initial stage, the purposes and expectations of the alliance are stated, membership criteria are established, and group norms begin to evolve. It is important that expectations be realistic and that mechanisms for assessment of benefits and costs be established early. Membership criteria are selective, designed to assure homogeneity among members. Furthermore, by limiting overlap in market areas, such criteria seek to minimize competition among members and avoid antitrust issues.

It might be recognized that the purposes of an alliance may shift somewhat over time; in recent years, for example, there is indication of movement away from association-type interests and toward business-type

purposes. Nevertheless, an issue that continues to arise and require attention is the degree to which an alliance remains true to its fundamental purposes, which revolve around the needs of its members.

Transition

In the second or transition stage, the alliance establishes mechanisms for coordination, control, and decision making. This stage can be somewhat difficult in that it is here that the management group is formed to oversee the activities of the alliance. While recognizing the need for such coordination, members may be reluctant to grant authority to management or sacrifice their own individual autonomy. It thus becomes incumbent on management to assure that alliance activities are responsive to member needs; on the other hand, members must deal with the necessity to commit to the alliance in order for it to achieve its purposes.

In this transition stage, the governance structure takes shape. As noted earlier, it is typical that the CEOs of the member hospitals or hospital systems form the governing body. There develops something of a dilemma with regard to board size, especially as alliances grow, between the interest of members in participating directly in the governance function and the need for more rapid and timely decision making. Some alliances have created executive boards or executive committees in an attempt to resolve the dilemma.

Governing bodies of alliances, composed of CEOs, are clearly insider-dominated boards. This is in contrast to developments in some other industries that appear to be moving toward more externally focused boards. It is also apparently a logic different from that used to constitute hospital or hospital system boards: They are characterized by the selection of individuals representing key stakeholders or constituencies or individuals who bring to the board particular expertise or knowledge. This issue may become more important for those alliances moving toward "business" rather than "association" purposes.

The general absence of physicians from responsible posts in either alliance governance or management suggests that successful accomplishment of some alliance objectives might be problematic. Physician involvement in relevant policy formulation and management decision making could prove to be essential to achieve some of the intended objectives of alliances, such as vertical integration, regional networking, and effective linkage of financing and delivery of services.

Maturity

The third stage of an alliance's life cycle is that of maturity and growth. In this stage, it becomes important that the alliance begin to achieve its objectives and aid members in dealing with environmental and competitive threats. Such success, or the perception thereof, enables the alliance to grow. Furthermore, it is central that members be willing to put the interests of the alliance, at least in several areas of activity, ahead of their own individual interests. It becomes incumbent on the members to recognize that they will not necessarily benefit equally from all alliance activities; it is essential, however, that they benefit equitably.

As alliances seek to attain their objectives and sustain member commitment, a number of issues arise. For example, as alliances continue to grow, it becomes increasingly difficult to maintain the criterion of avoiding overlapping market areas among member organizations. If such overlap occurs, with the attendant competition between members, then the question arises of what role the alliance should play in resolving the resultant conflict and what mechanisms are most appropriate in mediating such intermember relationships. Tension related to the issue of commitment is being exacerbated by growing competition among alliances for new members, members switching between alliances, and mergers of organizations that belong to different alliances.

It is central that members be willing to put the interests of the alliance, at least in several areas of activity, ahead of their own individual interests.

There are also matters of relationships between the members and the alliance corporate management. For instance, are new programs to be initiated through the corporate office, individual members, or both? If primarily through the corporate office, then what happens to similar programs already developed by individual members for use by their own organizations? Are there, or should there be, incentives to individual members for innovations that might then be shared on some basis among the balance of the alliance membership? To what extent should participation in alliance programs be mandatory, versus voluntary? Thus a number of issues centering around relationships among the members and between the membership and the corporate office are highlighted in this stage.

Critical crossroads

As they evolve into a fourth stage of development, alliances move to what may be a critical crossroads. To this point, we find members becoming increasingly dependent on the alliance for needed resources, growing pressure for greater member commitment to the alliance, and more centralization in decision making. In many ways, these developments run counter to the reasons for which hospitals initially joined the alliance. That is, an alliance was attractive because it appeared to provide a relatively low-cost vehicle to reduce resource dependence while maintaining organizational autonomy. Thus, this stage may well be a critical crossroads at which some members may conclude that the price of belonging to the alliance is too high, and withdraw. Indeed, it would appear that at least one alliance has collapsed precisely on this point.[33] Conversely, others may conclude that it is necessary to move toward more hierarchical, more tightly coupled types of arrangements, akin to corporate models.

The underlying issue is whether there is sufficient glue to hold alliances together over time. While there is a degree of commonality in goals, ideology, and values, and while inducements to members have been offered (e.g., equity positions, shared risks), alliances remain relatively loosely coupled arrangements. At issue is whether the degree of commitment required will be secured and whether members will be willing to sacrifice autonomy and allow greater discipline in decision making. The requisite balance calls for alliances to become sufficiently integrated to secure the synergies of collective action while retaining adequate differentiation to satisfy the membership. In a sense, this crossroads may represent a test of the alliance or federation model versus the corporate model.

While this fourth stage has been cast in dichotomous terms, it is of course quite likely that there is a range of possible outcomes within the extremes. For example, one could envision a scenario within which alliances remain broadly based umbrellas under which members are involved in a variety of interorganizational linkages. Such a scenario might evolve to include loosely coupled alliances serving multiple sets of more tightly coupled regional, state, and local systems. This scenario is premised on the belief that health care delivery is primarily a local, state, and regional phenomenon. Effective responses to changing environmental conditions will require horizontally and vertically integrated systems operating in defined market areas and linking financing with delivery. The role of the alliance, in this context, will be to serve these integrated systems through focused areas of activity, capitalizing on the collective strength of the alliance and enhancing the position of the members in the markets within which they operate.

The proposed life cycle model could be useful as a blueprint for managers concerned with forming, joining, or guiding an alliance. Such utility, however, first calls for empirical testing of the model to verify its validity and reliability. Such testing would also allow us to modify, refine, and extend the model and add to our understanding of alliances as a form of interorganizational strategy.

EFFECTS OF ALLIANCES

The performance of alliances is of importance and interest to managers, policymakers, purchasers, and consumers. Such performance might be assessed along several dimensions and should enable us to assess the extent to which alliances achieve their goals and objectives, demonstrate their ability to secure needed resources, satisfy key stakeholders, and add value to the membership.

Economic effects

In this area, it would be important to examine the effects of programs designed to secure economies of scale. Such programs might include joint purchasing, pooled insurance, and other shared services. It would also be interesting to assess the extent to which dollar savings generated by the programs are passed along to buyers. Furthermore, the economic impact of alliances using population-based measures such as cost per capita would be especially interesting. To the extent that data permitted, comparisons of economic effects prior to and following the introduction of prospective payment would be interesting. The ability of alliances to improve financial resources for members, such as generating new sources of revenue and enhancing access to capital, should be tested.

Organizational effects

Organizational effects may be viewed in several ways. A key impact is the extent to which alliances benefit members with regard to their market position. The role of alliance programs and products in facilitating member penetration in new markets and maintaining or improving their share in current markets would be an important focus. Effects on referral networks would also warrant attention. Another avenue of exploration lies in the management and technical services and their effects on member organizations. Of particular interest would be indication of the impact of such services on utilization of resources and productivity in member organizations. Still another area of interest would be performance in the recruitment and retention of human resources, an area to which alliances devote a good deal of programmatic attention.

Social and political effects

Social and political effects likewise have several dimensions. Social effects could center on the role of alliances with regard to access to care, availability of services, and quality. That is, can we observe changes in access, availability, and quality of those served by alliance members that may be attributable or related to alliance activities? The political impact, though difficult to measure, might involve the influence of alliances as it relates to public policy, legislation, and regulation. Of particular concern would be the benefits and costs to alliance members, the degree of influence exerted by alliances on decision making and policy formulation within traditional trade associations, the effects on the role of and relationships with such trade associations, and the political impact on the field at large.

• • •

Although this approach to assessment must be considered preliminary, it is clear that there is much to be done to systematically evaluate the benefits and costs of alliances along several important dimensions and in terms of several key stakeholders.

Alliances are clearly part of a restructuring of the hospital industry, leading toward greater concentration and consolidation. The life cycle model provides a useful framework for further exploration of the organizational dynamics of alliance formation, development, and growth. Furthermore, it is evident that significant research questions remain with regard to the economic, political, social, and organizational impact of alliances.

REFERENCES

1. Provan, K.G. "Interorganizational Cooperative and Decision Making Autonomy in a Consortium Multihospital System." *Academy of Management Review* 9 (1984): 494–504.
2. Fottler, M.D., et al. "Multi-institutional Arrangements in Health Care: Review, Analysis, and a Proposal for Future Research." *Academy of Management Review* 7, no. 1 (1982): 67–79.
3. Provan, K.G. "The Federation as an Interorganizational Linkage Network." *Academy of Management Review* 8, no. 1 (1983): 79–89.
4. American Hospital Association. *Data Book on Multihospital Systems and Alliances, 1984-1987.* Chicago, Ill.: AHA, 1988.
5. Herriott, S.R. "The Economic Foundations of Cooperative Strategy: Three Examples of Partnership Organization." Paper presented at the annual meeting of the Academy of Management, Chicago, 1986.
6. D'Aunno, T., and Zuckerman, H. "A Life–Cycle Model of Organizational Federations: The Case of Hospitals." *Academy of Management Review* 12 (1987): 534–35.
7. Pfeffer, J., and Leong, A. "Resource Allocations in United Funds: An Examination of Power and Dependence." *Social Forces* 55 (1977): 775–90.
8. Pfeffer, J., and Salancik, G.R. *The External Control of Organizations: A Resource Dependence Perspective.* New

York: Harper & Row, 1978.
9. Provan, K.G. "Interorganizational Linkages and Influence Over Decision Making." *Academy of Management Journal* 25 (1982): 443–51.
10. Provan, K.G., Beyer, J.M., and Kruytbosch, C. "Environmental Linkages and Power in Resource Dependence Relations Between Organizations." *Administrative Science Quarterly* 25 (1980): 200–25.
11. Thompson, J.D. *Organizations in Action.* New York: McGraw-Hill, 1967.
12. Pfeffer, J. "Merger as a Response to Organizational Interdependence." *Administrative Science Quarterly* 18 (1972): 218–28.
13. Pfeffer, J., and Nowack, P. "Joint Ventures and Interorganizational Dependence." *Administrative Science Quarterly* 21 (1986): 398–418.
14. Pfeffer, J. "Size and Composition of Corporate Boards of Directors: The Organization and Its Environment." *Administrative Science Quarterly* 17 (1972): 382–94.
15. Pfeffer, J. "Size, Composition and Function of Hospital Boards of Directors: A Study of Organization–Environment Linkage." *Administrative Science Quarterly* 18 (1973): 349–64.
16. Tibbetts, S. "New American Healthcare Sees a Key Role for Members in Restructuring Health Care System." *Federation of American Hospitals Review* 24 (1984).
17. Punch, L. "VHA Seeks 'Viable' Role as Alternative to For-Profit Multihospital Systems." *Modern Healthcare* 12 (1982): 60–61.
18. Barkholz, D. "SunHealth Alliance Plans Entry into Healthcare Insurance Arena." *Modern Healthcare* 16 (1986): 48–50.
19. LaViolette, S. "VHA Pushes Regional 'Clones' That Could Add 300 Hospitals to the Cooperative." *Modern Healthcare* 13, no. 12 (1983): 84, 86.
20. Cassak, D. "The Voluntary Hospitals of America." *Health Industry Today* (April 1984).
21. Johnson, D.E.L. "American Healthcare Systems." *Modern Healthcare* 16 (1986): 78–82.
22. Punch, L. "Hospital Alliance Forays Widen the Realm of Shared Services." *Modern Healthcare* 13 (1983): 136,138.
23. Anderson, H.J. "Premier Becomes National Alliance While Emphasizing Local Approach." *Modern Healthcare* 17 (1987): 78.
24. Southwick, K. "Two Hospital Chains See Profit in Clinical Research." *Federation of American Hospitals Review* 24 (1984).
25. Barkholz, D. "VHA Hoping Deals Will Create Its 'Brand' of National Healthcare." *Modern Healthcare* 15 (1985): 82–83, 86.
26. Barkholz, D. "AHS, Two Insurance Firms Enter Venture to Market Alternative Health Plans." *Modern Healthcare* 15 (1985): 28.
27. Greene, J. "Alliances Soon May Face Their Day of Reckoning." *Modern Healthcare* 17, no. 26 (1987): 24–26, 30, 32, 37.

28. Gray, B., and Ariss, S.S. "Politics and Strategic Change Across Organizational Life Cycles." *Academy of Management Review* 10 (1985): 702–23.

29. Kimberly, J.R., et al., eds. *The Organizational Life Cycle.* San Francisco: Jossey-Bass, 1980.

30. Quinn, R.E., and Cameron, K. "Organizational Life Cycles and Shifting Criteria of Effectiveness: Some Preliminary Evidence." *Management Science* 29, no. 1 (1983): 33–51.

31. Barrett, D. "Multihospital Systems: The Process of Development." *Health Care Management Review* 4, no. 3 (1979): 49–59.

32. Sheldon, A., and Barrett, D. "The Janus Principle." *Health Care Management Review* 2, no. 2 (1987): 77–87.

33. Johnson, D.E.L. "Board's Lack of Consensus Blamed for Failing of NORAM Enterprises." *Modern Healthcare* 16 (1986): 60.

Twelve laws of hospital interaction

David M. Kinzer

A strong case can be made for restructuring the health care delivery system using a vertically integrated model. The difficulties with such a voluntary effort surface with a review of 12 laws of hospital interaction.

Joining a system has recently been the "in thing" for health care provider organizations to do. The for-profit hospital systems started this movement, then the non-profits, with their Catholic, Jewish, and nonaligned subsets, and some but not many mixtures of the above followed. We have had horizontally integrated systems, vertically integrated systems, and nearly everything in between. And a distinction must be made between medical care systems, such as the Kaiser Permanente and Puget Sound medical groups, and management systems, which are predominant. In some cases, the physicians who practice in these management systems have little reason to know or care that the systems exist.

And we also have networks, alliances, consortia, and holding companies carry out functions and perform services similar to those in many of the so-called systems. In fact, one of the problems with the systems movement is the lack of consensus on the definition of what a system is.

Over the past 10 or 12 years a significant body of experience has built up around the systems movement, including substantial trial and error. It would seem that this experience deserves a review in the context of the suddenly revived public interest in laws that would make basic medical services a citizen right.

HOSPITALS AND PUBLIC NEED

When George Bush became president, the pendulum was swinging away from the Reagan-era competition and deregulation cycle toward more focused concern on access, quality, and cost issues.[1] Numerous polls documented that large majorities of citizens favored more central government initiatives and leadership in health, not fewer.[2]

One of the early surprises of 1989 was a poll that found that 89% of Americans "see the U.S. health care system requiring fundamental change in its direction and structure."[3(p.3)] Only 10% saw their health care arrangements as "working reasonably well."[3(p.3)] The poll compared American attitudes with those of Canadian and British citizens. Canadian and British respondents expressed higher levels of satisfaction with their

David M. Kinzer *spent 30 of his years as the chief executive officer of two state hospital associations, Illinois and Massachusetts. Most recently he has been active as a faculty member of the Harvard School of Public Health and the Duke University Medical Center.*

Health Care Manage Rev, 1990, 15(2), 15–19

health care systems than did American respondents. In fact, the majority of the Canadians (56%) thought their system was "working reasonably well." The poll reported even more support in Britain for a system that has been under very tight financial constraints than was found in the United States, where costs have been a prime issue. Also noteworthy is that 61% of U.S. respondents stated a positive preference for the Canadian system over the U.S. system.[3,4] Although the Americans who were polled may not have known enough about the Canadian system to support such judgments, they expressed an astonishingly high level of dissatisfaction with U.S. health care.

So what does this poll say to the ever-increasing number of people involved in health systems development in the United States? It seems to suggest that what they have been trying to do over the last several years does not relate very clearly to broad citizen health concerns. Whatever the accomplishments of systems, networks, chains, and alliances to date, we are not getting many supportable chains of positive impacts on the cost–quality–access issues.

Some of my best friends in the health world are members of some system or other. I know why most of them joined. They wanted economic protection. Some joined a system because of fears of a competing neighbor who had just joined another system. Some joined because they liked the people in it.

This is not to suggest that these motives are sinful; rather, that institutional financial health and the public interest are two quite different things.

The American Heritage Dictionary defines a system as a "regularly interacting or interdependent group of items forming a unified whole."[5(p.1306)] Under that definition, the nation's total of conforming nonprofit systems is much diminished. Even the Catholic hospitals that are owned by a single religious order often do not have tight mother-house control and have not been able to integrate their scattered parts successfully.

The least kind way of describing many of our not-for-profit systems is to say they would not exist if for-profit chains had not presented a competitive threat. In the process of building systems, not-for-profits have created another level of bureaucracy at which hospital managers gather to share ideas about the salvation of their institutions without making any binding commitments to help each other with money. The for-profits are different, of course, with motives that are more clear-cut: However, their managers cannot claim either that their systems have had significant impacts on access, quality, or cost.

All systems, for-profit and nonprofit, have a limited public constituency. Conventional wisdom is that in health care more than in other fields, local citizens feel little allegiance to hospitals with national headquarters and bosses in a distant place like Nashville or Irving, Texas. As Blendon put it, "The public would rather have Mother Teresa running their hospitals than Lee Iacocca. People don't like big business in a political sense. Hospitals have aggressively positioned themselves in the worst possible political box."[6(p.36)]

There are at least two more areas where we do not have a good match between what our systems are doing and what the public seems to want. First, while most of our systems concentrate on acute care or specialties thereof, there are strong indications that the public likes one-ticket–entry systems where no hassles inhibit movement in the care continuum and where the provider has clear incentives for rational and prudent use of limited resources. As the lobby for the elderly gains numbers and power, pressure is mounting to bring primary, acute, and chronic care under one organizational umbrella. Vertical integration is gaining support as the health care system becomes more pluralistic, segmented, and complicated. Consigning most of chronic care to a welfare program (Medicaid) and most of acute care to private sector and governmental entitlements never made much sense, anyway.

Institutional financial health and the public interest are two quite different things.

The second area in which the fit between system practice and public desire is not good relates to cost control in the macro sense. Whatever systems have saved through group purchasing and pooled management services is now dwarfed by governmental health budget–cutting on a grand scale. There will be more of this before there is less. The organizations that will be able to deal with cuts on this scale will be the larger, vertically integrated ones with the capacity to distribute their services more rationally and efficiently than is possible under the present uncoordinated pluralism. No surviving system will be able to afford any redundancy of lithotriptors, trauma centers, or units doing coronary bypass surgery. Capacity in the different levels of care will be ordained by the number of patients needing the service and not by its assumed profitability.

A strong case can be made for restructuring the health care delivery system using a vertically integrated model.[7] Is designing such a model possible in the present environment, through more voluntary systems initiatives of the kind we now have? It would seem to be worth a try; but the difficulty of this kind of "voluntary effort" needs to be recognized in advance.

TWELVE LAWS OF HOSPITAL INTERACTION

The difficulties with such a voluntary effort surface with a review of 12 laws of hospital interaction. These laws are a byproduct of the author's 30 years as a hospital association chief executive officer (CEO) trying to catalyze the development of regional health care systems and sometimes as a behind-the-scenes promoter of institutional weddings that usually did not quite come off.

1. The law of protective risk sharing

The health care journals have been giving much space to the glorification of risk takers in the health-provider and financing sectors. The implication of this is that they represent the new wave of health care managers. If this implication is correct, perhaps it explains why the CEO attrition rate is now rising steadily. I think risk taking is no more popular now than it ever was: The operational environment is just getting riskier. A more accurate way of describing our current situation is that it has become much easier to find parties who are glad to share their risks with you. We are into a scenario that can be called the "risk shift." Government is trying to share more of its risks with providers, employers with their employees, health maintenance organizations (HMOs) and other "managed care" enterprises with physicians, and on and on it goes. The big problem now is that there are too many players on the health care scene that are bent on unloading the risks they have. The phenomenon is very much on the increase among the different levels of care (medical center, community hospital, physician, nursing home, and home care agency). The workings of this law are mostly adverse to systems development. The prospect of sharing someone else's increasing risks is rarely viewed with enthusiasm.

2. The law of dollar displacement

You do not need to be a management genius to know that for every dollar you lose rendering one service you need to make it up someplace else. This explains why so many hospitals jumped on the "corporate diversification" bandwagon. They are getting criticized for this and it is threatening their tax exempt status, but running a fitness center, a weight loss clinic, or seminars on self-hypnosis, even travel agencies or community laundries—all seem like sensible moves to many hospital boards, at least compared to merging with another financially moribund hospital or neighborhood health center.

3. The law of voluntary motivation

The real meaning of the word "voluntary" is that you are going to do it only if you feel like it and it gives reasonable promise of helping your own cause. The hospital world learned this both when it tried cost control on a voluntary basis and earlier when it gave its blessings to voluntary health planning. The physician community is now learning this lesson in its attempts to encourage maximum physician participation in Medicaid as an alternative to laws that mandate participation. Attempts to bring together the elements of a vertically integrated system face this same problem. Even when the idea has rewards for all parties involved, it is certain that, going in, a lot of the parties will not believe it.

4. The law of proximate polarity

The closer hospitals are geographically, the more likely that the main themes of their relationships will be mutual distrust, secretiveness, and competitiveness. Effecting meaningful sharing between hospitals 40 miles or more apart has always been easier than between hospitals only a few blocks apart.

5. The law of dissonant motivation

Being in favor of profits has never been considered un-American, but that does not mean that the for-profit hospital world can blend in well with the not-for-profits and the governmentals. This bad fit is also the primary explanation for difficulties over the years in building a collaborative relationship between primarily for-profit nursing homes and primarily not-for-profit hospitals. In the public mind, this collaboration creates a basic conflict of interest. If an organization has been talking about and delivering on "charitable purposes" for a while, has an endowment, and periodically goes to the public with a capital-fund drive, then its constituency feels comfortable making demands on that organization that are quite different from those made on the investor-owned institution across town.

The coming together of the for-profits and non-profits or publics has mainly been one of acquisition by the for-profit chains of weak sisters under a now-outdated horizontal integration strategy. Now these chains are trying to get rid of the institutions they have been unable to make profitable. Lately they have been having trouble finding takers.

6.   The law of interfaith disunity

There is always a problem of coming together when the hospitals involved have different religious sponsorship. The feelings that led the towns of America to have a Catholic hospital and an "other" even when the town never needed more than one hospital—they are all still with us. This law has been broken with some frequency lately but it still is not easy to pull off consolidations that lead to the disappearance of the Catholic hospital identity. The abortion issue is only one of the reasons.

7.   The law of diminishing allegiance

Complicating the long-standing divisiveness identified in the laws identified above is the fact that health care providers are joining more organizations than ever before. Not only are they joining the new systems, networks, and alliances referred to earlier: They are also joining HMOs, preferred provider organizations (PPOs), and other managed care enterprises. Some hospitals seem to be connecting with any and all HMOs and PPOs that come along and encourage the fee-for-service physicians on their staffs to do the same. Joint ventures with groups of physicians or private corporate entities are another example of organizations joined by health care providers.

This proliferation of systems has made life more difficult for the traditional metropolitan, state, and national hospital associations. They are having trouble even getting the attention of the CEOs of their member hospitals, not to mention getting meaningful support from them on crucial political issues. The fact is, leaders of institutions that are a part of vertically integrated systems rarely have time to give that complex job the time it needs.

When the money begins to get tight, the reflex response is usually to intensify competition, share less information, and give less cooperation.

8.   The law of mutual noncooperation

When hospitals and other provider organizations are equals, or when their administrators think of their organizations as equals, their first instinct is to compete, not to share. When the money begins to get tight, the reflex response is usually to intensify competition, share less information, and give less cooperation. This situation seldom turns around until at least one of the parties is in a situation of dire necessity, verging on extinction.

9.   The law of relative inequality

While there can be few systems consolidations of true equals, there are also serious hangups when you try to bring together "unequals." The more "unequal" they are, we often have greater difficulty. There is too much of this in the hospital world with attempts at horizontal integration by acute care hospitals. The stronger hospital begins to feel that it is doing the weaker one a favor, so it tries to drive a hard bargain that can be accepted without the weaker party losing face. Often, more diplomacy is required than the larger institution can muster to make the weaker institution feel wanted and needed.

The nation seems to be moving into an era of having many hospitals that are willing to give themselves away; but they are finding more givers than takers. The big and strong in the institutional world have become chary about picking up any more liabilities.

10.   The law of diffused motivation

One problem frequently encountered in the hospital world is that, even when consultants report that consolidation is desirable or even a condition for survival and the report is supported by the hospital board, it should not be assumed that the proposal can never be made acceptable to all of the vested interests involved. You start with institutional management that is nearly always threatened by consolidation. Then you get the lawyers into the act, bringing with them the specter of antitrust. Then there are the medical staff pecking orders and the subsurface rivalries of the physicians in the hospitals being consolidated. Similar concerns affect department heads and other employees. Beyond that, there are the auxiliaries and other volunteer groups that sometimes behave like private social clubs, and you may have a situation where one hospital is unionized and the other not, or they have contracts with different unions. It goes on from there.

11.   The law of negative unity

Bringing institutions together to advance a common cause is always easier when they have a common enemy. The Massachusetts Hospital Association organized some active hospital councils in territory conterminous with that of the state's six health systems agencies (HSAs). Threatened with having plans dictated to them by the HSAs, some of the hospital councils started successful collaborative ventures of their own. Sometimes fear of a common enemy is strong enough to negate any "Law of Proximate Polarity," but this happens only rarely.

One reason systems consolidation efforts are so difficult today is that within each level of care—and between them, too—there is no common enemy. The enemies are now all around.

12.   The law of conflicting public expectations

From one arm of the national government has come the push by the Federal Trade Commission to prevent health care monopolies. From the Department of Health and Human Services (and from private-sector purchasers of service as well) comes pressure to prevent wasteful duplication of services. Medicare has become an exercise in governmental price fixing, but other areas of government are quick to persecute health care providers that try to do the same thing. One Massachusetts law requires hospitals to give "free care," but another department of that state's government has regulations that require those same hospitals to tighten their collection policies. These and other inconsistencies in governmental policy make it that much more difficult to put together viable health care systems.

PROGNOSIS FOR THE FUTURE

A reasonable expectation is that health care organizations will continue to evolve and experiment with more systems of care. Ever-building economic pressure seems to guarantee this response. However, as this pressure builds, one can also reasonably expect that the major initiatives will be economically driven and not necessarily responsive to the mainly social expectations of the public.

Assuming a continuation of our patchwork governmental commitment to pay for the health care of its citizens, the systems we have, present and future, will not and cannot give the public what it says it wants. Instead, we are into an accelerating process that Ginzberg has described as "destabilization."[8] There

already have been abundant indications that the groups trying hardest to be publicly responsive are having the heaviest trouble.

If some kind of national universal health care entitlement is adopted, the situation on systems of care will, of course, change radically. Then the main question will be: What kind of systems of care should the national government decide to do business with? It seems that it would be a mistake to enact a universal health entitlement without any decision on what kind of provider organizations can deliver on the quality, access, and cost promises of such a law. Demonstration projects with comprehensive, vertically integrated health care delivery organizations are needed now in order to determine their potential for being responsive to public wishes and needs. These projects need the support of big government, with front-end financial guarantees and enough time to support judgments about their feasibility under a national entitlement. A continuation of the present pluralistic provider establishment can only guarantee continued instability.

REFERENCES

1. Kinzer, D.M. "The Decline and Fall of Deregulation." *New England Journal of Medicine* 318, no. 2 (1988):112–16.
2. Blendon, R.J. "Public Perceptions for the Changing Health Care Delivery System." Paper presented at Harvard School of Public Health Colloquium, Boston, Mass., 27 March 1987.
3. Blendon, R.J. "Three Systems: A Comparative Survey." *Health Management Quarterly* 11, no. 1 (1989): 3–8.
4. Evans, R. "Perspectives: Canada." *Health Affairs* 7, no. 5 (1988): 17–25.
5. *The American Heritage Dictionary*, 1975, s.v. "System."
6. Larkin, H. "Image Problems Expand CEO Role." *Hospitals* 63, no. 5 (1989): 36–42.
7. Mick, S.S., and Conrad, D.A. "The Decision to Integrate Vertically in Health Care Organizations." *Hospital and Health Services Administration* (Fall 1988): 345–61.
8. Ginzberg, E. "The Destabilization of Health Care." *New England Journal of Medicine* 315 (1986):757–61.

Warfare or partnership: Which way for health care?

R. Scott MacStravic

There are many voices urging health care organizations to adopt aggressive competitive warfare, but a careful look at the dynamics affecting health care suggests that partnership may be at least as promising a strategy as warfare to promote mission and survival.

There seem to be two philosophies of marketing vying for favor in health care. One is an extension of traditional health service values in which marketing is seen as a way to improve and add dimension to health care services, increasing their value to the customer. The second is an adoption of commercial business values in which marketing is seen as warfare among competitors, with only the fittest surviving. These views are not truly opposites, since they have different frames of reference; one focuses on customers and the other on competitors. On the other hand, they represent widely differing philosophies regarding how health care organizations should examine, plan, and conduct their activities.

The contention of this discussion is that health care organizations should adopt a philosophy in which they seek to establish and maintain working partnerships rather than strive to win battles and wars. There are risks involved in adopting such a philosophy, but they are not as severe as those attending conscious belligerence. The benefits to the organization—and more important, to the communities served—seem far greater in the partnership approach, despite the substantial attractions of competitive warfare.

WARFARE VERSUS PARTNERSHIP

Warfare

Despite—or perhaps because of—a growing disenchantment with warfare as a means of settling international differences, a growing body of literature has arisen extolling the virtues of warfare as a marketing philosophy. Kotler and Singh championed consideration of a variety of offensive and defensive strategies as essential for effective marketing in the 1980s.[1] Ries and Trout authored a book on marketing warfare dedicated to the gurus of military strategy throughout history.[2]

The focus in warfare is on the enemy: competitors in the same markets. The goal is to win battles through carefully selected offensive or defensive strategies. The minds and behavior patterns of customers represent the battleground and objectives of particular campaigns, while the strategies and tactics chosen are based on competitors' strengths and vulnerabilities. All the idioms and images of war are used not only to examine

Robin Scott MacStravic, *Ph.D., formerly Vice President for Planning and Marketing at Health and Hospital Services, Bellevue, Washington, is now an independent consultant in Mercer Island, Washington.*

Health Care Manage Rev, 1990, 15(1), 37–45

and plan the combative situation, but also to motivate the troops who will go out there to fight and win.

These authors advocate a belligerent philosophy for business in general; now health care authors are advocating the same philosophy. Kessler, a health care administrator, advocates battlefield strategies as a basis for power management and strategic success in health care.[3] Malhotra outlines a range of attack and defense strategies available to health care organizations that hope to survive in the increasingly competitive and constricted health care marketplace. He concludes that "health care institutions that survive—or thrive—will do so at the expense of others."[4]

Others in health care, while not direct advocates of warfare as a philosophy, have sensed the need for a departure from traditional ways of doing business. Abrahamson describes the new breed hospital administrator as "entrepreneurial" and "profit motivated."[5] Fallucchi asserts that health care is essentially a competitive business in which management must strive to stay ahead of the pack.[6]

Others are less enthusiastic about belligerence. Lovelock points out the critical difference between influencing consumers' behavior for their own and the community's benefit versus doing it for the good of the organization.[7] Mauet warns of the dangers of a marketing mindset that focuses too much on the organization and its success, at the expense of customers and service.[8] The author of *Business Week* review of Reis and Trout's book feared that businesses would "forget satisfying the customer—just outfox the other guy."[9]

Studies in health care suggest that competition drives costs higher, a dangerous effect in an increasingly price-sensitive and payment-restricted market.[10] Mourning reminds health care organizations of the many stakeholders upon whom they are dependent and of the extent to which competition can interfere with maintaining good relations with those stakeholders.[11]

The attraction of the belligerent philosophy may come from its emphasis on winning and surviving. Certainly everyone has been taught that winning is far better than losing, and that being first is inestimably superior to being second. As the marketplace becomes more pressured and survival less assured, there is a natural tendency to focus more on being a survivor.

Yet most health care organizations are in business to serve a purpose and carry out a mission, not to survive or beat out their competitors. It should be the fervent hope of many health care providers that the need for their services should diminish, or even disappear, through people becoming healthier. There are sure to be times when providers long for a good epidemic or disaster to help fill beds and waiting rooms, but such longings should be passing fancies rather than organizational policies.

The key is to retain a focus on the ends sought rather than on the means used. Even warfare advocates stress that the purpose of war is to produce an improved peace. Warfare does not justify war: It is a means rather than an end. If the purpose of the survival of a health care organization—the patient's health—is stressed over the survival itself, then warfare as a philosophy may be counterproductive rather than advantageous.

Anyone with direct or vicarious experience of warfare should recall the corrupting effects it can have on the behavior of armies. There is a tendency—almost a necessity—for warriors and noncombatants to dehumanize their human enemies. Warfare not only accepts expediency, it elevates it to honored status. Whatever will produce a victory in skirmishes, battles, and campaigns is automatically good.

There are clear delights in war: its effect on mobilizing the will of warring peoples, its excitement, and its economic effects especially for the winners. Yet, looking back over recent wars, we rarely conclude that they were the best option. There is a strong tradition in this country that favors warfare in sports and competition in everyday life, but there is also a tradition of mutual cooperation toward important community goals.

Partnership

An alternative philosophy to war is one in which health care organizations see themselves as seeking and maintaining partnerships with others in pursuit of shared goals. Such partnerships may be formal or informal, implicit or explicit, with few or with many. The partnership philosophy clearly fits better with traditional health care values; an argument can be made that it also fits better with marketing realities.

Marketing prides itself on being customer focused and customer driven. The notion is that those who do a better job at identifying and serving the needs of customers will thereby prosper and survive. Even if the desired end is to survive and prosper rather than to serve, the idea is that by focusing on service, the desired end comes about naturally. As Ohmae put it, "strategy isn't beating the competition, it's serving customers' real needs."[12]

Partnerships with customers are strongly advocated in the marketing and sales literature. Albrecht and Zemke stress the importance of customers as providers of feedback to improve the success of marketing efforts.[13] Gronroos cites the importance of customers in service development, because of the need to constantly focus on how customers gain from their interactions with service providers, and because of the need to discover how they can best participate in the service process.[14] Pottruck emphasizes the importance of building and maintaining customer loyalty in a lifetime relationship.[15]

Others have insisted that selling be oriented toward serving the customer's interests, not the seller's. Carew advocates that sales professionals become members of their customers' teams, focusing on how they can help, instead of on how much they can sell.[16] Hanan describes how sales forces should become their customers' partners in achieving their customers' goals and contributing to their customers' bottom lines.[17]

A partnership philosophy differs vastly from a belligerent approach. It focuses on the purposes of the organization more than on its survival. It looks for ways to link with others rather than to defeat them and for shared goals and interests rather than for ways to exploit situations for the organization's own gain. However more attractive a partnership approach may seem in the rhetorical sense, however, the test is how well it works in the practical arena. Will it truly contribute more to the purposes of health care organizations and enable them to achieve their goals better, than will belligerence?

PARTNERSHIPS WITH WHOM?

Just as in warfare it is necessary to know one's enemy, in partnership it is essential to determine who one's potential partners are. In health care, there appear to be at least eight categories: the community, patients, physicians, purchasers, the organization's own employees, internal departments, suppliers, and peers. Whether the organization can establish and maintain effective working partnerships with each will determine how well it succeeds and survives and whether it has to resort to warfare in order to do so.

Community partnerships

The basis for partnership with the community as a whole is the fact that health care providers and the community share an interest in the health of residents. Not all interests are shared, of course; providers often wish to be compensated somewhat more than communities desire to compensate them. Barring this financial

snag, however, the interests and commitments of providers and the community should overlap.

Mourning has suggested that provider organizations develop stakeholder strategies by identifying everyone who has an interest in the organization's survival and mission. Attempts should then be made to network with all stakeholders in pursuit of shared goals. Competition can easily interfere with stakeholder relations, as when hospitals open up pharmacies or home health services that compete with existing firms, or when physicians start their own ambulatory surgery or after-hours urgent care centers.[11]

However more attractive a partnership approach may seem in the rhetorical sense, the test is how well it works in the practical arena.

Hill-Chin describes how some communities have organized cooperative efforts to avoid the negative effects of competition and to improve the key components of health care success: quality, access, and cost containment. The Community Program for Affordable Health Care, sponsored by The Robert Wood Johnson Foundation, the American Hospital Association, and Blue Cross/Blue Shield, is an attempt to create community partnerships among providers, purchasers, consumers, and government in pursuit of shared commitments.[18]

Poniatowski describes how a rural hospital strove to keep elderly people out of the hospital by developing senior housing and support services to promote independent living and the health of elderly people. Lifeline emergency response links enable elderly and handicapped citizens to live independently while being assured of aid in an emergency. The hospital supports and networks with other community agencies in pursuit of health objectives and promotes economic development in the area.[19]

While partnerships with the community are aimed primarily at improving service and health, they also add to the strength of the organization. High levels of involvement in the community promote public awareness of the organization's services at a cost that is likely to be lower than that of advertising. Such involvement is also likely to prove advantageous when consideration of tax-exempt status arises.[20]

Clearly, health care organizations should be in partnership with the communities they serve. The purpose of health care demands such a partnership, and its goals can be far better accomplished when alliances exist with community organizations and the public at large. Since this is true for all health care organizations, it suggests a possible dilemma: How can health care organizations be partners with each other's community organizations and the public, and yet be at war with each other? How can we be at war with our partners' partners?

Patient partnerships

However much the tradition of a physician's paternal advocacy for patients may endure, there are powerful reasons to replace it.[21] Yet, partnership with patients is under attack by purchasers and provider corporations, who demand that physicians be champions of economical use of resources, protecting the welfare of the organization even at the expense of the patient.[22] The physicians' own interests may conflict with those of their patients.

It is fairly well understood that providing health care creates partnerships with patients in many if not most cases. Patients must actively participate in the curing process, both during and following care encounters. Patients enable providers to succeed in many ways, including contributing useful information, cooperating in care processes, complying with advice, paying bills, and encouraging their friends to use the same provider.

The active participation of patients in the care process is becoming increasingly essential, as well as desirable. For instance, providers must obtain informed consent to treatment, and life-and-death decisions regarding heroic measures must be made in concert with patients or their surrogates. Patients are more and more often being held to have legal or moral rights to participate in care decisions.

In addition, such participation has significant therapeutic and marketing benefit. Lazare has described the advantages of a negotiated approach in the relationship between providers and psychiatric patients.[23] Quill has described a similar mutual contracting approach to caring for medical patients in which providers and patients share responsibility for care.[24] The Planetree Project has demonstrated how a partnership approach to inpatient care both saves money and promotes patient satisfaction.[25]

Although there may be some conflicts, clearly patients and providers share essential interests. Providers and patients should in most cases agree on the desired outcomes of care, even if they disagree on how best to achieve them or on how much should be paid for them. Partnerships have the potential to galvanize the patient to pursue desired outcomes and to reduce complaints and malpractice suits.

Physician partnerships

It is becoming increasingly essential for hospitals to create and sustain partnerships with physicians. As Abrahamson has pointed out, the traditional workshop model of the hospital–physician relationship is obsolete. He has described how hospitals and physicians should supplement their already-significant shared interests by sharing financial risks and benefits through arrangements such as health maintenance organizations (HMOs) and preferred provider organizations (PPOs).[5]

Payne suggests that hospitals must partner with physicians in order to improve the efficiency of care. While the environment and patient–family factors have some impact on hospital efficiency, physician-controlled factors account for 75% of the difference between efficient and inefficient care. For both surviving under tighter government payment systems and competing for increasingly price-sensitive purchaser contracts, provider efficiency is essential to survival.[26]

Partnerships between hospitals and their medical staffs are by no means easy to establish and maintain. Gill and Meighan have described five significant roadblocks to effective partnerships between institutions and their medical staff members. They also suggest how these barriers can be overcome, and argue that they must be overcome to enable both parties to succeed and survive.[27]

Ideally, there will be a powerful set of shared interests between hospitals and physicians, enough to provide at least a starting point for effective partnerships. Both should be committed to the same health and patient outcomes, though their economic interests often diverge. Shared risks and benefits through HMOs and PPOs may strengthen the mutuality of interests, though they may also make clearer the conflicts that remain. Mutual malpractice insurance, marketing, and management assistance may serve to strengthen relations with physicians as well.

Purchaser partnerships

It is unusual to think of purchasers as partners in marketing situations, although such a relationship is possible in most cases. The exchange process that underlies all marketing transactions creates a kind of partnership between buyers and sellers. Both parties wish to consummate a deal and share an interest in at least achieving an exchange. Sellers hope that buyers will come back, or refer others, thus sellers and buyers share an interest in the exchange turning out to be satisfactory to the buyer.[28]

In health care, the major purchasers of health care are HMOs, employers, unions, government, and private insurance. They may have a dominant interest in minimizing their outlay for health care, in conflict with what providers feel is fair or essential payment, but there are still significant shared interests. Employers, HMOs and unions want to obtain prompt, high quality, and satisfactory service. Both providers and purchasers want patients to be restored to full, or at least optimal, functioning as soon as is practical.

In partnerships with purchasers, providers may find themselves necessarily at odds with their peers.

Purchasers and providers share a commitment to promoting the health of people, preventing disease and injury, minimizing the damage from each when it occurs, and improving the quality of life for all. Both are at least rhetorically committed to promoting high quality, fair access, and reasonable cost. HMOs and hospitals, for example, may find ways of becoming partners rather than adversaries in their negotiations, according to one article.[29]

Divergence of interests may be promoted or reduced by the strategic choices of providers. The hospital wishing to fill its beds may do battle with purchasers, or instead it may offer such high quality and efficiency of care that it secures larger shares of the market and higher occupancy by helping purchasers achieve their goals. Kenkel has reported an example of providers and purchasers jointly developing an HMO in order to solve cost and access problems in the community.[30]

In partnerships with purchasers, providers may find themselves necessarily at odds with their peers. Adopting a responsive or even proactive approach to a buy right strategy by purchasers will tend to benefit the effective and efficient providers at the expense of others.[31] Assuming that there is indeed a surplus of providers, not all will survive as purchaser interests become more dominant, and some form of warfare may be inevitable.

On the other hand, there are many health-related needs available for providers to serve. Those who fail to survive in one market are free to look for other markets to serve. Those who fall behind in one year are free to improve their quality, efficiency, access, or other performance factors of interest to purchasers, and thereby do better in the next year.

Employee partnerships

The provider's own employees are not often discussed as potential partners, but they have a lot to recommend them. While some employees may come to work merely in order to receive a paycheck, most presumably had a reason for choosing health care as a career. To the extent that they are committed to providing high quality and satisfying and efficient care, they are potentially the most important of all partners. Providers are either constrained or enabled by the quantity and quality of the employees they are able to recruit and retain.

In Drucker's "New Organization," employees are more important and managers less so.[32] In the service organization, managers should be coaches, motivators, and supporters; they should either be serving customers or serving those who do.[12] In health care, employees often deliver the first impression that patients have, and thereby influence or determine the marketing success of the organization.

Employees may act as partners in several basic marketing functions. They may supply useful intelligence about customers; in fact, they have been shown to be better at supplying such intelligence than are their supervisors.[33] They can supply practical ideas for ways to improve quality, efficiency, and customer satisfaction that strategists and managers could only guess at. They can be active ambassadors and word-of-mouth advertisers.[34]

Hospitals are more likely to be successful if they mobilize employees as partners in the pursuit of organizational goals than if they have to coerce, cajole, or otherwise manipulate participation. Whether such partnerships are best based on shared financial risks and rewards, shared philosophies and values, or some combination of the two remains to be learned, but the potential has been well established.

Interdepartmental partnerships

In addition to partnerships with employees in general, there exists the possibility of creating more effective partnerships among the organization's basic departments. Marketing is new in most health care organizations and has not always been warmly welcomed. Becoming an active and accepted partner rather than a skeptically adopted outsider may be an aspiration for many marketing professionals and departments.

As Roodman points out, a fishing boat is a good analogy of how marketing fits in to an organization: Finance is responsible for keeping the boat fueled, operations sets and recovers the nets, and marketing finds the fish and baits the hook.[35] While this is not a particularly savory analogy in relation to health care patients, it does suggest the partnership among basic organizational functions.

Frommelt has described in detail how finance and marketing can be partners; he calls for greater mutual understanding and cooperation between these functions in health care organizations. Too frequently, finance serves merely to judge marketing efforts. Finance can assist marketing efforts by ensuring that personnel dealing with admitting and business office contacts promote patient satisfaction. Finance can also supply useful data for marketing strategy and find ways to enable the organization to set prices that are acceptable and attractive to purchasers.[36]

Supplier partnerships

Suppliers of goods and services can greatly help or hinder the organization's mission and survival. Insurers can force providers to eliminate services, for example, by refusing to insure them.[37] Hospital supply companies may partner with hospitals to develop new products and services, improve quality and productivity. They may offer marketing advice and suggest ways to improve service to patients.[38]

More recently, suppliers have partnered with hospitals in cooperative advertising. General Electric promotes mammography in its advertising, thereby increasing volumes at hospitals offering the service, if also promoting sales of its mammography equipment. Bayfront Medical Center in St. Petersburg, Florida recently launched an advertising campaign in cooperation with its medical equipment and supplies vendors. Each advertisement highlights both the vendor's product and the hospital.[39]

Peer provider partnerships

It is in the area of peer relationships that the choice between partnership and warfare is clearest and most significant. While health care tradition has emphasized cooperation among providers, there has always been a recognition that providers compete for personnel, re-

sources, patients, and prestige. At the same time, as providers recognize and engage more often in conscious competition, they can remember the potential for partnerships in striving toward mutually desired goals.

Devine has discussed the conflict between traditional health care values and the growing adoption of hard-headed, businesslike strategies in health care. While recognizing that old-time administrators may have lacked some business skills, he suggests that new wave administrators may be lacking some important values. He advocates that providers with like values, specifically Catholic hospitals, strive to collaborate rather than compete with each other.[40]

While pressures exist for hospitals to find additional sources of revenue, find alternative uses for empty beds, and diversify into new lines of income-producing business, the tendency is to compete rather than collaborate. On the other hand, all of these strategies may be carried out through joint ventures, networking, and other peer alliances instead of through warfare.

As purchasers increasingly look for single sources of comprehensive service contracts, for example, networking with high quality, efficient peers may be the best way to compete. A comprehensive set of services developed in competition with experienced and successful peers already serving the same market may be doomed to poor quality and marketing failure, whereas a partnership could have strengthened all participants.

Antitrust constraints set clear limits on direct partnering with peers. However, there are many examples of partnerships with peers who serve slightly different markets, or offer slightly different services. General acute hospitals have invited children's hospitals or psychiatric institutions to place a dedicated unit within their facility, for example, rather than develop their own units.[41] Rural hospitals may network with a large urban referral center rather than take it on in competition.

Competing provider organizations may cooperate indirectly by simply choosing to focus on a market where the other is not competing. Peers may select markets and services that complement each other simply by recognizing where the other is well entrenched, offers superior quality, and enjoys marketing advantages. Even warfare advocates recommend avoiding direct competition where the enemy is strongest.

As long as complementary strategies are arrived at without collusion, there should be no antitrust problem. If the strategies are chosen well, the community should benefit. Moreover, peers that have followed complementary competitive strategies will be well prepared for merger, networking, or other formal partnership arrangements when they become desirable or necessary.

Warfare assume a zero-sum game: Survival and mission accomplishments can be achieved only at the expense of peers. There are parts of the health care market that are close to a zero-sum game, but there are many other parts that are not. There are still many populations that are not getting enough care, where economic barriers, lack of information, or negative attitudes prevent people from seeking services that would benefit them. There are still quality-of-life-enhancing services that are yet to be developed, people with undiscovered conditions who are yet to be served. The market potential for health services has by no means been exhausted, although the willingness of government and industry to pay for them is close to exhausted.

Looking at all the stakeholders involved in health care, it is clear that partnership makes sense with the vast majority—with patients, the community, purchasers, and physicians in particular. There are reasons and situations favoring both warfare and partnership with peers. The risks in choosing partnership come from the possibilities that partners may choose warfare. Physicians may choose to compete with the hospital in ambulatory surgery, diagnostic imaging, laboratory services, urgent care, and any number of services that are essential to hospital survival. Other hospitals may duplicate its most profitable services or win away patient volumes that make the difference between high quality, efficient, financially rewarding operations and disaster.

The rewards of partnership can be in both survival and mission achievement. It is not only possible but likely that any provider organization can achieve more, both qualitatively and quantitatively, in partnership with selected peers than in warfare with all or by going it alone. Survival as part of a larger alliance may be more possible than survival as a lonely warrior. The more successful partners may become the hubs or leaders of coalitions and consortiums, alliances and systems that do far more in extending and achieving their missions than they could ever have accomplished alone.

Partnerships require the deliberate identification and conscious reinforcement of common interests. Provider organizations that see themselves clearly and behave as though they are in partnership with key stakeholders are likely to retain a more effective focus on those interests. Organizations that are at war may tend to see such interests as momentary opportunities for exploitation rather than as bases for permanent relationships. Warfare tends to make it harder to achieve and maintain lasting relationships with anyone.

The rewards in warfare are potentially great. By defeating the enemy, successful competitors may win the field. Driving a competitor to bankruptcy can drive down the price of acquisition or leave the market unsullied by competition. Of course, it can also result in the acquisition of a competitor by another firm that will be even better at warfare. Defeating a competitor in battle may also sour relations with the competitor's partners and stakeholders.

Perhaps the greatest risk in choosing warfare is that it closes off so many other choices. Once warfare begins, battle lines are drawn, and sides are clearly established. Even small partnerships or collaborative arrangements may become difficult or impossible because they require treating with the enemy. The warfare mentality may extend further than desired; physicians, purchasers, and even patients and the community may be treated as battlegrounds rather than as customers or partners, and even employees may become cannon fodder.

The risk is that the deliberate choice of warfare and its rhetoric may make competition inefficient or ineffective. The goal in war is victory, and the mission may be lost in the furor. Survival becomes such a key concern that the purpose of being may be lost in the shuffle, and the organization may become changed beyond recognition.

Warfare tends to make it harder to achieve and maintain lasting relationships with anyone.

Partnerships are driven primarily by mission concerns. We choose to partner, and with whom, based on who can contribute most and best to achievement of mission. Survival will still be a major goal in most cases, but changes in form and role become more acceptable if they will promote the mission. To the extent that the organization's stakeholders are motivated more by its mission than by its survival, partnerships can galvanize the effort needed to survive and succeed.

Warfare is driven primarily by survival concerns. Everyone that can harm the organization tends to become the enemy, even if some are capable of contributing to its mission, even its survival, as well. Everyone who is not an ally tends to be thought of as an enemy.

To the extent that the organization's stakeholders are committed more to its mission than to its survival, warfare may actually threaten its survival, regardless of what the enemy does.

Partnership seems to have a stronger basis than warfare for motivating and organizing the efforts of stakeholders. Employees, physicians, patients, and purchasers may not like the idea of warfare; they may prefer preserving their options rather than wiping them out. They may object to the obvious signs of warfare in terms of advertising and marketing expenditures that do not benefit customers. Moreover, competitors may respond to belligerence by adopting a warrior stance, and prove better at it than expected.

The government not only forbids anticompetitive collusion by peers in the same market, it also discourages what are called predatory marketing practices. Where destroying the enemy in warfare is encouraged, destroying a competitor in business is frowned upon. The communities may not take kindly to losing a choice of health care providers or the jobs and other contributions to the economy that a former competitor represented.

• • •

Since the purpose even of warfare is a better peace, it makes more sense to delineate what that better peace is and choose the best means to achieve it than to prefer either warfare or partnership for its own sake. Partnership should be considered a possible means to the organization's basic ends, mission, and survival. It would be naive to ignore competitive realities when competitors are not doing the same. Partnership offers no guarantees of success and no head start for being morally superior.

On the other hand, consciously choosing war without considering its total consequences would be equally naive. The champions of warfare do a disservice when they make rhetoric to make warfare appear so attractive or inescapable that it is chosen as an end in itself. In health care, at least, the mission should be more important than competitive victory. Providers should always be willing to look for the best means to carry out the mission, even if those means necessitate change and cooperation, instead of resorting to battle and warfare.

There are ample signs that warfare is not universally accepted as a superior or even acceptable strategy in commercial business. While there may be advantages to those who first adopt an effective strategy and risks to those who wait and see, there are many questions yet to be answered regarding warfare's place in health care. Health care has a nurturing mission, and in the long run, it may be incompatible with war's destructive animus.

REFERENCES

1. Kotler, P., and Singh, R. "Marketing Warfare in the 1980s." *Journal of Business Strategy* 1, no. 3 (1981): 30—41.
2. Ries, A., and Trout, J. *Marketing Warfare*. New York: McGraw-Hill, 1986.
3. Kessler, D.M. "Viewing Health Care as a War Theater." *Health Care Strategic Management* 6 (March 1988): 5–9.
4. Malhotra, N. "Health Care Marketing Warfare." *Journal of Health Care Marketing* 8 (March 1988): 17.
5. Abrahamson, L. "Batting 1,000 in Medical Staff Marketing." *Topics in Health Care Finance* 14 (Spring 1988): 14.
6. Fallucchi, A. "Health Care in a Competitive Business." *Facilities Design and Management*. Northfield, Ill.: Mitchell International, March 1987.
7. Lovelock, C., and Weinberg, C. *Marketing for Public and Non-Profit Managers*. New York: Wiley, 1984, p. 567.
8. Mauet, A., and Burns, M. "The Marketing Mindset: A Cautionary Note." *Journal of Health and Human Resources Administration* 10 (Fall 1987): 189–205.
9. "Forget Satisfying the Customer—Just Outfox the Other Guy." *Business Week* (7 October 1985):
10. Robson, J., and Luft, H. "Competition and the Cost of Hospital Care 1972–1982." *JAMA* 257 (19 June 1987): 244.
11. Mourning, S. "Networking Strategies for Hospitals." *Topics in Health Care Finance* 14 (Spring 1988): 56–61.
12. Ohmae, K. "Getting Back to Strategy." *Harvard Business Review* 88 (September/October 1988): 149.
13. Albrecht, K., and Zemke, R. *Service America*. Homewood, Ill.: Dow Jones–Irwin, 1985.
14. Gronroos, C. "Developing the Service Offering." In *Add Value to Your Service*, edited by C. Surprenant. Chicago: American Marketing Association, 1987, pp. 81–85.
15. Pottruck, D. "Building Company Loyalty and Retention through Direct Marketing." *Journal of Services Marketing* 1 (Fall 1987): 53–58.
16. Carew, J. *You'll Never Get No For An Answer*. New York: Simon & Schuster, 1988.
17. Hanan, M. *Successful Market Penetration*. New York: American Management Association, 1988.
18. Hill-Chin, L. "Add Cooperation to Regulation and Competition." *Hospitals* 62 (5 December 1987): 88.
19. Poniatowski, L. "Doing Everything Right." *Health Management Quarterly* 10, no. 2 (1988): 3–5.
20. Greene, J. "Not-for-Profit Tax Exemption Under Fire." *Modern Healthcare* (22 July 1988): 76, 84.
21. Levy, S., and Hill, J. "Advocacy Reconsidered: Progress and Prospects." *Hospital and Health Services Administrators* 33 (Winter 1988): 467–79.

22. Pozos, R. "The End Game Strategy." *HealthWeek* (27 July 1987): 35–38.
23. Lazare, A., et al. "The Customer Approach to Patienthood." *Archives of General Psychiatry* 32 (May 1975): 553–53.
24. Quill, T. "Partnerships in Patient Care: A Contractual Approach." *Annals of Internal Medicine* 98 (1983): 228–34.
25. Jenna, J. "Toward the Patient Driven Hospital." *Healthcare Forum* 29 (May/June 1986): 8.
26. Payne, S. "Identifying and Managing Inappropriate Hospital Utilization." *Health Services Research* 24 (December 1987): 407–18.
27. Gill, S., and Meighan, S. "Five Roadblocks to Effective Partnership in a Competitive Health Care Environment." *Hospital and Health Services Administrators* 33 (Winter 1988): 505–20.
28. Kotler, P., and Clarke, P. *Marketing for Health Care Organizations*. Englewood Cliffs, N.J.: Prentice-Hall, 1987.
29. "Hospital Contracting: Adversaries Become Partners." *GHAA News* 29 (May/June 1988): 15–17.
30. Kenkel, P. "Providers, Local Businesses Form Partnership to Contain Health Costs." *Modern Healthcare* (27 May 1988): 132.
31. Kenkel, P. "Seeking a Rational System." *Modern Healthcare* (4 November 1988): 64.
32. Drucker, P. "The Coming of the New Organization." *Harvard Business Review* 66, no. 1 (1988): 45–53.
33. Marr, J., and Andrews, J. "Employee Feedback Regarding Customer Service Quality, Problems and Solutions." In *Add Value to Your Service*, edited by C. Surprenant. Chicago: American Marketing Association, 1987, pp. 153–55.
34. Grossi, P. "Employee Volunteerism...A Natural Extension of Human Relations." *Healthcare Marketing Report* 6 (June 1988): 16–18.
35. Roodman,R."Innovative Marketing Strategies." In *Medical Staff Marketing Third National Forum Proceedings*. Chicago: American Hospital Association, 1987, pp. 73–83.
36. Frommelt, J., et al. "Finance and Marketing: Birth of a Profitable Relationship." *Healthcare Financial Management* (December 1987): 25–32.
37. "Nonprofit Organizations Grapple with the Vagaries of Liability Insurance." *The Wall Street Journal* 70 (20 June 1989), p. 1.
38. Doyle, S., and Boudreau, J. "Hospital/Supplier Partnership." *Journal of Health Care Marketing* 9 (Mar 1989): 42–47.
39. Droste, T. "Hospital Shares Print Ads—and Costs—with Vendor." *Hospitals* 63 (20 July 1989): 48.
40. Devine, R. "Catholic Healthcare's New Crisis." *Health Progress* 69 (April 1988): 71–73.
41. "Marketing Children's Hospitals Isn't Child's Play." *Healthcare Marketing Report* 4 (June 1986): 1–4.

PART III

PROCESS

Total quality management in health: Making it work

Curtis P. McLaughlin
and
Arnold D. Kaluzny

Many health organizations are trying total quality management (TQM). This approach represents a total paradigm shift in health care management and presents a series of potential conflict areas in the way health organizations are managed. These areas include TQM's participatory approach versus professional and managerial authority, collective versus individual responsibility, quality assurance and standards versus continuous improvement, and flexible versus rigid objectives and plans. This article reviews the areas of conflict and suggests a number of action guidelines for the successful implementation of TQM.

Health Care Manage Rev, 1990, 15(3), 7-14
© 1990 Aspen Publishers, Inc.

Interest in total quality management (TQM), a major managerial innovation, is running high. The Joint Commission on Accreditation of Healthcare Organizations (Joint Commission) has placed its "agenda for change" squarely within the philosophical context of TQM.[1] The Hospital Research and Educational Trust of the American Hospital Association has recently published a report to help hospitals "organize for, communicate about, monitor and continuously improve all aspects of health care delivery."[2(p.2)] This report is part of a three-year quality improvement initiative sponsored by fifteen hospital systems and alliances.

TQM, first developed in the United States and successfully implemented in Japan, is obviously receiving serious attention by U.S. health service organizations as they try to improve quality with fewer resources.[3-5] A growing number of hospitals and health maintenance organizations (HMOs) are implementing TQM. Some will succeed; many will fail. This article argues that TQM represents a fundamental paradigm shift in health care management and explores a series of potential conflicts between TQM and the way that health care institutions normally are managed. A number of action guidelines are suggested to better ensure that TQM fulfills its potential and functions effectively within health service organizations.

TQM AS A PARADIGM SHIFT

Total quality management is a conceptual approach different from quality assurance (QA) and quality inspection and runs counter to many underlying assumptions of professional bureaucracies. It calls for continuous and relentless improvement in the total process that provides care, not simply in the improved actions of individual professionals. Improvement is thus based on both outcome and process.

Batalden et al.[6] outline what the health leadership must learn to implement TQM successfully.

- Management must learn the meaning of quality, including an understanding of the importance of

Curtis P. McLaughlin, *D.B.A., is Professor of Health Policy and Administration, School of Public Health, and Professor of Business Administration, School of Business, at the University of North Carolina in Chapel Hill, North Carolina.*

Arnold D. Kaluzny, *Ph.D., is Professor of Health Policy and Administration at the School of Public Health, University of North Carolina in Chapel Hill, North Carolina.*

the customer, and that there are multiple customers in the production process.

- Top management must sponsor and encourage the continuous improvement of quality, including the wise use of teams that can work together effectively to improve systems and of other processes, including group processes and organization and system change skills.
- Management must learn the meaning of statistical thinking: how to speak with data and manage with facts; how to take the guesswork out of decision making; how to reduce variation and unnecessary complexity through the use of the seven standard tools of data analysis and display (cause-and-effect diagram, Pareto chart, histogram, scatter diagram, flow chart, run or trend chart, and control chart); and how to link the results of the use of these tools with appropriate management action.[6]

TQM demands that change be based on the needs of the customer, not the values of the providers. It requires the meaningful participation of all personnel and a rapid and thoughtful response from top management to suggestions made by participating personnel. Management is no longer able to stifle the suggestions of personnel by requiring additional study or by requiring that all decisions be reviewed by a higher level of management.

TQM is more than a change in values and responsiveness by top management. It requires rigorous process flow and statistical analysis, evaluation of all ongoing activities, and the recognition and application of underlying psychosocial principles affecting individuals and groups within an organization. It requires accepting the fundamental assumption that most problems encountered in a health care organization are the result of not errors by administrative or clinical professionals, but the inability of the structure—within which all personnel function—to perform adequately.

An obvious conflict is between the relentless inquiry of TQM and the established norms of professional autonomy. This is not merely a conflict between administrators and clinical professionals: It is a fundamental challenge to the way all professionals think about quality, evaluate and regulate themselves, and gain and protect their professional domains and autonomy. TQM does not respect existing professional standards; it is continually demanding new ones.

TQM places primary emphasis for problem characterization on the system rather than the individual. Deming[7] estimates that 85% of errors introduced into a

process are the result of problems with the system rather than the type of random errors and mistakes introduced by individuals. This runs counter to the prevailing assumption in health services that a problem is a result of one individual's error rather than of the larger structure or system within which the individual functions. For example, one of the authors was hospitalized briefly last summer and experienced a number of scheduling and coordination difficulties that unnecessarily complicated the stay. In an effort to provide constructive feedback to management, the author described his experience and displeasure to a staff member, suggesting that these problems could be improved, if not eliminated. A few weeks later at a social occasion, the supervisor of one of the departments involved approached him and started asking questions such as, "What did the person look like? Was the employee short or tall? I checked the records the day you were in, and the person who was on duty was the one least likely to do that." Unfortunately, the normal response to complaints is to "take names and kick butts."

Similarly, at a recent executive training program, a group of midlevel managers was asked to consider programmatic issues such as "Why does it take one to two hours to get a discharged patient from the floor to the front door?" Obviously, the solution to this problem lies in coordinating several departments, and the group members agreed that they could resolve the problem. However, they argued that upper management had not asked them to solve the problem. They knew it was a systems problem, but they felt responsible for managing only their own functions, not a system; therefore, the problem continued.

Finally, TQM challenges the prevailing model of who the customer is. The customer in TQM is not only the patient, but also the many users of a department's output. Here again, the criterion is not whether or not the work meets professional standards, but whether the user, often a member of a different profession, is satisfied with its timeliness and utility.

The reality is that both models—TQM and the professional bureaucracy—must be accommodated if TQM is to make a difference in health care organizations. For example, Galbraith[8] outlines the importance of the professional model in handling the flood of technical information that medical research has developed. He suggests that specialization is a way of handling information overload, especially in the absence of other information-processing alternatives such as a common management information system or lateral linkages for information coordination. In fact, one can see TQM as a methodology for developing lateral linkages in the health care organization that transfer information between disciplines as needed. It is a powerful method of lateral technology transfer in the traditionally highly compartmentalized organization.

CONFLICTS BETWEEN THE TWO MODELS

The nature of the organizational change required to implement TQM can be outlined by contrasting the two models and evaluating points of conflict (see Figure 1). While they are not mutually exclusive and while the observed points of conflict will vary between organizations, each of the models requires explicit recognition.

Individual versus collective responsibility

The professional model places the responsibility for performance squarely on the individual professional. As described by Mintzberg, "the Professional Bureaucracy...hires duly trained and indoctrinated specialists—professionals—and then gives them control over their own work."[9(p.349)] He goes on to state that such control means that the professional works independently of colleagues but closely with clients. If the professional makes a mistake, then that professional is primarily liable for damages. If the error is blatant, a QA committee, and the professional society in the very worst cases, sanctions the individual. Only in the most

grievous cases is the organization itself at risk for damages.

The TQM model focuses on the system. If errors or problems occur (e.g., if individuals were not properly trained, key information was not transferred, or procedures were not adequate to the variety of possible situations), the TQM model focuses on the process, not the individual provider. To correct problems and errors, a group—usually interdisciplinary—of individuals in the organization is asked to assume ownership of each process and joint responsibility for its improvement.

Clinical versus managerial leadership

In the health service organization, a continuing source of conflict is the relationship between the various levels of administrative management and the clini-

Managers are required to involve clinical professionals in the decision-making process, leaving it up to them to solve quality problems as they arise.

cal professional leadership. At a time when the management is trying to gain more control over the clinical

FIGURE 1

AREAS OF CONFLICT BETWEEN TWO ORGANIZATIONAL MODELS: PROFESSIONAL AND TQM

Professional		TQM
Individual responsibilities		Collective responsibilities
Professional leadership		Managerial leadership
Autonomy		Accountability
Administrative authority		Participation
Professional authority	◄—Versus—►	Participation
Goal expectations		Performance and process expectations
Rigid planning		Flexible planning
Response to complaints		Benchmarking
Retrospective performance appraisal		Concurrent performance appraisal
Quality assurance		Continuous improvement

professional in the face of pressures for cost-containment purposes, TQM comes along and demands that management take a more participative approach. Managers are required to involve clinical professionals in the decision-making process, leaving it up to them to solve quality problems as they arise. Yet, while this is a participative program, it is clearly a managerial initiative. Paradoxically, participation may be perceived as a threat to professional autonomy while at the same time contributing to individual and group autonomy.

Autonomy versus accountability

Autonomy is central to the clinical professional model. Under this model, clinical professionals have the special privilege of freedom from the control of outsiders. This privilege is justified by three claims:

1. Unusual degrees of skill and knowledge are involved in clinical professional work, and administrative professionals are not equipped to evaluate or regulate it.
2. Clinicians are responsible, and they may be trusted to work conscientiously without supervision.
3. Clinical professionals themselves may be trusted to undertake the proper regulatory action on those rare occasions where an individual does not perform work competently or ethically.[10]

Clinical professionals are thus suspicious of managerial actions in the areas of cost control and QA, and TQM may look like another in a progression of management steps designed to reduce their professional autonomy. TQM is a technique that is likely to increase personal autonomy in undertaking task-oriented change. It does not, however, respect professional autonomy as much as it respects personal autonomy. At the same time, it demands that clinical professionals hold themselves accountable for both outcome and process performance on a continuous basis.

Administrative authority versus participation

TQM, through the use of quality circles, puts responsibility for quality control in the province of the front-line managers and employees. Quality circles are small groups of employees from the same area who work on a range of problems to increase productivity and efficiency. Maintaining quality no longer means taking names and booting bottoms; it means monitoring and teaching employees to monitor their own performance and taking corrective action.

Professional authority versus participation

The TQM approach diffuses responsibility for quality among the members of the team responsible for the delivery of care. The criteria are not necessarily those selected by physicians and other professional groups. TQM emphasizes that criteria are selected by the users of the output. It was best described by the director of a major teaching hospital, who defined his objective in starting a TQM program as wanting to "make this a customer-driven instead of a doctor-dominated hospital." Teams are likely to be multidisciplinary, and the creativity and worth of every team member must be respected equally. This has been reported frequently as a perceived threat to the status of middle managers. The same is quite likely to be the case with high-status professionals.

Goal versus process and performance expectations

The usual expectation in health care is that one has an objective goal for every act; that there is a "gold standard" for care. This means that each activity has a protocol for behavior and an expected outcome, and that the protocol remains in effect until a technological change makes it obsolete. That is not the case with TQM. The objective for TQM is one of continuous improvement. While this is not totally foreign to health care (e.g., the history of organ transplants has been one of continuous improvement), the hospital does not measure the success ratios of many of its basic procedures, such as getting the discharged patient out the door more quickly.

Rigid versus flexible planning

A major teaching hospital tried forming quality circles and, like many other hospitals, developed a series of major cost-saving actions. As might be expected, these proposals often had associated capital requirements, and the hospital had already planned its capital investments for three or more years. The proposals were not implemented quickly, and the quality circles lost interest.

TQM requires that management be responsive to quality improvement suggestions. New priorities are necessary, and they must be addressed aggressively through flexible, ongoing planning rather than through rigid, preprogrammed activities.

TQM includes a concept called *benchmarking* of products and processes. This involves comparing current activities and performance against the best of the competition, the idea being to develop a product and process that significantly betters the competition. This implies several changes to existing approaches in health care, where the primary stimulus for change is the recognition of a problem vis-à-vis the established norm. First, TQM explicitly acknowledges that there is a competition to be studied and surpassed. Second, it recognizes the customer's experience as the basis of comparison. Third, it expects that the organization and its processes should be improving all the time, regardless of whether or not a complaint is registered or a problem identified. It means that the accepted way of doing things does not last long. It requires continuous growth and learning on the part of everyone, no matter how old or how educated.

Retrospective versus concurrent performance appraisal systems

Most performance appraisal systems are based on setting goals and then meeting them. TQM appraisals focus on gaining skills to contribute to the process of quality improvement. Therefore, the reward system is based on contribution to a team effort to improve outcomes rather than on whether specific set objectives have been met. If TQM is in effect, the objectives will be changing almost daily: as some are achieved, new ones are immediately set. This case illustrates the concept of TQM.

A European company won a contract to deliver headlamps to a Japanese car manufacturer. The initial contract allowed 50 defective lamps per 100,000. The lamp manufacturer modified its process to meet that standard painlessly. The next contract called for 20 defective lamps per 100,000. The lamp manufacturer managed to meet that too, so the next contract called for 5 per 100,000. Once again, the supplier struggled and met the new requirement. The next contract called for 10 per 1,000,000. This time the lamp manufacturer complained, "Why didn't you ask for that standard the first time?" "We didn't know what you could do, when we started," the Japanese replied.

The concept of Kaizen,[11] or "continuous improvement," is what drives a TQM program. No matter how well one does, one should be preparing and attempting to do better.

Quality assurance versus continuous improvement

The underlying premise of QA has been to identify human errors in the process, to follow established protocols, and to search for failures to meet the gold standard. This is the traditional Joint Commission approach: Either the standard is met or it is not. TQM emphasizes system errors and the continuous nature of improvement. Moreover, it requires that improvement be the responsibility of all personnel, not just those designated as "QA" personnel. Fortunately, the new Joint Commission standards are planned to reflect the TQM approach, emphasizing a process for continuous improvement rather than a go versus no-go measure.

PREPARING FOR CHANGE

The implementation of TQM requires that administrative and medical managers mediate areas of conflict. How well management functions during the transition will depend on its ability to follow the action guidelines presented below.

Action 1: Redefine the role of the professional

Most health care organizations have hired professionals on the basis of their possession of technical skills and standards certified by the training programs from which they were hired. Management has had relatively little control over professionals once they are hired, so they must have the right work habits, standards, and methods when hired. It has been assumed that the possession of this training and these work habits would lead to decision making that would meet the gold standard for an extended period of time.

The new set of decision-making skills required by TQM will have to include not only technical skills, but also the ability and flexibility to be guided by a quest for continuous improvement. This requires fundamental skills for statistical analysis of procedures and the ability to work with and in multidisciplinary teams. In essence, the routine tasks of the physician, nurse, and other providers will have to include basic epidemiology, statistics, and a variety of group process skills.

Action 2: Redefine the corporate culture

Americans tend to look for the quick fix, the home run, and the Nobel Prize. While TQM may yield a home run early on, the basic philosophy is one of incessant change, the hitting of lots of singles, and the tortoise over the hare. Imai observes that Westerners are concerned with performance, while Easterners are concerned with both performance and process.[11] The Eastern philosophy calls for continuous employee training to assist with continuous improvement. This means that there must be a change in what Kilmann[12] refers to as culture, management skills, team-building strategy, structure, and reward system. Failure to address each in a systematic effort will greatly limit the implementation of TQM.

Action 3: Redefine the role of management

In TQM, the manager becomes a symphony conductor, orchestrating the independent actions of a variety of professionals and project-oriented teams. This change really modifies current leadership roles at the top, middle, and bottom of the management hierar-

---

The top managers will do less of the decision making, leaving it to lower and middle levels of management to make the majority of the decisions, often on a consensual basis among the departments involved.

---

chy.[13] The top managers will do less of the decision making, leaving it to lower and middle levels of management to make the majority of the decisions, often on a consensual basis among the departments involved. The role of top management, then, is to manage the culture and to allocate resources to support the change process. Top management will have to establish a planning process that is flexible enough to adapt to the propositions that the TQM process develops. Top management will have to be the spokespersons for the clients who are not represented in the system, especially the patients. Middle management has responsibility for monitoring the process of TQM and authorizing the implementation of the process changes that are identified for improvement of both quality and cost. Front-line management acquires the key role in TQM. The first-line manager has to lead the process and at the same time give people enough room to make it work. All levels of management must be evaluated as role models for TQM, and top managers have especially key roles in modeling, teaching, and providing feedback as part of the TQM process.

Action 4: Empower the staff to analyze and solve problems

The most important challenge for management is to empower the staff to gather data, analyze it, and make recommendations. This involves convincing the staff that it is safe to collect data and do something with the results. This means that management must overcome

status barriers; must be diligent in convincing people to try out statistical quality control techniques, making sure that people get rapid feedback to their proposals; and must be diplomatic. Supervisors also have to act as liaisons if problems turn out to have multiple causation (as they so often do). They have to be able to see the system in a systems way, focusing not first on their own units but on a component in a complex system. Most of all, they must all be supporters of the massive social changes that TQM can require.

Action 5: Change organizational objectives

The organization's objectives need to be expressed in terms of both performance objectives and process objectives. This means that programs will have to set their own quality objectives period by period as they develop the capacity to measure, follow, and modify their own processes.

Action 6: Develop mentoring capacity

The professionals and the managers will both perceive the changes as risky to implement and threatening to their professional identity. They will need models of behavior to follow and mentors with whom they can discuss their plans and feelings about the risks involved. Senior executives who are convinced of the importance of TQM are going to provide advice and support. In fact, in one industrial organization, a criterion for promotion among mid- and upper-level managers is how subordinates judge their abilities to function as role models.

Action 7: Drive the benchmarking process from the top

The hardest process step will be the benchmarking process, a process that must be led from the top of the organization. Top management is the group responsible for assessing the outside environment. They have the capacity to identify the best performance of competitive organizations and compare internal operations with these high-performance organizations. This will not happen effectively without strong leadership from the top down.

The unit of analysis for benchmarking is critical. It is not just "Do we have the best radiology department in the country?" It is also "Do we give our patients the best experience? Do we serve the attending physicians better than anyone else? Are we making fewer processing errors and fewer delayed reports than last month, and are we working to make this the best in the world?"

Action 8: Modify the reward system

The reward system of health care is constrained to a high degree by professional status and prerogatives. The health care institution, however, must reserve some rewards for those who cooperate most whole-heartedly and effectively. The rewards are most likely to be psychic rather than financial payments. They can effectively include travel, entertainment, employee recognition (best used for teams), and vacation time. For example, one major U.S. company that is very successful at TQM has eliminated all financial awards in its suggestion system. It now gives books on how to improve job performance and trips to continuing education programs instead. The ideal reward system should reward both performance and process development.

Action 9: Go outside the health industry for models

Xerox Corporation of Stamford, Connecticut, has been one of the most successful adherents of TQM. TQM has helped the company to thrive in the highly competitive copier market and to compete well enough to recover some of its market from the Japanese. David T. Kearns, Chairman and Chief Executive Officer of Xerox, has suggested that the next benchmark for Xerox copiers after Japanese copiers is the telephone, with its attributes of both high reliability and low cost. Health managers should not hesitate to go outside of the health industry for its models of consumer-driven quality. The obvious future targets are highly successful consumer service organizations such as Walt Disney, American Airlines, Marriott, and American Express.

Action 10: Set realistic time expectations

The process of adopting and institutionalizing TQM, like all organizational change processes, takes time under the best of circumstances, most likely three to five years. It is likely to take longer in a large, complex organization like a teaching hospital. People will have to start with a realistic estimate of the time required. Two types of time are required—hours of input by already busy managers and professionals and calendar time required to implement the program. The latter is illustrated even in the case of a very tightly controlled organization such as Xerox, where new issues concerning TQM institutionalization continue to surface five years after implementation. For example, employee evaluation systems were not changed to include management commitment and role modeling for TQM, and college employment recruiters were not using TQM-related selection criteria until shortly before the firm received the Malcolm Baldridge Prize in 1989 in recognition of its successful implementation of TQM.

Action 11: Make the TQM program a model for continuous improvement

The cases cited above highlight possibilities for using the TQM program to model a continuous improvement orientation for the total organization. Those who are responsible for program oversight must consciously challenge the TQM staff to suggest improvements in the program and respond rapidly and effectively. The professionals will be especially sensitive to any gaps between what is preached and what is practiced by those associated with this program. They have already seen many programs come and go in recent years, and they must be convinced that management is serious about TQM. Here actions will truly speak louder than words.

•　　•　　•

Health service organizations are facing new challenges, challenges that require a new look at how and why resources are organized and managed. The expectations are high for TQM. A recent survey by Peat, Marwick, Main & Co. of Chicago reports that 69% of institutional providers and 78% of physicians, purchasers, and third party payers believe that the cost of poor quality is so great that quality improvement should pay for itself.[14] Industrial organizations have reduced their operating expenses by 20% to 40%. If health care organizations can do half as well, quality improvement programs will have a major impact on the field.

TQM represents an approach with a great deal of potential, yet it presents some basic conflicts with underlying norms and expectations that guide professional bureaucracies. While the conflict exists, the problems are not intractable and, if recognized, represent opportunities not only to improve quality of care but also improve the system designed to provide quality care.

REFERENCES

1. Ente, B.H. *Brief Overview of the Joint Commission's "Agenda for Change."* Chicago, Ill.: Joint Commission, 1989.
2. James, B.C. *Quality Management for Health Care Delivery.* Chicago, Ill.: The Hospital Research and Educational Trust of the American Hospital Association, 1989.

3. Berwick, D. "Continuous Improvement as an Ideal in Health Care." *New England Journal of Medicine* 320, no. 1 (1989): 53–56.
4. Berwick, D. "Health Services Research and Quality of Care." *Medical Care* 27, no. 8 (1989): 763–71.
5. Goldfield, N., and Nash, D.B. *Providing Quality Care: The Challenge to Clinicians*. Philadelphia, Pa.: American College of Physicians, 1989.
6. Batalden, P., et al. "Quality Improvement: The Role and Application of Research Methods." *The Journal of Health Administration Education* 7, no. 3 (1989): 577–83.
7. Deming, W.E. *Out of Crisis*. Cambridge, Mass.: MIT Press, 1986.
8. Galbraith, J. *Designing Complex Organizations*. Reading, Mass.: Addison-Wesley, 1973.
9. Mintzberg, H. *The Structuring of Organizations*. Englewood Cliffs, N.J.: Prentice Hall, 1979.
10. Freidson, E. *Profession of Medicine*. New York, N.Y.: Dodd, Mead, 1975.
11. Imai, M. Kaizen: *The Key to Japan's Competitive Success*. New York, N.Y.: Random House, 1986.
12. Kilmann, R. *Beyond the Quick Fix*. San Francisco, Calif.: Jossey-Bass, 1989.
13. Kaluzny, A.D. "Revitalizing Decision-making at the Middle Management Level." *Hospital and Health Services Administration* 34, no. 1 (1989): 39–51.
14. Peat, Marwick, Main & Co. *Setting Quality Standards in Health Care: Balancing Purchaser, Provider and Patient Expectations*. Chicago, Ill.: KMPG Peat Marwick, 1988.

Health care quality: The new marketing challenge

Carl W. Nelson
and
Arnold S. Goldstein

More and more buyers of health care are evaluating the quality of care as well as the cost. To stay competitive, providers must now learn how to sell quality.

Now that the health care industry leaves behind a decade of preoccupation with cost containment, the focus is again returning to the quality of care. Health care providers faced with sharply increased competition, reduced demand for inpatient care, new and alternative delivery systems, and an evolving revolution in how health services are being purchased are looking for new ways to capture their share of business. Coupled with strong marketing programs, many health care providers are trying to take advantage of this new consumer interest in the quality of health care by touting the superiority of their services.[1] Using various means, these providers promote the clinical quality of their services as a selling tool.

Quality of care will become a major marketing issue in the decade ahead. Much of the thrust is because the industry is dealing with increasingly sophisticated consumers, employees, government agencies, and other buyers of health services. With heightened awareness of quality issues, these groups seek ways to define and measure quality and will make decisions about where to obtain health care based on both objective evidence and perceptions of quality.[2]

EMERGING APPROACHES TO QUALITY ASSESSMENT

While there are many emerging approaches to quality assessment, it would appear that consumers of health services have taken the lead from providers in coalescing efforts to define quality as a criterion for buying health care.

- The federal government, the largest buyer of health services, has undertaken perhaps the most ambitious quality assessment initiatives through its Health Care Financing Administration (HCFA). HCFA has publicly released hospital mortality data for Medicare recipients and is expected to release physician specific performance data. With these first steps toward broader

Carl W. Nelson, *Ph.D., is an Associate Professor and Area Coordinator for Health Care Management at Northeastern University, College of Business Administration in Boston, Massachusetts. He also serves as a consultant to the health care industry.*

Arnold S. Goldstein, *M.B.A., LL.M., is a Professor of Pharmacy Administration at Northeastern University in Boston, Massachusetts. He teaches health care law and administration and has authored numerous articles and several books on health care management.*

Health Care Manage Rev, 1989, 14(2), 87–95
© 1989 Aspen Publishers, Inc.

disclosure of quality performance data, HCFA's quality assessment program may well establish quality standards that will dictate where the billions of dollars in federal health care funds will be channeled. Moreover, HCFA benchmarks may create standards that set the pace for the private sector as well.

- The Joint Commission on the Accreditation of Healthcare Organizations (Joint Commission) is actively involved in its own quality assessment program. The Joint Commission plan focuses quality review under the accreditation process on clinical performance measures and outcomes (adjusted for the severity of patient illness) in 25 clinical areas.[3] Ultimately, the Joint Commission envisions a full menu of measures across all clinical categories resulting in data that clearly highlight areas of potential quality problems. The Joint Commission's approach to quality depends on professional medical consensus and data on provider's actual experience, outlining indicators of acceptable performance and referring for special evaluation cases that fall outside the acceptable range. While many see the Joint Commission initiative more as a matter of quality specification rather than quality assessment, others are concerned that the data can lead to the ranking of hospitals and therefore have a significant competitive influence.

- Employer groups, equally concerned about the quality of care, are designing their own quality assessment systems for participating providers. General Motors and the United Auto Workers, as prime examples, now require the 140 participating health maintenance organizations (HMOs) that service their million-plus members to submit to intensive quality review audits. While the automobile makers are in the vanguard, large employers within virtually every industry are developing quality specifications for participating providers. For example, Ryder System, a transportation and truck rental firm, is now compiling data on operations and the number of times a surgeon performs a given procedure. Through its own Medfacts System, Ryder can now give employees who are looking for a physician detailed information about a local practitioner's training and fees. "What we are trying to do is make our employees more intelligent consumers," says Joseph Charles

who oversees employee benefits for Ryder. Adds Princeton University health care economist Uwe Reinhardt, "Ten years from now programs such as Medfacts will be routine."[4] Other employers gather information from insurance companies, fiscal intermediaries, data consortia, and other sources to help them define quality and are using this information to acquire health services. If hospitals and other providers expect to win business from large firms, they must be able to supply the information on quality sought by these employers.

- The "Blues"—Blue Cross and Blue Shield—have expressed a long-standing concern about quality measurement. In an all-out effort to improve assessment techniques, Blue Cross/Blue Shield has embarked on a variety of programs. For example, Blue Cross/Blue Shield of Minnesota now uses the Medigroups's quality review software package (Mediqual Systems) to monitor and measure provider performance. Through the Medigroups System, Blue Cross can more precisely detect deviations from accepted norms, define practice standards, and negotiate more advantageous provider contracts. Its use of the system could set a precedent for other Blue Cross plans and establish a new standard for other insurance underwriters to adopt.

- Professional Review Organizations (PROs), the ordained watchdogs of health care quality under Medicare, are now in search of more advanced tools to measure the quality of care. Several promising approaches are being pursued by various PROs investigating variations in medical practice patterns within their state. PROs also are working closely with the HCFA to find measures of potential quality problems other than traditional indicators such as mortality rates.

With such a broad base of activity, the health care industry is unquestionably entering an era in which the quality of services will be measured and scrutinized far more closely than in the past. And to help with the task there is a new and burgeoning support industry introducing the capabilities of computer technology. The Medigroup Software System now in use by Blue Cross of Minnesota is only one of many such firms offering sophisticated quality assessment programs. Another prototype system is marketed to health care purchasers by San Francisco's National Medical Audit, which is-

This groundswell of activity has the potential to create an enormous database of quality measures that eventually can be used by purchasers, regulators, and providers alike to define "value" in medical practice.

sues "report cards" to hospitals, HMOs, preferred provider organizations (PPOs), and other providers, ranking their performance (on a 1–7 scale) based on the frequency and severity of adverse incidents in selected clinical areas. Other producers of software that measures quality of care are rapidly being organized to satisfy the growing demand. Systemetics (Santa Barbara, California); Health Systems International (New Haven, Connecticut); Commission on Professional Hospital Activities (Ann Arbor, Michigan); and Pittsburgh Research Institute (Pittsburgh, Pennsylvania) are but a few innovators in the field offering a formi-

dable array of quality measurement systems. Although each takes a somewhat different approach toward quality assessment, their very existence points out the strong commitment to quality measurement now existing within the industry.

Many additional researchers and health care organizations are searching for a practical definition of quality. A two-year study by Dr. Barry Bleidt of the University of Texas suggests the number of separate groups engaged in the design of quality standards could easily number in the thousands.[5]

Developments in data acquisition and processing have stimulated the use of comparative assessment and monitoring and greatly amplify their usefulness in defining criteria for buying health services. This groundswell of activity has the potential to create an enormous database of quality measures that eventually can be used by purchasers, regulators, and providers alike to define "value" in medical practice. Unfortunately, it also has the possibility of creating a vast amount of confusion in the health care marketplace

Nosocomial Infection Rates

The June 2, 1987, headline of *The Tab* (a Brookline, Massachusetts, weekly newspaper) read: "Infections Await Many at Local Hospitals." In the accompanying article, the nosocomial infection rates of a total of 15 hospitals (5 community hospitals, 5 large general hospitals, and 5 smaller general hospitals) used by town residents were presented. Raw data had been drawn from hospital medical reports filed with a private medical data clearinghouse under contract to the state Rate Setting Commission. The newspaper purchased the data from the Commission, and its reporters subsequently analyzed the data for the article.

Six of the 15 hospitals were reported to have nosocomial infection rates that exceeded a national average of 0.5% of admissions. Two community hospitals had rates nearly double the national average, while one widely respected Brookline teaching hospital had the highest infection rate in its hospital's category. The article further alluded to the general impact of hospital cost-cutting measures on quality.

Hospital responses appeared two weeks later, along with a second article. One letter to the editor from the chief of infectious diseases at a hospital with reported infection rates at double the national average disputed

the accuracy of the figures and the methodology employed by the authors. He also strongly faulted the editorial policies of the paper. Another physician responsible for infection control admitted that hospitals could be dangerous but warned against scaring sick patients away with such statistics. The physician president of one hospital questioned the ability of drawing real conclusions from the data.

Subsequent private discussions with administrators from a cross section of these hospitals suggest that many believed that the original data were flawed because of coding errors on the part of overworked or poorly trained medical record personnel. Diagnostic coding errors are said to be in the range of 15% to 20%. One institution suspected that the problem arose because medical record personnel interpreted "n.s.," used for nonspecified infection, as an indicator of nosocomial infection. None wanted to risk acknowledging this quality problem, since those data were included in submissions to third party payers.

Administrators also revealed that their hospitals did not notice any change in admissions as a result of the bad publicity. Those with high occupancy levels remained "full, fat, and happy," while those with slipping levels were unable to say how they were affected.

until common criteria and methodologies are validated and accepted.

PERSPECTIVES OF QUALITY

While the industry continues to grapple with the underlying question of how quality of care can best be measured, progressive marketing-oriented providers are already at work selling "quality" to an increasingly responsive market.

One significant unknown is the relationship between the utilization of health care services and the quality of care. "The best providers do not always attract the most patients," comments Bleidt. "So far there is little correlation between 'quality' and patronage," he adds. "Providers must learn how to communicate the quality of their services if they are to compete."

Yet more market-sensitive providers agree that merely communicating data that illustrate an institution's quality of care will not in itself ensure a successful marketing program. A more important variable is the perception of quality of service, which may vary greatly between market segments. Though patients, physicians, and payers each speak in terms of "quality," the term takes on very different meanings to each group when used as a marketing tool. The greater challenge to the provider is to express "quality" in terms to which payers, physicians, and patients can relate and which each can understand. "Hospitals and other providers must begin to understand that very distinct buyer groups are emerging in the health care fields, and each group looks for different attributes in a provider," says Benson Fishman of Philadelphia's Professional Marketing Associates. "Essentially, providers need the right stimuli to attract the three major segments: patients, physicians, and cost underwriters," he adds.

In other industries, studies of the relationship between consumer perceptions of the quality of goods and services and a firm's market share indicate that changes in perceived quality are associated with changes in market share.[6] Furthermore, decision theorists and cognitive scientists now believe that individual decisions in situations involving risk and uncertainty are influenced more by new information than by the repetition of what is already known.[7]

The current situation in the health care industry remains somewhat contradictory. Hospital occupancy rates in competitive markets have generally so far been unaffected by public disclosure of high mortality and infection rates. (See the case summary "Nosocomial Infection Rates" in the box.) Yet continuing dramatic press reports of significant lapses in patient care can have a significant impact upon a hospital's image and occupancy levels. (See the case summary "Unexpected Hospital Related Mortality" in the box.) Up to now deeply ingrained public perceptions of an institution's good or bad quality have not been easily altered, without overwhelming evidence.

Unexpected Hospital-Related Mortality

On February 22, 1987, less than twenty-four hours after a routine operation to remove an infected gallbladder, the 58-year-old artist Andy Wharhol was unexpectedly found dead in his bed at a respected New York hospital medical center. Almost three years previously, Libby Zion, the 18-year-old daughter of a prominent attorney and writer for *The New York Times*, died unexpectedly after admission through the same hospital's emergency department. A highly publicized grand jury investigation and numerous other investigations had found routinely expected care deficient in the case of Libby Zion and focused upon the long shift hours and problems of continuity of care delivered by hospital residents. In another publicized case, a 39-year-old vice-president of Empire Blue Shield, Michael Gannon, died of a cardiac arrest at home after returning from an incomplete workup in the same hospital's emergency department. The hospital's hematology and nursing staffs were also cited by the state for substandard care of a 24-year-old leukemia patient who was related to the hospital's chief endocrinologist.

In the face of such continuing bad publicity over these cases and other investigations, the hospital's occupancy dropped by over 5% while other similar hospitals experienced little or no decline. The hospital changed its leadership and many senior administrators have been replaced. New admitting procedures and a revamped quality assurance program have been put into place. New cardiothoracic surgical talent has been recruited to improve the hospital's faded reputation and rebuild occupancy levels. Malpractice suits over the Wharhol and other cases are expected to continue for years.

Patient perspectives

To illustrate the importance of buyer group differences, consider the results of a comprehensive survey on how consumers, physicians, and third party payers view quality care as recently undertaken by Voluntary Hospitals of America (VHA), a nationwide alliance of 740 not-for-profit hospitals. The survey included 4,000 consumers, 1,600 physicians, and 1,600 employers who reported widely varying criteria when asked to identify the key elements of high quality hospitals.[8]

The VHA study disclosed, for instance, that more than one-half of the consumers surveyed say they can identify high-quality hospitals in their community. The most important criterion of quality cited by patients was the caring attitude of employees (mentioned by 52% of consumers) followed by a highly qualified medical staff (38%). Advanced technological services and a wide range of services was cited by 20% of the consumer respondents, while 15% equated quality with the hospital's general reputation. Consumers less frequently mentioned competent administration, cost efficiency, and efficient billing procedures as indicators of quality.

However, PMA's Ben Fishman pointed out that consumers cannot be expected to evaluate complex clinical data to define quality. "Consumers will always base quality on the factors they can assess. Typically, a 'good' hospital is a hospital that offers good meals, good accommodations, and good service. In short, patients will always judge a hospital much like they would judge a hotel because those are the features they understand. Ambiance is always easier to sell than clinical quality."[9]

This reality has not been lost on hospitals that have turned to Madison Avenue techniques to help them draw more patients. In 1983, health care professionals, led by hospitals, spent $41 million on television spots, up more than 11 times from the $3.7 million spent in 1977. In 1985, hospitals employed 2,000 marketing executives, compared to 6 in 1978.[10]

With an eye on consumer motivation, the Greater Southeast Community Hospital in Washington, D.C., for example, ran radio advertisements, complete with a musical jingle, advertising reduced rates for "comfortable homelike rooms" and "overnight guest" privileges. Methodist Medical Center in Illinois promotes its valet parking, while other hospitals advertise cash rebates to patients who have to wait more than a few minutes in an emergency department or in situations where floor nurses do not respond within one or two minutes to a patient's call.[11] Still other hospitals feature gourmet menus, enlarged libraries and game room facilities, and even free "recuperative" vacation trips in an all-out effort to fill empty hospital beds.

Despite the difficulty of interpreting outcome strategies, a number of hospitals throughout the United States have been quick to advertise their mortality statistics and other quality indicators. Both Eisenhower Medical Center in Rancho Mirage, California, and St. Lukes Medical Center in Phoenix, Arizona, have promoted low death rates in their cardiac surgery services.[12] Most other hospitals, however, express caution in utilizing crude measures of mortality unadjusted for acuity, comorbidity, age, sex, race, and other variables.

Despite the hoopla, hospitals have done a poor job of selling themselves to consumers based on medical performance. "Patients just assume that a major teaching hospital must be good," says Charlotte Kirsch a health care specialist for Coopers and Lybrand. "And if a hospital makes headlines for a heart transplant," she adds, "the public automatically assumes the obstetrics department is equally skilled." Therefore, hospitals rely on public relations and broad brush imagery to create the perception of quality.

"The crux of the problem is that a hospital cannot credibly say it performs a gall bladder operation better than another hospital," says Ben Fishman. "So hospitals are forced to turn to more tangible if less meaningful criteria."

Other hospital administrators defend their avoidance of promoting clinical quality to consumers on the basis that physicians—not patients—are their primary markets, as patients inevitably go to hospitals with which their physicians are affiliated. However, there is an unmistakable trend toward patient selection of hospitals as more discerning patients no longer blindly follow their physicians' preferences. Some patients go so far as to select their physicians based on their hospital affiliations (see the box, "Unexpected Hospital-Related Mortality").

Although hospitals appear slow to sell consumers on the basis of clinical quality, other providers who cannot depend on physician referrals are less reluctant to share clinical data with prospective patients. For example, Cleveland Clinic Administrators plan to select common diagnosis related groups (DRGs) of illnesses, such as cardiac care or hip replacements, as areas of clinical strength. They will gather data to show patient morbidity, mortality, discharge, and return to productive life style and use the results as selling tools. Similarly, the Harvard Community Health Plan (HCHP), a Boston-based HMO, has developed a comprehensive 11-point quality assurance program to attract new members in a pitched battle with Massachusetts Blue Cross/Blue Shield. In addition to tracking the clinical components of care, the HCHP system also reports on patient access, interpersonal care, integration of services, and overall patient satisfaction.

For most physicians the most important single factor associated with the quality of hospital care is the nature of the hospital itself.

Health care specialists Victor and Ruth Sidel remind us that most people in the United States are abysmally ignorant [about health care], and therefore, criteria requiring even basic medical knowledge may be self-defeating.[13] However, in today's marketplace, the typical quality-conscious consumer is young, well-educated, and better informed as a result of health care advertising combined with efforts by consumer groups and the media to educate the public. Therefore, patient perceptions of quality are bound to change to the extent that they learn to differentiate among competing providers by using meaningful clinical quality criteria.

Physician views

Physicians certainly can be expected to pay considerably more attention to clinical criteria than can lay consumers. In fact, the VHA survey disclosed physicians, in contrast to consumers, attached significant importance to technology, facilities, and the quality of the medical and support services. Physicians further reported teaching and research functions as important to quality.[14]

However, as with patients, physicians tend to equate quality with the structure of the institution. Structure means the material and social instrumentalities that are used to provide care. These include the number, mix, and qualifications of the staff; the manner in which the staff is organized and governed; and space, equipment, and other physical facilities. The assessment of structure is a judgment on whether care is being provided under conditions that are either conducive or inimical to the provision of good care.

Although physicians express interest in the processes by which a hospital controls and monitors quality of care, so much of the health care process is under the control of physicians that it is seldom a viable marketing tool for hospitals to use in attracting or retaining physician support.

Yet, a number of hospitals now are successfully marketing themselves to physicians based on the availability of more advanced quality control systems. Many hospitals are creating systems that collect information about variations in medical practice patterns and they relay that data to the medical staff. They believe that physicians who receive comprehensive information will make better decisions about the care they provide and be able to improve their performance. But a number of physicians resist providing clinical data claiming data are intrusive, and others are unwilling to share information for fear it may expose poor medical practice and even encourage malpractice suits.

For most physicians, however, the most important single factor associated with the quality of hospital care is the nature of the hospital itself. Physicians surveyed by the New York City Teamsters Union overwhelmingly expressed the view that the quality of care is best in large, urban, university-affiliated hospitals and worst in proprietary urban hospitals and other hospitals, whether urban or rural.[15]

Perhaps it is this unshakeable preconception among physicians coupled with career-long institutional loyalties that discourage hospitals in their attempt to attract new physicians to their ranks. "A physician rarely changes hospital affiliations," comments James Rice, a marketing consultant to New England-based hospitals. "Hospitals must instead place their marketing focus on physicians who share affiliations with several hospitals and coax the physician to send patients their way."

While physicians continue to choose from among several competing hospitals on the basis of geographic convenience or patient preference, there is a sharp upturn in physician selection based on the perceived quality of care for the particular illness. "Hospitals must define their niche and concentrate on what it is they do best," says Jim Rice. "Hospitals who foolishly pretend they're the best in every area lose the opportunity to differentiate themselves."

Third party payer views

More than any other group, those who pay the bills are exerting increased pressure on health care providers to develop meaningful quality criteria and particularly criteria based on clinical outcomes.

Employers, for example, are particularly concerned about the rate, speed, and extent of recovery as a way to gauge the ability of employees to regain employment. Health underwriters that provide disability coverage are equally concerned about this variable.

Third party payers (government agencies, employers, unions, and insurance companies) continue to be concerned about costs but appear more confident about the effectiveness of their cost containment strategies than they did a few years ago. The new interest of third party payers is in value, which requires fine-honed data to balance the quality of care against costs. Among third party payers the notion of quality at any cost has been replaced by a concern for appropriate care at the best available price.[16] A number of third party payers have discovered that quality and cost containment are simultaneously achievable, and in fact, high-quality services often cost less than inferior services.

To attain their objectives, large third party underwriters and employer groups are developing "quality" specifications for providers. These typically include patient satisfaction surveys, physician training, hospital certifications, and the range of services offered. Providers wanting to sell their services to smaller third party sponsors also now commonly focus on the same type of criteria in their marketing campaigns.

While third party payer dissatisfaction with the more traditional measures relating to the process of care has led to better ways of measuring clinical outcome, they continue to discover with frustration that the outcome of care is also vague and difficult to determine, even if one limits the measurement to short-term outcome under specific conditions. Factors such as severity of illness and quality of life are exceptionally difficult to quantify. Moreover, it is frequently impossible to relate outcome to any specific element of the process of medical care; and often the outcome, influenced by other factors, may not be related to the quality of medical care at all. Still, to the extent clinical outcomes can be accurately measured, third party payers will be the first to welcome these data.

Providers who are most successful in selling to employer groups and other third-party payers do so on their ability to design specifications that best meet the individual needs of each group. "Specification," in health care, is the process of deciding what the client wants and needs, and what the provider must then deliver.[17]

Specification typically encompasses both technical and nontechnical aspects of health care. Third party payers, for example, will be particularly concerned with guidelines that express *when* and *whether* surgery should be performed under certain circumstances instead of *how* surgery should be performed.

If the primary characteristic in marketing health services to large cost underwriters is the flexibility to work closely with the prospective clients in tailoring specific programs to match both their budget and their needs, many more providers must develop a market-driven, consumer-oriented philosophy. Up to now health care providers put their wares on the table and expected to sell. Under the new marketing theme, providers must first ask what it is a particular customer wants to buy.

SIX CHALLENGES

Because quality of care can be categorized in so many ways, and the clustering of attributes are so distinct from one consumer group to another, it has thus far been impossible to devise a singularly successful approach to quality as a meaningful marketing tool. And there are those who claim quality will remain only so much rhetoric in an industry that cannot possibly measure performance with any degree of confidence. Others argue that even if a coherent quality assessment system does emerge, it will do little to influence how health services are bought and sold. Quality, they suggest, will remain an ever-illusive objective but never become a significant factor in the marketplace. It is too early to tell whether the skeptics are correct; and according to Paul Batalden, M.D., Vice-President for Medical Care at Hospital Corporation of America, it may take another decade before workable methods to measure and ensure quality in health care institutions will come about.[18]

Admittedly, there is much about the determinants of performance that we do not understand; and considering the nature of health services, measurements will always remain faulty. However, to the extent that consumers demand quality of care information and to the extent providers are anxious to use it in their marketing efforts, we must meet other challenges before quality issues can be taken seriously.

- Quality of care must be measured with both consistency and comparability. The one major underlying danger to a coherent approach of quality assessment in America is due to the diverse efforts of so many different groups. The proliferation of measurements can only create confusion and disarray in the marketplace and throw into question the validity of any one approach. There is great need for close coordination between the various organizations, each presently in search of its own quality benchmarks. The ultimate goal must be to develop uniform data reporting systems as a universal language by which quality can be spoken with one tongue by all groups. Defining, measuring, monitoring, and managing the quality of health care services will remain the major challenge to the industry. Arriving at a sound and consistent approach will take a concerted effort among providers, consumers, employees, underwriters, physicians, the government, and others rightfully concerned with health care issues.

- Within any universal data reporting system, the industry must establish modules or bundles of data most meaningful to the respective consumer groups that must each assess and respond to quality criteria from their own perspective. Providers, in turn, must learn how to package and promote the right quality measurements to the appropriate groups if they are to effectively compete in the years ahead.

- To provide a more balanced approach to quality assessment, the power to define and review quality, now resting solely in the hands of medical professionals (through PROs and "peer review audit committees"), must be shared by both health care administrators, who are ultimately accountable for the delivery of quality care, and by the communities served by the institution, who are the ultimate beneficiaries of quality care. Therefore, quality review mechanisms must include the active involvement of administrators and community-elected consumer representatives.

- Quality assessment must be undertaken with far more precise accountability then presently exists. Quality must be measurable as to department (obstetrics, cardiac, and so forth), specific services (coronary bypass, hip replacement, and so on), and staff category (nursing, pharmacy, and so forth). Of particular importance, hospitals and other institutions must discover and then disclose the performance of their medical staff who most

influence overall institutional standards. Hazy institutional rankings must give way to the reality that any hospital is a composite of various strengths and weaknesses and that each must be identified.

- Aggressively marketed claims of quality carry with them the potential for abuse that must be anticipated and prevented. Internal data used in marketing efforts must be verifiable and accurate and closely monitored by the provider and outside groups to prevent misleading claims. Moreover, claims of quality must be tempered to encourage only needed treatment rather than to create a demand for unwarranted or baseless services.

- Those involved in buying health services—patients, physicians, and third party payers—must become both quality conscious and quality educated if the new marketing imperative is to take hold. Buyers of health care must assume neither that quality exists nor that it cannot be identified but instead must be oriented to search for excellence.

Finally, and most subtly, is the question of who should take the lead in designing a coherent quality assessment program for the American people. If providers do not accept the responsibility, the initiative will continue to be with consumers of health services whose demands for quality of care data can only increase with time.

Supporting this theme, at the recent 99th Shattuck Lecture to the Annual Meeting of the Massachusetts Medical Society, Paul Ellwood urged development of what he terms "outcomes management."[19] Outcomes management is to consist of:

- a patient-understood language of health outcomes;
- a national database of information and analysis of medical interventions and health outcomes;
- a national database of information and analysis of health outcomes and health expenditures; and
- open access to the information and analyses relevant to patient, payer, and provider decisions.

Although Ellwood's prescription for rational decision making will be long in coming, it will be in the interest of many hospitals to seriously consider the merits of his proposal at the local level. Health care managers, marketing personnel, and medical staffs can independently develop profiles of medical interventions, outcomes, and expenditures that are meaningful to patients, physicians, and third party payers. We see this proactive effort as the most logical way of meeting the challenge of health care in the 1990s.

REFERENCES

1. Super, K. "Providers Tout Quality to Get Edge in Marketing." *Modern Healthcare* 17 (1987): 27.
2. Ibid.
3. Graham, J. "Quality Gets a Closer Look." *Modern Healthcare* (February 27, 1987): 20.
4. Ricks, T. "New Corporate Program Lets Employees Compare Local Doctors' Fees and Training," *The Wall Street Journal*, 4 August 1987, p. 1.
5. Bleidt, B. Assessing Quality of Care in Pharmacy Practice, unpublished study, 1988.
6. Garvin, D.A. *Managing Quality*. Glencoe, Ill.: Free Press, 1988.
7. Viscuoi, W.K., and Magat, W.A. *Learning about Risk.* Boston: Harvard University Press, 1987.
8. Hays, M. "Consumers Base Quality Perceptions on Patient Relations." *Modern Healthcare* 17 (February 27, 1987): 33.
9. Fishman, B. *Marketing Health Services*. Philadelphia: PMA Press, 1985, p. 36.
10. Califano, J. *America's Healthcare Revolution* . New York: Random House, 1986.
11. Ibid.
12. *The Wall Street Journal*, 28 July 1987.
13. Sidel, V., and Sidel, R. *A Healthy State*. New York: Pantheon Books, 1983.
14. Viscuoi and Magat, *Learning about Risk.*
15. Donabedian, A. "Quality of Medical Care." In *Health Care: Regulation, Economics, Ethics, and Practice,* edited by P.H. Abelson. Washington, D.C.: American Association for the Advancement of Science, 1978, pp. 12–20.
16. Nelson, C. "The Administrator's Role in Quality Assessment." *Health Care Management Review* 2, no. 1 (1977): 7–18.
17. Ibid.
18. Graham, "Quality Gets a Closer Look."
19. Ellwood, P.M. "Shattuck Lecture—Outcomes Management." *New England Journal of Medicine*, 318 (1988): 1549–56.

Creating a total quality health care environment

Michael E. Milakovich

Until recently, health professionals lacked incentives to integrate internal management processes, depending instead on external quality assurance and regulatory standards. Competitive markets and increased regulatory pressures now encourage managers to reorient systems from a cost-driven reimbursement approach to the implementation of **Total Quality Care** *as a management strategy.*

This article defines the emerging concept of *total quality health care*, discusses problems with identifying costs associated with continuing poor-quality management practices, suggests ways to more accurately measure costs, and offers action guidelines for health professionals seeking to implement continuous quality improvement. Results reflect recent research application of service quality improvement techniques and how they can be integrated into a hospital or health care environment.[1-3]

THE NEW ENVIRONMENT OF CONTINUOUS QUALITY IMPROVEMENT

The continuous improvement of all facets of health and medical care service quality has received renewed attention recently with the shift in emphasis from distribution of resources through cost reimbursement policies to the present regulated cost-competitive system. This change and its impact on the health care profession has been detailed by several authors.[4-9] During the last decade, federal health policies encouraged the use of competitive markets to allocate resources, yet simultaneously increased regulations in an effort to control costs. Free-enterprise policies have fostered entrepreneurism and corporate ownership of health care facilities, and accelerated the change in U.S. medicine from a locally controlled, fee-for-service cottage industry to a heavily subsidized and regulated national industry. Questions remain, however, as to whether procompetitive (Win-Lose) policies are best suited to achieve the transformation to a total quality health care environment.

Continuing corporate acquisition and restructuring of health care facilities, particularly hospitals, have contributed to increased efficiencies in delivering care. Expensive high-tech equipment such as nuclear magnetic resonance imagers (NMRs) and laser scanners has improved the overall technical quality of medical care. Yet, the increased costs of these innovations have limited access for the uninsured. Consistent with accepted standards of medical care, continuing centralization of health care facilities encourages consumers

Michael E. Milakovich, *Ph.D., is an Associate Professor of Political Science at the School of Business Administration, University of Miami, Coral Gables, Florida.*

The author wishes to thank Dr. Howard Gitlow, Director, University of Miami Institute for the Study of Quality in Manufacturing and Service, for his patience and willingness to teach total quality control theories and techniques to non-statisticians.

and third-party providers to become ever more vigilant about the quality and costs of services provided.

Changes in government policies, marketing strategies that emphasize delivery of quality care, and increased patient awareness of costs have focused greater attention on the need to create an integrated medical–managerial–consumer total quality improvement environment. Insurance companies, health maintenance organizations (HMOs), preferred provider organizations (PPOs), corporations with large medical bills, and government reimbursement agencies have supported efforts to discipline primary care providers to begin thinking in a more "business-like" manner. In addition, hospitals have recently begun to adopt and implement total quality care (TQC) improvement systems based on industrial models to meet special needs and control costs.[10,11]

Leading theorists and researchers in the field of quality improvement stress the need for total system change, not just tinkering with the current system.[12-21] The new regulated-cost competitive health care service delivery environment offers opportunities for managers to market and manage systems on the basis of TQC (Win-Win) strategies as well as lower cost and strict external quality assurance standards.

THE FAILURE OF EXTERNAL REGULATION TO IMPROVE QUALITY

The past decade has brought about significant changes in both the service economy and health delivery systems in the United States. In an effort to mandate procedures and contain costs, most policies designed to implement these changes have been financial or regulatory, including increases in fixed-price insurance contracts and the imposition of strict payment rules covering specific medical procedures under Medicare's diagnosis related groups (DRGs). Initiated by external regulators, most of these policies have failed to stem rising aggregate health care costs, reduce expenses per procedure, increase access, or improve the quality of *internal* system processes.

In practice, external regulation provides a poor model for improving total system quality. Enforcing stricter legislation or regulations by accrediting associations such as the Joint Commission on Accreditation of Healthcare Organizations (Joint Commission), physician review organizations (PROs), or state departments of human resources only risks increased cooperative opposition or passive resistance from primary care providers, especially physicians and hospi-

tal staff.[9,22] This occurs because of institutional control over admission to the allied health and medical care professions and individual control of quality assurance standards. It is reinforced by the self-serving association, real or imagined, between cost containment and a "necessary" reduction in care provided. When outside attempts are made to regulate system procedures or reduce resources, health professionals frequently respond not by seeking improved internal management system efficiencies, but by real or threatened restrictions in the quality of services provided.

Quality is often perceived as a fixed commodity only health care professionals can define, rather than as a strategic mission shared by the entire organization.

Under these circumstances, quality is often perceived as a fixed commodity only health care professionals can define, rather than a strategic mission shared by the entire organization. Those who stress the importance of strategically managing quality see the concept as a variable necessity based upon performance, durability, customer satisfaction, or improved system capacity.[16,23] Other health care experts have pointed out that quality care and cost containment can exist simultaneously and are not necessarily incompatible.[22,24-26] Moreover, stressing both need not result in lower-quality care or higher costs, if hard statistical evidence is provided that the level of care provided in a quality-assured (licensed) facility meets or exceeds customer expectations.

Thus, rather than depending solely on regulatory standards and cost-containment measures to ensure professional standards of care, health professionals are encouraged to design and implement total quality improvement systems capable of improving all aspects of quality care.[27] The difficulty of measuring quality of care has been previously identified as a critical institutional and attitudinal obstacle to quality improvement.[28] If adopted, a continuous commitment to customer-driven internal process improvement, through a TQC strategy of quality management, would begin to shift professional attitudes away from dependence on cost control and external regulation as the only means to achieve higher levels of quality. The implementation of a TQC system based on conformance to valid customer requirements would provide

FIGURE 1

THE EXTENDED HEALTH CARE ORGANIZATION.

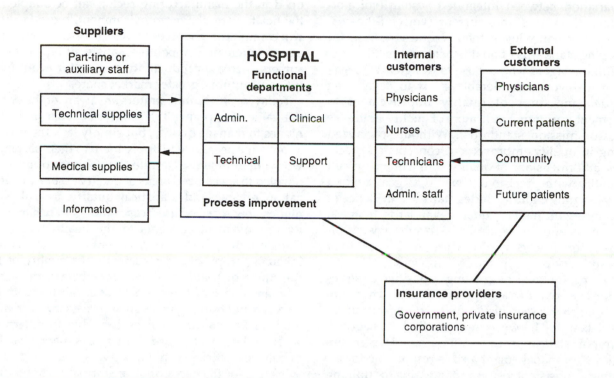

Reprinted with permission from Greebler, C., and Rosen, R. *Solving the Problems Facing Health Care: From the Individual Physician to the Large Hospital*. San Diego, Calif.: Total Quality Management Plus, 1989. In-house publication.

the statistical evidence that customer expectations are being met and that levels of quality are continuously improving.

WHAT IS TOTAL QUALITY HEALTH CARE?

Total quality care is a unique combination of applied modern high technology, access to facilities at reasonable costs, patient-centered quality primary and specialized clinical care, and low-tech holistic human healing skills. It is important to monitor all these dimensions of care, so as much effort must be devoted to designing measurement systems that assess perceived quality of care as has been previously expended in assuring the quality of medical laboratories, suppliers' services, patient billing systems, or clinical care.

In other sectors of the U.S. service economy, TQC is emerging as a strategic resource management technique, an accepted and viable alternative to both regulation and cost containment.[21,29] TQC stresses continued process improvement and the participation of all stakeholders in meeting extended customer requirements by doing the correct things right, the first time. Thus, TQC is based on prevention rather than inspection. Moreover, the concept of customer involves more than patients. In the extended definition of a health care organization, everyone affected by an organization's actions is either an internal or external customer (Figure 1).

In order to implement TQC, measures must be broader than traditional definitions of quality assurance, which focus on professional (i.e., clinical or medical) definitions of the quality of services provided.[30] Before health care managers can deploy quality as a strategic management tool, a service-oriented quality culture must be created,[31] and measures of clinical or medical care must be integrated with financial, cost-control, *and* patient-satisfaction measures. The variation between integrated system (voice-of-the-process) indices and current (voice-of-the-customer) performance levels then becomes the basis for developing standards of quality achievement.[32]

Health managers who choose to design a TQC system must devote considerable effort to developing expanded measures of quality improvement to supplement traditional indicators of quality assurance (Joint Commission standards). Without specialized training in quality improvement concepts and techniques, all dimensions of quality care will be difficult to quantify with precision. Thus, TQC goes beyond quality assurance and includes statistical evidence of compliance with medical quality standards, financial management and cost-control data, results of voice-of-the-customer surveys, and measures of the quality of goods and services provided by suppliers.

Achieving the goal of creating a positive environment for TQC requires a far greater degree of horizontal *cross-functional coordination* and *vertical integration*[33] than exists today between most medical, managerial, and support staffs in many quality-assured health care facilities. Top management also is responsible for articulating a consistent vision and initiating the training to change attitudes and behavior. Managers must themselves recognize the diseases and obstacles preventing a transformation to a TQC culture, and then change their behavior to reflect this new, quality-oriented culture. For example, traditional management may view the organization as a loose collection of separate, highly specialized, individual performers and units, linked together by levels within a functional hierarchy. The new culture of TQC views the institution as an interconnected network of interdependent processes, linked laterally, over time, through a network of cooperating (internal and external) suppliers and customers. How these new principles are articulated and supported by top management will determine the success or failure of institutionalized TQC efforts.

Equally important, TQC must develop from the bottom up within the organization, not be imposed from the top down. Everyone must be included because everything in the facility is subject to continuous improvement. This top down–bottom up strategy must be guided by a consistent, statistically based quality improvement philosophy, and supported by a retraining effort along the lines suggested by quality gurus such as Deming,[13,14] Crosby,[12,34] Juran,[20] or Sherkenbach.[21] As more managers, suppliers, nurses, and physicians realize that tools and techniques developed in the manufacturing sector can be adapted to the health care delivery environment, more facilities will commit the resources to design TQC systems necessary to remain competitive, satisfy all types of consumers, increase productivity and, in for-profit institutions, capture a greater market share.

Today, health administrators are aware of the potential value of applying TQC concepts, tools, and techniques to manage quality, but simply lack the time or knowledge necessary to apply them to their particular work environments. Despite the volumes of research devoted to specialized areas of quality assurance, utilization review, and statistical quality control techniques, few service-based case studies translate quality improvement concepts to the health care field. Compounding the lack of pertinent case studies is the inherent complexity of measuring the quality of the full range of health services. Nonetheless, managers who are aware of the obstacles, yet fail to make the research and training investment necessary to create a total quality culture, will be less able to determine whether their systems are producing at maximal levels of both cost efficiency and quality.

In sum, for the necessary transformation to occur in thinking about total quality health care management, the technical language and concepts of statistical quality control, quality assurance, and TQC must be merged into a common set of applicable health care examples, illustrating the use of statistical tools and guided by quality improvement principles. This new process-oriented way of thinking about managing quality has several essential elements.

- All actions are guided by principles of continuous quality improvement.
- Decisions are based on facts, data, and statistical information.
- Everyone in the organization is dedicated to serving extended customers, broadly defined as anyone affected by its actions.
- Quality progress is measured against valid customer requirements, not externally imposed standards.
- Teamwork is rewarded as a means to break down barriers to communication and enhance interdepartmental cooperation.

Creating a Total Quality Health Care Environment   205

FIGURE 2

HIDDEN COSTS OF POOR QUALITY.

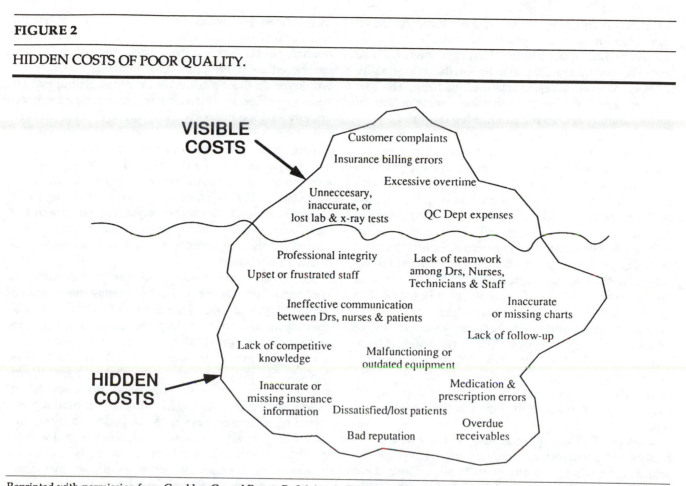

Reprinted with permission from Greebler, C., and Rosen, R. *Solving the Problems Facing Health Care: From the Individual Physician to the Large Hospital.* San Diego, Calif.: Total Quality Management Plus, 1989. In-house publication.

WHAT ARE THE REAL COSTS OF POOR QUALITY?

In order to realize total quality as a strategic management vision, the costs of poor quality must be acknowledged, measurement systems must be designed to accurately translate these costs, and team-based quality indicators must be established. This recognition phase precedes the quality implementation phase and involves the entire organization—medical, nursing, support staff, and suppliers—in the critical task of identifying system indicators to be monitored. Established techniques previously used in health care—such as Pareto analysis, fishbone diagrams, control charts, quality control (QC) circles, and brainstorming in team sessions,[35]—as well as extended surveys of internal and external customers can be used to identify process-improvement opportunities. In addition, hum sensors must be carefully trained to monitor process improvement using statistical quality-improvement techniques.[20] It is important to employ these modern theory-based techniques to collect appropriate baseline data for managers to use in determining quality trends.[14,20]

In manufacturing, costs associated with poor quality are typically used to establish guarantees and warranty charges. More recently, managers of health care organizations have recognized that they, too, make continuous service delivery errors requiring substantial and costly rework to meet customer expectations.

Administrative errors, increasing malpractice insurance premiums, and duplicate appraisals are all expensive results of poor internal process control.

Administrative errors, increasing malpractice insurance premiums, and duplicate appraisals are all expensive results of poor internal process control. These costs, however, are only the tip of the poor-quality iceberg. Without a TQC system to go below the surface, many of the most damaging consequences of poor-quality practices remain hidden (Figure 2).

There are economic as well as strategic management implications of not knowing how many resources are lost because of poor quality control. As suggested in the earlier section, more than measurement systems are needed to understand the costs of poor quality. With an understanding of total quality, perceptions of the causes of variable costs will also change. For example, one physician may perform a cholecystectomy for $3,000 and another, for $5,000. Other factors being equal, the $2,000 cost differential becomes a cost of poor quality. Health professionals must be exposed to reality, which places losses from inefficiency, unnecessary procedures, and waste between 25% and 30% of all health care expenditures. Despite these general estimates,[36] most facilities still lack TQC systems capable of providing specific knowledge of how poor quality affects their services and what steps are necessary to eliminate the causes from their internal system processes.

A simple five-step process can be used to address quality requirements at each customer–supplier link within an extended health care facility. Once these requirements are established for all customers, then top management can proceed with the elimination of poor-quality costs by integrating financial, customer service, and quality assurance measures.

1. What is your major product or service?
2. Who are your major users or customers?
3. What quality requirements are demanded by your users or customers?
4. What is the most competitive product or service offered by your competitors?
5. What kinds of comparative studies do you conduct to compare your product or service with those of your competitors for the quality requirements of your customers?[1]

Eliminating Poor-Quality Costs

In general terms, losses can be broken down into direct (visible) and indirect (hidden) quality costs. Direct quality costs can be further subdivided into controllable costs, which include prevention and appraisal costs, and resultant costs, which include internal and external error costs. Management has direct control over controllable (or assignable) poor-quality costs that result from "systemic" causes. They can be either prevention costs necessary to help an employee do the job correctly every time, or appraisal costs expended to determine whether a standardized activity is done properly every time. Typical prevention costs are those incurred for developing quality data collection and reporting systems, vendor surveys, and preparation and documentation for Joint Commission inspections. All health care facilities can benefit from a TQC system designed to uncover these costs. However, in organizations larger than about 100 employees, it is absolutely necessary to provide a statistical monitoring and control system to manage data and assess results.

Statistical thinking for quality improvement and cost reduction also provides top management with a better understanding of the nature of variation within their system. Understanding the distinction between common variation (under management control) and special or random variation (outside its control) is basic to any statistical process-control system.[17] When common variation is distinguished from special or random variation, management can stop blaming external regulators or employees for poor-quality results and focus instead on the elimination of internal system quality barriers. When fully operational, TQC internal management systems can define valid customer quality requirements; establish measurement indicators, standards, or benchmarks for improvement; monitor progress; and provide continuous statistical feedback to eliminate the underlying causes of poor quality.

Emphasizing Prevention Costs

All organizations tend to deny the existence of quality problems or to define quality narrowly as conformance to accepted external professional standards (i.e., quality is what doctors and hospital administrators say it is). To minimize this tendency, the costs of quality can be conceptually divided into the price of nonconformance and the price of conformance. The price of nonconformance is all expenses involved in doing things wrong, often repeatedly. Examples run the gamut of activities, from routine corrections of incomplete purchase orders to the need to duplicate physician orders for a second or third time to the more time-consuming and damaging liability costs and subsequent litigation resulting from administering the wrong medication to a patient. Joseph M. Juran offers a chilling example of the possible consequences of not having a TQC system in place to discover the underlying causes of these costs.

> For years the hospital industry had only the vaguest idea of the extent of errors in the process of giving medication to patients. All hospitals posted rules requiring nurses to report medication errors promptly...however, in many hospitals the nurses had learned that when they made such reports they were often subjected to unwarranted blame. Hence they stopped making such reports. In due course a classic study made by a qualified outsider showed that (1) about seven percent of the medications involved errors, some quite serious, and, (2) the bulk of the errors were management-controllable, not worker-controllable.[20(p.85)]

The price of conformance is what it would cost to do things right in the first place. Examples here include most professional quality assurance functions, education and training, and actions to improve leadership skills. In attempting to more accurately gauge the total costs of poor quality, organizations have been classified as being at different points on the quality–cost spectrum ranging from total uncertainty to absolute certainty.[34] Most hospitals are typically at the first stages (uncertainty), where there is little comprehension of total quality as a management tool; quality costs are hidden; total quality measures do not exist; and problems are resolved as they occur, or their existence is denied in the first place. To eliminate losses due to poor quality, the costs of repairing defective work must be analyzed.[18] In organizations with a high degree of certainty about quality costs, the price of conformance represents between 3 percent and 5 percent of total expenses.[12]

An organization can most effectively eliminate these costs by investing in preventive actions. Unfortunately, these investments are time-consuming and, as opposed to equipment or personnel costs, difficult to tie to a tangible return on investment. Again, the underlying problem is too much concern about numbers, and not enough about service quality. Once the customer–supplier relationship for all internal and external customers is defined, then problem-solving techniques can be applied to identify and prevent the root causes of system problems.

Results of Poor-Quality Costs

Resultant poor-quality costs include all expenses that occur because of errors or because activities were not done right every time. These are called *resultant* costs because they are directly related to management decisions made in the controllable poor-quality cost category. They may be further divided into internal and external error costs.

Internal error costs occur before a product or service is accepted by a patient, because everyone did not do the job right every time. They are preventable and under the control of management; examples include a patient's refusal to submit to a blood draw because it was not done according to an acceptable schedule; the billing system's not producing bills on time; or an employee's drawing a specimen from a patient for a second or third time because it was not performed properly the first time.

External error costs result from poor-quality work by health care professionals, often purchasing officers. They include the loss of health care delivery contracts and revenues owing to poor financial analysis of proposals, late delivery of supplies, or poor laboratory specimen recordkeeping.

More difficult to measure but equally important to monitor are those *indirect* or hidden costs depicted in Figure 2 reflecting poor quality practices in all facilities, yet independent of medical care provided, and not directly measurable on a profit–loss ledger. Most indirect poor-quality costs are related to lack of teamwork among physicians, nurses, and technicians; patient dissatisfaction with employee behavior; and loss of repeat visits from friends or relatives of dissatisfied patients. Not having TQC systems in place to monitor and correct even relatively minor inconveniences at critical times in a patient's treatment can cause major problems. For example, something as simple as how a patient is greeted by an admissions clerk can negatively affect patient satisfaction levels, totally apart from the technical quality of services rendered.

Regardless of the quality control or assurance systems in existence, if service levels do not meet or exceed customer expectations, then any facility can incur expensive indirect costs from excessive staff turnover, absenteeism, poor morale, or loss of patients to competitive providers. This could create a negative ripple effect with dissatisfied former staff and patients telling others about their experiences. As many as 10 potential customers, immediate family members, or friends can be influenced by a single negative evaluation. This can devastate the reputations of small- or medium-sized facilities and dramatically increase costs and reduce repeat visits. These word-of-mouth evaluations affect attitudes about and perceptions of the facility as a whole, so loss of a good reputation negates all other positive services provided by a facility. Most of the

> *Most of the negative results of patient dissatisfaction can be prevented with carefully designed voice-of-the-patient surveys.*

negative results of hidden patient dissatisfaction can be prevented with carefully designed voice-of-the-patient surveys, administered at appropriate intervals following treatment.

An accurate measure of total quality reveals the price of nonconformity, or the costs of continually doing things wrong. With a better understanding of the relationship between costs and quality, these costs can be divided into traditional categories of prevention, appraisal, or failure to comply with standards. They may have either a direct or indirect impact on various health care services. Conceptual guidelines and methodologies for process flow charting are available to managers seeking to establish TQC measurement systems to eliminate the hidden costs of poor quality.[37,38] Before implementation can proceed, health service organizations must develop and integrate *behavioral* quality indicators with traditional technical quality-of-conformance or quality-assurance measures. These integrated measures can be used initially to guide administrators to target areas for quality improvement, then refined for use in marketing and management actions as visible proof of the commitment to achieving continuous quality improvement.

IMPLEMENTING A TQC IMPROVEMENT SYSTEM

The best quality-improvement systems are only as good as their organizationwide implementation. This is especially true in services where the problems of measuring behavioral quality, as well as the technical quality of clinical care, facilities, or equipment, are generally more complex. Measuring quality in labor-intensive services is often more difficult because no tangible product results from various internal processes, and the service is usually consumed when it is rendered.

FIGURE 3

THE PDSA CYCLE AND THE SEVEN GRAPHIC TOOLS.

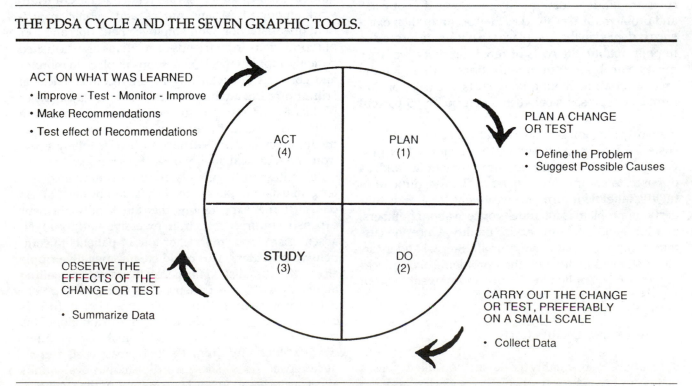

ACT ON WHAT WAS LEARNED
• Improve - Test - Monitor - Improve
• Make Recommendations
• Test effect of Recommendations

PLAN A CHANGE OR TEST
• Define the Problem
• Suggest Possible Causes

OBSERVE THE EFFECTS OF THE CHANGE OR TEST
• Summarize Data

CARRY OUT THE CHANGE OR TEST, PREFERABLY ON A SMALL SCALE
• Collect Data

ACT (4)   PLAN (1)   STUDY (3)   DO (2)

Reprinted with permission from Greebler, C., and Rosen, R. *Solving the Problems Facing Health Care: From the Individual Physician to the Large Hospital.* San Diego, Calif.: Total Quality Management Plus, 1989. In-house publication.

Developing Service Quality Measures

In service organizations, measures are also more difficult to define and accurately monitor because of the independence of discretionary decision makers such as physicians, nurses, and lab technicians. Health care facilities depend on human sensors rather than scientific instruments for data collection. Human sensors must be more sophisticated and sensitive, and capable of overcoming the natural tendencies of all individuals to make judgments according to their biases. Careful and continuous training is the key to overcoming these biases. Creating an environment of trust and removing fear are critical. All employees must be assured that no retaliation will result when poor-quality costs are uncovered.

Before implementation can proceed, all departments in a health service organization must be involved from the bottom up in strategic planning for quality, but one person should initially act as quality coordinator. Ideally, this person should be at or near the top management level within the organization, preferably the chief executive officer (CEO) or president. As a practical matter, and in view of various routine quality-assurance data-collection efforts required of most accredited facilities, a senior vice president or comparable appointee will typically initiate, coordinate, and monitor the quality-review process. So long as the effort has the full support of top management, and the person assigned the task has authority commensurate with his or her responsibilities, then department wide actions can begin.

Mission Statement, Teams, and Quality Functions

After the development or updating of an organization's mission statement, the next step in the implementation process is the formation and training of teams of 8 to 12 persons representing each work unit. These teams will meet initially to discuss the goals of the quality review, identify problems that inhibit work efforts, and develop measures appropriate for each quality function within the work unit. Quality functions are the critical links between customer requirements and system quality measures. Maximal benefit will be achieved from quality improvement *only if* the implementation process is focused on items of importance to the customer. As the true experts in their particular skills or services, team members must develop a set of quality indicators, measures that are directly related to the improvement of the work unit, based on the quality requirements of their customers.

All members of the department, workgroup, or subunit must be included in the process and everyone must accept the responsibility to examine their jobs and find better ways to do them. Such involvement can identify problems using established techniques and develop quality function measures to complement both financial and clinical care indicators.[11,17] To identify quality-improvement opportunities, every employee will be taught basic statistical quality concepts and problem-solving techniques based on the Plan-Do-Check-Act (PDCA) cycle of continuous quality improvement shown in Figure 3.

Next, team leaders will be selected and given additional training in quality-improvement theory and techniques. They must be carefully chosen and trained to communicate the purposes and goals of the activity to their work units. Team leaders must understand TQC concepts, explain the necessity of developing customer-driven measures, and facilitate the identification and collection of data from each department. Some quality measures may already be available through existing information-collection systems, while others may have to be developed. In a patient accounts payable department, for example, the number of patient inquiries about mischarges may be an appropriate quality-function measure. Team leaders must explain the TQC concept at the departmental level, conduct brainstorming sessions with all members to develop complete lists of quality functions, and represent departments or subunits in coordinated planning with other units. Until TQC and management become a routine part of information-collection processes, top management must actively support departmental quality projects by encouraging small-group quality efforts. New group problem-solving actions such as nominal group technique, quality stories, quality circles and the PDCA cycle have been used successfully in other large service organizations to overcome resistance, gain participation, motivate employees, achieve top management goals, and sustain the total quality-improvement effort.[3]

Data Collection and Cross-Functional Management

It is possible for most medium- to large-sized facilities to automate much of the data collection and reporting effort required to reduce added paperwork burdens on employees. As important as the change in thinking required of all employees is the development of fact-based information-processing systems and the availability of a statistician–systems person capable of accurately assessing the validity and reliability of various quality indicators proposed by team members.

After a few months of dedicated work, departmental liaisons or team leaders will condense the lists and provide a summary of indicators, then meet with other departmental representatives during a cross-functional coordination exercise to discuss strategies for identifying the costs associated with each quality indicator. Representatives from such staff areas as admissions, finance, and payroll could also be involved in these exercises. All departmental team leaders will discuss quality indicators with the project coordinator, who, in turn, will devise a monthly reporting system using the feedback from each of the departmental reporting team sessions. Team members will then meet and discuss progress in quality improvement on a continuous basis and review the statistics generated by each department. Fine-tuning adjustments to the process will be made as necessary, based on these data. In this way, all members of the organization become quality conscious and at the same time begin to develop fact-based approaches to the solution of departmental and organization-wide quality problems.

Collecting data on the costs of poor quality is not inherently difficult, but it is rarely done in the hospital or health care setting, as clinical care and financial requirements dominate data-collection efforts. In fact, with the support of qualified outside consultants, and the outline of a TQC system can be put together in just a few months of team effort. The first data-collection effort may yield only 70 percent to 80 percent of the total data required, but analysis of these data will provide sufficient shock value that most facilities will not need the remainder of the data for some time. Over the next few months, as more data are collected, the quality review process can be expanded as necessary.

To some employees in any organization, the data collection and reporting steps outlined above may initially appear to be overly detailed and time consuming. In all likelihood, most line workers, especially nurses, are already overburdened with required meetings, paperwork, charts, data to collect, and other procedures to be monitored. Skilled white-collar service employees will not be unfamiliar with techniques such as QC circles and control charts, yet they may be dubious of the need to attend meetings or fill out another form, if they do not fully comprehend the purpose of the exercise. For this reason, the mission of TQC as a bottom-up exercise in total organizational quality im-

The mission of TQC as a bottom-up exercise in total organizational quality improvement must be clearly communicated to everyone . . . .

provement must be clearly communicated to everyone in order to gain cooperation.

Action Guidelines for Quality Improvement

In different types of health care organizations, TQC implementation plans will vary from the more conceptual and philosophical to the more detailed and pragmatic approaches. Following the organizationwide commitment to quality, decisions on the scope of the TQC effort are made by top management. While the specific plan depends on the size, mission, and function of a particular facility, there are several common elements in any effort to strategically manage quality.

1. Develop, publish, read, videotape, and utilize case studies of total quality improvement experiences in health care facilities. Unfortunately, there are relatively few applied studies in the area, as TQC methods and techniques have only been applied to service industries since the mid-1980s.
2. Create a culture conducive to quality improvement by active personal involvement of top management to initiate and sustain the process of top down–bottom up implementation.
3. Recognize cost as a necessary transition step toward the development of a TQC implementation plan. Cost measures must be integrated with patient-care and medical data to develop quality-function indicators. Here, top management must support small-group, quality-improvement efforts as part of the routine information-collection processes, but never emphasize cost control as a means to achieve quality improvement.
4. Ensure patient privacy as well as the professional autonomy of physicians, psychologists, nurses, and other state-licensed professionals, while at the same time involving all professionals in the design of TQC implementation plans.
5. Develop bottom-up work unit–based measures consistent with professional discretion and patient privacy requirements, designed to meet a wider range of extended definitions of customer quality expectations.

6. Break down structural barriers inhibiting cross-functional coordination both vertically and horizontally between line and staff functions, using training, teamwork, deployment flow charting, and small-group, problem-identification techniques.

7. Implement Quality Function Deployment (QFD). In today's competitive market, providers must show improved services on the basis of results from quality function measures designed to meet valid customer satisfaction requirements. QFD is an advanced technique to merge valid customer requirements, organizational process controls, and quality-assurance standards.[39] It has been used in other industries to deploy TQC-improvement systems and has produced better design of products and processes in far less time.[40]

8. Use gainsharing, benchmarking, and other motivational techniques to provide incentives for participation, minimize costly resistance during the critical start-up phase, establish quality standards based on the best industrywide processes, and sustain continuous TQC process-improvement efforts.[41]

• • •

In addition to these general guidelines, administrators must define precisely how TQC differs from other management strategies, reexamine annual employee merit review procedures to reward quality improvement efforts, include teams as units of analysis, stress extended definitions of customer satisfaction, provide incentives for training *all* employees, and develop valid customer-defined multiple measures of quality. Those who master these new quality management skills will become invaluable assets to facilities seeking greater productivity, reduced costs, increased market share, and enhanced profits in the ultra-competitive regulated health care market of the 1990s.

REFERENCES

1. Kano, N., and Gitlow, H. *Lectures on Total Quality Control and the Deming Management Method.* Coral Gables, Fla.: University of Miami Quality Program, 1988–89.

2. Milakovich, M. "Total Quality Management for Public Service Productivity Improvement." *Public Productivity and Management Review* 14 (1990a): 19–32.

3. Milakovich, M. "Florida Power and Light: Lessons on Quality Improvement in Services." University of Miami, 1990. Case study draft in process.

4. Berwick, D.M. "Continuous Improvement As An Ideal in Health Care." *New England Journal of Medicine* 320 (1989): 53–7.

5. Ginzberg, E. *American Medicine.* Totowa, N.J.: Rowman and Allanheld, 1985.

6. Ginzberg, E. "For-Profit Medicine." *New England Journal of Medicine* 319 (1988): 757–61.

7. Relman, A. "Practicing Medicine in the New Business Climate." *New England Journal of Medicine* 316 (1987): 1150–51.

8. Starr, P. *The Social Transformation of American Medicine.* New York, N.Y.: Basic Books, 1982.

9. Thompson, F. *Health Policy and the Bureaucracy: Politics and Implementation.* Cambridge, Mass: MIT Press, 1983.

10. Burda, D. "Vermont Hopes Improved Quality Can Control Costs." *Modern Healthcare* (1989): 38.

11. Goldfield, N., and Nash, D. (Eds.) *Providing Quality Care: The Challenge to Clinicians.* Philadelphia, Pa.: The American College of Physicians, 1989.

12. Crosby, P. *The Eternally Successful Organization.* New York, N.Y.: McGraw-Hill, 1988.

13. Deming, W.E. *Quality, Productivity and Competitive Position.* Cambridge, Mass.: Massachusetts Institute of Technology Center for Advanced Engineering Study, 1982.

14. Deming, W.E. *Out of the Crisis.* Cambridge, Mass.: Massachusetts Institute of Technology Center for Advanced Engineering Study, 1986.

15. Fiegenbaum, A.V. *Total Quality Control.* 3rd ed. New York, N.Y.: McGraw-Hill, 1984.

16. Garvin, D.A. *Managing Quality.* New York, N.Y.: Free Press, 1988.

17. Gitlow, H., et al. *Tools and Methods for the Improvement of Quality.* Homewood, Ill.: Irwin, 1989.

18. Harrington, H.J. *Poor Quality Costs.* New York, N.Y.: Marcel Dekker-ASQC Press, 1987.

19. Ishikawa, K. *What is Quality Control? The Japanese Way.* New York, N.Y.: Free Press, 1985.

20. Juran, J.M. *Juran on Planning for Quality.* New York, N.Y.: Free Press, 1988.

21. Scherkenbach, W.W. *The Deming Route to Quality and Productivity.* Rockville, Md.: Mercury Press, 1986.

22. Donabedian, A. *The Definition of Quality and Approaches to Its Assessment.* Ann Arbor, Mich.: Health Administration Press, 1980.

23. Caper, P. "Defining Quality in Medical Care." *Health Affairs* 7 (1988): 49–61.

24. Batchelor, G.J., and Esmond, T.H., Jr. "Maintaining High Quality Patient Care While Controlling Costs."

Healthcare Financial Management 43, no. 2 (1989): 20–30.

25. Donabedian, A. "Quality and Cost: Choices and Responsibilities." *Inquiry* 25 (1988): 90–99.

26. Ullmann, S.G. "The Impact of Quality on Cost in the Provision of Long-Term Care." *Inquiry* 33 (1985): 292–306.

27. Wyszewianski, L. "The Emphasis on Measurement in Quality Assurance: Reasons and Implications." *Inquiry* 25 (1988): 424–36.

28. Schmacher, D.N. "Organizing for Quality Competition: The Coming Paradigm Shift." *Frontiers of Health Services Management* 5, no. 4 (1989): 4–30.

29. Rosander, A.C. *The Quest for Quality in Services.* Milwaukee, Wis.: ASQC Press, 1989.

30. Joint Commission on Accreditation of Healthcare Organizations. *Guide to Quality Assurance.* Chicago, Ill.: Joint Commission, 1988.

31. Albert, M. "Developing a Service-Oriented Health Care Culture." *Hospital and Health Services Administration* 34 (1989): 167–83.

32. Scherkenbach, W.W. "How to Put the Deming Philosophy to Work in Your Organization." Seminar; 18 January, 1990; Newport Beach, Calif.

33. Clement, J.P. "Vertical Integration and Diversification of Acute Care Hospitals: Conceptual Definitions." *Hospital and Health Services Administration* 33 (1988): 99–110.

34. Crosby, P. *Quality is Free: The Art of Making Quality Certain.* New York, N.Y.: McGraw-Hill, 1979.

35. Goldberg, A., and Pegles, C. *Quality Circles in Health Care Facilities.* Rockville, Md.: Aspen Systems, 1984.

36. Califano, J.A., Jr. "Billions Wasted: At Least a Fourth of American Health Care Dollars Are Misspent." *New York Times*, 16 April 1989, 10.

37. King, C. "A Framework for a Service Quality Assurance System." *Quality Progress* 3 (1987): 27–32.

38. Tribus, M. *Deployment Flow Charting*, 2 vols. Los Angeles, Calif.: Quality and Productivity 1989. Workbook to accompany videotapes.

39. Hauser, J.R., and Clausing, D. "The House of Quality." *Harvard Business Review* 66 no. 3 (1988): 63–73.

40. King, B. "Better Designs in Half the Time: Implementing QFD in America," Methuen, Mass.: GOAL/QPC, 1987.

41. Camp, R. *Benchmarking: The Search for Industry Best Practices that Lead to Superior Performance.* Milwaukee, Wis.: ASQC Press, 1989.

Index

About the Editor

Montague Brown is a consultant and Director of Strategic Management Services, Inc. a national management consulting firm, with offices in Shawnee Mission, Kansas and Washington, D.C. Brown is Of Counsel with the law firm of Calligaro and Mutryn, Washington, D.C. and is also Editor of *Health Care Management Review.*

Dr. Brown's practice focuses on strategic issues and policies including mergers, vision and strategy, active aging, and building comprehensive vertically integrated systems of health service.

He has served as a hospital trustee and is currently on the boards of the Johnson County Foundation on Aging, the Consumer Health Information and Research Institute, and the Forum for Health Care Planning. He also serves as founding director of the Florida Foundation on Active Aging.

Dr. Brown's work in health care includes service with the New Jersey Hospital Association, Director of the Program and Associate Professor in the W.K. Kellogg School of Management, Northwestern University, and Professor, Department of Health Administration, Duke University. Dr. Brown also serves as adjunct professor, University of Kansas. He has held numerous voluntary positions over the years and has written many books, articles, and reports on issues dealing with the profession of health administration and ways of improving organizational performance.

Dr. Brown holds an AB and a MBA from the University of Chicago, a Doctor of Public Health (Dr PH) and a Juris Doctor (JD) from the University of North Carolina. He has lectured at dozens of universities and participated in international workshops in Canada, Austria, Germany, and England. He continues to lecture, write and participate actively in ongoing research and education programs.